# Pregnancy Cooking & Nutrition

FOR

**Pregnancy Cooking & Nutrition For Dummies®**

Published by
**John Wiley & Sons, Inc.**
111 River St.
Hoboken, NJ 07030-5774
www.wiley.com

WILEY

# *About the Author*

**Tara Gidus** is a registered dietitian (RD) and recognized expert in nutrition and health promotion. She appears biweekly as the "Diet Diva" on the national morning television show *The Daily Buzz*. Tara is also the Healthy Eating Expert and blogger on `www.health line.com` and the nutrition advisor for *American Baby* magazine.

Along with being an expert in pregnancy nutrition, Tara specializes in performance nutrition for athletes and busy professionals, teaching them how to eat right to excel in their careers. She's the team dietitian for the NBA's Orlando Magic and a sports nutrition consultant to the athletes at the University of Central Florida.

As a past spokesperson for the American Dietetic Association, Tara acts as a resource for the media. Her expert quotes appear frequently in various newspapers, websites, and magazines and on television and radio. Tara owns her own nutrition consulting business in which she's a speaker, spokesperson, writer, and consultant.

Tara earned a bachelor's degree with a double major in dietetics and nutrition, fitness, and health and a master's degree in health promotion from Purdue University. She's a Board Certified Specialist in Sports Dietetics (CSSD).

Tara is wife to husband, Stephen, and mother to two boys, Basil and Levi. She loves to run, cook nutritious meals for her family, and eat her daily dose of chocolate. She lives in sunny Florida.

# Dedication

This book is dedicated to every pregnant woman who strives to fill her body with nutritious food to provide the gift of good health to her child.

# Author's Acknowledgments

Writing this book has been an amazing experience, and I was helped and encouraged by a few folks in particular.

Thanks to my agent, Margot Maley Hutchison, who came to me with this project and had faith in me from the beginning. Special thanks to my project editor, Jennifer Tebbe, who could not have been a better sounding board as she literally lived as my target audience as she edited the book while going through her first pregnancy. And I couldn't have done it all without the rest of the editing team at John Wiley & Sons, Inc., especially acquisitions editor Michael Lewis, copy editor Amanda Langferman, recipe tester Emily Nolan, nutritional analyst Patty Santelli, and technical editor Elizabeth Ward, RD. I truly appreciate your thoughtful oversight and suggestions.

I was lucky enough to have lots of help from other places, as well. Thanks to Kristina LaRue, RD, and Evie Lyras for the fun and laughs we had while developing recipes for this book. Stephanie Matos, you kept me stocked with good research along the way, and I appreciate it all! I'm blessed to have many friends, relatives, and colleagues who contributed their fabulous recipes, and I enjoyed tasting them as I wrote this book!

I have been inspired by many amazing people in my career as a nutrition professional and would like to especially thank Cindy Heroux, RD, Heidi Hanna, PhD, Dawn Jackson Blatner, RD, Bonnie Taub-Dix, RD, Keri Gans, RD, Cynthia Sass, RD, Elisa Zied, RD, and Raquel Malo, RD, for your solicited (and sometimes unsolicited) advice and encouragement throughout the years.

Finally, I would like to thank my family. Thank you Mom and Dad, Don and Jean Timpel, for the incredible support and love you showed me as I grew from a child to an adult. One of my greatest pleasures in life is seeing the joy your grandchildren bring to your lives. Christine "Chia" Kindell, you are the second mother to my children when I am not there, and I am incredibly grateful for the special care and love you give my boys on a daily basis. I would not be able to "do it all" without you!

Of course, a book on pregnancy nutrition would not have been possible for me to write so thoroughly without having gone through the experience myself (twice!). I thank God every day for blessing me with my two beautiful boys, Basil and Levi. I couldn't ask for a better partner and best friend in their wonderful father and my devoted and supportive husband, Stephen. I'm sorry that I missed out on so much fun on Saturdays while working on this book, and I'm ready now to get back to sharing those days with my three boys!

## Publisher's Acknowledgments

We're proud of this book; please send us your comments at http://dummies.custhelp.com. For other comments, please contact our Customer Care Department within the U.S. at 877-762-2974, outside the U.S. at 317-572-3993, or fax 317-572-4002.

Some of the people who helped bring this book to market include the following:

**Acquisitions, Editorial, and Vertical Websites**

**Project Editor:** Jennifer Tebbe

**Senior Project Editor:** Christina Guthrie

**Acquisitions Editor:** Michael Lewis

**Copy Editor:** Amanda M. Langferman

**Assistant Editor:** David Lutton

**Editorial Program Coordinator:** Joe Niesen

**Technical Editor:** Elizabeth Ward, RD

**Recipe Tester:** Emily Nolan

**Nutritional Analyst:** Patty Santelli

**Editorial Manager:** Christine Meloy Beck

**Editorial Assistant:** Rachelle S. Amick

**Art Coordinator:** Alicia B. South

**Cover Photos:** © iStockphoto.com/Valua Vitaly

**Cartoons:** Rich Tennant (www.the5thwave.com)

**Composition Services**

**Project Coordinator:** Katie Crocker

**Layout and Graphics:** Carl Byers, Samantha K. Cherolis, Corrie Socolovitch

**Proofreaders:** Lindsay Amones, Betty Kish

**Indexer:** Valerie Haynes Perry

**Illustrators:** Kathryn Born, Elizabeth Kurtzman

---

**Publishing and Editorial for Consumer Dummies**

    **Kathleen Nebenhaus,** Vice President and Executive Publisher

    **Kristin Ferguson-Wagstaffe,** Product Development Director

    **Ensley Eikenburg,** Associate Publisher, Travel

    **Kelly Regan,** Editorial Director, Travel

**Publishing for Technology Dummies**

    **Andy Cummings,** Vice President and Publisher

**Composition Services**

    **Debbie Stailey,** Director of Composition Services

# Contents at a Glance

Introduction ........................................................................... 1

## Part 1: In the Beginning: Growing a Baby Bump ............ 7

Chapter 1: Eating Right for You and Your Baby ..............................9
Chapter 2: Expecting to Expect: Good Nutrition before Pregnancy.......... 17
Chapter 3: Nourishing Your Bump: Proper Nutrition while Pregnant ...... 29
Chapter 4: Knowing What to Avoid during Pregnancy .................... 49
Chapter 5: Weighty Matters: Managing Pregnancy Pounds ................ 63
Chapter 6: Overcoming Embarrassment: The Unpleasant
    Unmentionables of Pregnancy.................................... 75

## Part 11: Eating Right for Pregnancy..................... 91

Chapter 7: Completing the Puzzle: Discovering How to Eat while Pregnant ... 93
Chapter 8: Making Safe and Healthy Choices When Dining Out............ 105
Chapter 9: This or That: Making Grocery Shopping Decisions.............. 117
Chapter 10: Presenting Baby-Bump-Friendly Kitchen Basics............... 135
Chapter 11: Meal Planning with Your Growing Belly in Mind ............. 149

## Part 111: Cooking for Pregnancy ..................... 157

Chapter 12: Rise and Shine: Breakfast and Smoothie Recipes.............. 159
Chapter 13: Adding Fuel to Your Day: Snack, Appetizer, and
    Salad Recipes................................................... 175
Chapter 14: The Land, Sea, and Air: Main Dish Recipes .................. 201
Chapter 15: Plants, Please! Meatless Side and Main Dishes................ 227
Chapter 16: How Sweet It Is: Dessert Recipes........................... 253
Chapter 17: Cook It Fast: Speedy Recipes Ready in 10 Minutes or Less..... 271

## Part 1V: What You May Not Be Thinking
about but Should ........................................ 285

Chapter 18: Help Me, Doc! Situations That Require Medical Attention........ 287
Chapter 19: Mommy-and-Me Food Allergies ............................ 297
Chapter 20: After the Arrival: Caring for You and Your Baby.............. 303
Chapter 21: Losing Those Lingering Pounds............................. 317

## Part V: The Part of Tens ................................................. 329

Chapter 22: More Than Ten Nourishing Foods for Your Whole Pregnancy........... 331
Chapter 23: Ten Tricks for Getting Back to Your Pre-Pregnancy Weight............... 337

## Appendix: Metric Conversion Guide ........................... 343

## Index .................................................................. 347

# Recipes at a Glance

## *Breakfast Foods*

↻ Apricot Oatmeal Bake .................................................................. 163
↻ Berries and Cream French Toast ................................................ 164
↻ Broccoli Hash-Brown Quiche ..................................................... 171
↻ Chocolate Banana Blast Smoothie ............................................. 173
↻ Cottage Cheese Pancakes .......................................................... 165
↻ Decaf Mocha Smoothie .............................................................. 274
↻ Greek Omelet .............................................................................. 170
↻ Homemade Maple Berry Crunch Granola ................................... 162
↻ Oh, Baby! Banana Chocolate Chip Muffins ............................... 161
↻ Pomegranate Power Smoothie .................................................... 174
Sausage Asparagus Frittata ........................................................... 169
↻ Southwest Avocado Breakfast Burrito ........................................ 167
↻ Spinach, Egg, and Cheese Sandwich .......................................... 168

## *Appetizers and Snacks*

↻ Apple Cinnamon Trail Mix .......................................................... 177
Asian-Style Chicken Wings ............................................................ 187
Avocado Shrimp Martinis ............................................................... 183
Chicken Lettuce Wraps ................................................................... 189
↻ Crunchy Garbanzo Beans ........................................................... 179
↻ Dill and Chive Veggie Dip .......................................................... 275
↻ Fig and Olive Bruschetta ............................................................ 184
↻ Minty Watermelon Salsa ............................................................ 181
↻ Quinoa Nut Mix .......................................................................... 178
Sausage-Stuffed Baked Potato Skins ............................................. 188
↻ Steamed Artichoke with Garlic-Herb Dipping Sauce .................. 185
↻ Sun-Dried Tomato and Ricotta Stuffed Mushrooms .................... 186
↻ Truffle-Flavored Popcorn ........................................................... 180
White Chicken and Pineapple Flatbread ......................................... 190

## *Salads*

Asian Chicken Spinach Salad ......................................................... 198
↻ Cranberry Gelatin Salad ............................................................. 200
↻ Creamy Grape Salad ................................................................... 199
↻ Deconstructed Greek Salad ........................................................ 197

↻ Fresh Mozzarella, Tomato, and Pepper Salad ................................195
↻ Fruity Poppy Seed Salad ...............................................................193
↻ Honey Orange Grapefruit Salad ...................................................276
Mixed Greens with Chicken, Cantaloupe, & Red Grapes Salad........192
↻ Roasted Beet and Pistachio Salad ................................................196
↻ Three-Bean Artichoke Salad .........................................................277
↻ White Bean and Portobello Salad ................................................194

## Soups and Chilis
↻ Black Bean Chili ...........................................................................232
↻ Broccoli Cheese Soup ...................................................................230
↻ Souped-Up Split Pea Soup ...........................................................231
↻ Tomato Bulgur Soup .....................................................................229

## Beef Entrees
Beef and Bean Quesadillas ...............................................................205
Beef Empanadas................................................................................204
Cocoa-Rubbed Grilled Steaks ...........................................................209
Good to the Last Lick Casserole .......................................................203
Indian Lentil Slow Cooker Beef Stew ...............................................207
Italian Stuffed Steak Rolls ................................................................208
Nana's Moussaka ..............................................................................206

## Poultry and Pork Entrees
Chicken Hummus Pita .......................................................................278
Chicken Kabobs ................................................................................224
Crispy Lime Chicken Tenders ...........................................................223
Curry Chicken Salad ..........................................................................222
Parmesan-Herb-Crusted Pork Chops................................................218
Peachy Chicken Barley Pilaf .............................................................225
Rosemary Chicken on Asparagus Risotto..........................................221
Sauerkraut and Turkey Sausage Pasta Bake......................................220
Spinach, Date, and Blue Cheese Chicken Panini...............................226
Super Easy Pulled Pork .....................................................................217
Turkey Cheeseburger Chowder .........................................................219

## Seafood Entrees
Garden Fresh Paella...........................................................................215
Mango Avocado Salmon....................................................................212
Pecan-Crusted Tilapia with Pear and Fig Chutney ...........................213
Spaghetti with Clam Sauce ...............................................................211
Thai Scallops with Noodles ..............................................................214

## Vegetarian Entrees and Side Dishes

Baked Ziti with Tofu ........................................................................ 240

Broccoli, Beans, and Feta Pasta ..................................................... 250

Giant Beans with Spinach and Feta ................................................ 237

Havarti Pear Grilled Cheese on Pumpernickel ............................... 280

Homemade Gnocchi with Pesto ...................................................... 249

Quinoa Tabbouleh with Garbanzo Beans ....................................... 235

Ratatouille with Cannellini Beans ................................................... 234

Roasted Eggplant, Olive, and Goat Cheese Homemade Pizza ......... 251

Sesame Asparagus .......................................................................... 281

Sesame Noodle Salad ..................................................................... 239

Sloppy Lentil Joes ........................................................................... 236

Spanakopita (Greek Spinach Pie) ................................................... 245

Steamed Broccoli with Mustard Sauce and Cashews ..................... 243

Sweet Potato Hash .......................................................................... 246

Tofu Vegetable Stir-Fry .................................................................. 238

Vegetable Lasagna .......................................................................... 248

Wheat Berry Edamame with Dried Fruit ......................................... 241

Zucchini Patties .............................................................................. 244

## Desserts

Apple Cinnamon Crêpes ................................................................. 269

Banana Mini Trifle .......................................................................... 257

Chocolate Butterscotch Chip Bundt Cake ....................................... 264

Chocolate Lover's Sippable Sundae ................................................ 262

Dark Chocolate Cherry Pistachio Bark ........................................... 261

Fruit Cookie Pizza ........................................................................... 266

Fudgy Peppermint Black Bean Brownies ........................................ 260

Grilled Bananas .............................................................................. 284

Kiwi Custard Pie ............................................................................. 256

Lemon Raspberry Cupcakes ........................................................... 268

Mango Coconut Rice Pudding ......................................................... 258

Mixed Berry Frozen Yogurt ............................................................ 255

Peanut Butter Chocolate Chip Pie .................................................. 263

Pineapple Spice Loaf with Cream Cheese Frosting ......................... 267

Ricotta Parfait ................................................................................ 283

Sautéed Summer Fruit over Ice Cream ........................................... 282

White Chocolate Berry Oatmeal Cookies ........................................ 270

# Table of Contents

*Introduction* ........................................................................... 1

    About This Book .............................................................. 1
    Conventions Used in This Book ...................................... 2
    What You're Not to Read ............................................... 3
    Foolish Assumptions ...................................................... 3
    How This Book Is Organized ......................................... 3
        Part I: In the Beginning: Growing a Baby Bump ................ 4
        Part II: Eating Right for Pregnancy ..................................... 4
        Part III: Cooking for Pregnancy ........................................... 4
        Part IV: What You May Not Be Thinking about but Should ...... 5
        Part V: The Part of Tens .................................................... 5
    Icons Used in This Book ................................................ 5
    Where to Go from Here .................................................. 6

*Part 1: In the Beginning: Growing a Baby Bump* ............. 7

**Chapter 1: Eating Right for You and Your Baby** ................... 9

    Delving into Pregnancy Nutrition ................................. 9
        Knowing which foods to avoid ........................................ 10
        Gaining your baby weight slowly and steadily ................. 11
    Overcoming Pregnancy's Not-So-Fun Side
      Effects with Simple Food Tricks ................................... 11
    Discovering How to Eat ................................................ 12
    Making Healthy Choices ............................................... 13
        Picking the nutritious options at restaurants
          and grocery stores ................................................ 13
        Preparing good-for-you-both meals ................................ 14
    Sticking to Good Nutrition When Faced with Unique Circumstances ...... 14
    Thinking Ahead to Life Post-Delivery ........................... 15
        Figuring out your body's post-pregnancy nutrition needs .... 15
        Getting back in shape .................................................... 16

**Chapter 2: Expecting to Expect: Good Nutrition before Pregnancy... 17**

Preparing for the Baby Bump ............................................................ 17
  Understanding why you should eat right (and exercise) now ....... 18
  Getting your body ready ............................................................ 19
  Managing current health conditions ........................................ 21
Conception Troubles: Recognizing How Diet Affects Fertility ............... 22
  Nutrients that may influence your fertility .............................. 22
  The controversies surrounding alcohol and caffeine .................... 24
Discovering Why Your Weight Matters ............................................ 26

**Chapter 3: Nourishing Your Bump: Proper Nutrition
while Pregnant** ............................................................ 29

Eating for Baby and You: Balancing Calories
  Eaten and Calories Burned ...................................................... 29
  First trimester (weeks 1–13): Don't
    purposely take in extra calories ............................................ 30
  Second trimester (weeks 14–27): Take
    in an extra 300–350 calories ................................................ 31
  Third trimester (weeks 28–40): Take
    in an extra 450–500 calories ................................................ 33
Figuring Out Where Your Calories Should Come from ....................... 34
  Carbohydrates: Energy for the body ........................................ 35
  Protein: Cell building and repair ............................................ 36
  Fat: Nervous system development and function .......................... 37
Getting the Nutrients You Need ...................................................... 38
  Folate (folic acid) .................................................................. 39
  Iron .................................................................................... 39
  Calcium ............................................................................. 40
  Choline ............................................................................. 40
  Omega-3 fatty acids ............................................................ 41
  The rest of the essential pregnancy nutrients ............................ 42
Discovering the Numerous Benefits of Fiber ...................................... 44
  Knowing how much fiber you need .......................................... 44
  Filling up on fiber-rich foods .................................................. 44
  Sneaking more fiber into your day .......................................... 45
Realizing Why Proper Hydration Matters ......................................... 46
  How much fluid do I need? ...................................................... 46
  Where should my fluid come from? .......................................... 46
  What if I can't stay hydrated? .................................................. 47
Living a Vegetarian Lifestyle while Pregnant ...................................... 47

**Chapter 4: Knowing What to Avoid during Pregnancy ............. 49**

Foods That Aren't Safe during Pregnancy ......................................... 49
A Warning on Herbals ...................................................................... 52

Focusing on Foodborne Illnesses Caused by Bugs ...................53
    *Campylobacter* ...................54
    *E. coli* ...................54
    *Listeria* ...................55
    *Salmonella* ...................55
    *Toxoplasma* ...................56
Tackling Food-Related Toxins ...................57
    Mercury ...................57
    Pesticides ...................58
    Plastics ...................58
Going without Your Daily Alcohol or Caffeine Fix ...................60
    Lose the booze ...................60
    Moderate your caffeine intake ...................61
    Coping strategies for life with less caffeine and no alcohol ...................61

**Chapter 5: Weighty Matters: Managing Pregnancy Pounds ........ 63**

Gaining Weight Gradually ...................63
    How much to gain ...................64
    What to do when you're not gaining enough ...................65
Preventing Excess Weight Gain ...................65
    Potential complications from gaining too much ...................66
    How not to gain the "Pregnancy 50+" ...................66
Adding Exercise to Your Routine:
   You've Got to Move It, Move It ...................67
    Safety guidelines to consider ...................69
    Suggested exercises for pregnancy ...................70
    Exercises to avoid ...................74

**Chapter 6: Overcoming Embarrassment: The Unpleasant Unmentionables of Pregnancy ............................... 75**

Morning Sickness Can Happen Morning, Noon, or Night ...................75
    Dealing with nausea ...................76
    Understanding how vomiting may prevent you from
      getting enough nutrients ...................78
    Determining when medical intervention is necessary ...................78
Your Digestive Tract Acquires a Mind of Its Own ...................80
    Avoiding heartburn with the help of some nutrition tricks ...................80
    Reducing gas with an antibloating diet ...................82
    Preventing pregnancy constipation ...................83
    Dealing with hemorrhoids ...................84
    Steering clear of urinary tract infections ...................85
Fatigue Drains Your Energy Dry ...................86
    Eating to have energy ...................87
    Getting the sleep you need ...................88

## Part II: Eating Right for Pregnancy ............................. 91

### Chapter 7: Completing the Puzzle: Discovering
### How to Eat while Pregnant ................................... 93
Adopting a New Dining Strategy: Eat Small Amounts Frequently ........... 93
    Using the hunger gauge to interpret your body's signals ................... 94
    Keeping your hunger from becoming ravenous ............................. 96
    Knowing when to stop ................................................ 97
Snacking Is Sensible ....................................................... 98
    Presenting guidelines for smart snacking ................................ 98
    Being prepared with a go-to pregnancy snack list ....................... 99
    Determining how many snacks you need ............................... 101
Get Me Some Ice Cream . . . NOW!: Understanding
  and Managing Cravings ............................................... 102
    Why am I craving this food, anyway? .................................. 102
    How can I get through my cravings without gaining 70 pounds? ..... 103

### Chapter 8: Making Safe and Healthy Choices When Dining Out ... 105
First Things First: Navigating the Menu ..................................... 105
    Spotting high-sodium foods .......................................... 106
    Picking out high-fat foods ............................................ 106
    Zeroing in on good-for-you descriptions .............................. 107
Placing Your Order ......................................................... 107
Standing Strong in the Face of Common Restaurant Temptations ....... 108
    Dealing with appetizers .............................................. 108
    Handling oversized portions .......................................... 109
    Being smart about beverages ......................................... 112
    Saving room for dessert .............................................. 113
Keeping Food Safety in Mind at Your Favorite Restaurant ................. 114
    Send back food that isn't right ....................................... 114
    Reheat takeout and delivery food before you eat it ................... 115
    Keep your leftovers safe .............................................. 115

### Chapter 9: This or That: Making Grocery Shopping Decisions ..... 117
Choosing to Go Organic .................................................... 117
    Organic food basics .................................................. 118
    What the different types of "organic" labels mean .................... 118
    Why some pregnant women consider going organic .................. 119
Being Selective with Sweeteners ........................................... 122
    Acesulfame K ........................................................ 122
    Agave nectar ......................................................... 123
    Aspartame ........................................................... 123
    High-fructose corn syrup ............................................. 123

Honey ..........................................................................124
Saccharin .....................................................................124
Sucralose.....................................................................124
Stevia ..........................................................................125
Hitting the Seafood Counter................................................125
Knowing which fish to be cautious of ..............................125
Discovering which fish are best........................................126
Going the Convenient Route with Convenience Foods ..........127
Selecting nutritious frozen meals ....................................127
Making sure grab-and-go items are safe to eat ...............128
Simplifying Your Next Trip to the Store .............................130
Deciphering food labels ..................................................131
Preparing your pregnancy grocery list............................133

**Chapter 10: Presenting Baby-Bump-Friendly Kitchen Basics .....135**
Stocking the Kitchen ..........................................................135
Out with the old .............................................................136
In with the nutritious......................................................138
Practicing Safety in the Kitchen.........................................139
Embracing cleanliness.....................................................139
Cooking foods to the appropriate temperatures...............140
Storing your food properly..............................................143
Cooking the Healthy Way ...................................................143
Modifying recipes to make them healthier.......................144
Trying healthier cooking techniques ...............................145
Making Cooking More Comfortable as Your Pregnancy Progresses ....147

**Chapter 11: Meal Planning with Your Growing Belly in Mind .....149**
The Importance of Having a Plan .........................................149
Taking charge of your meals and snacks.........................150
Making meal planning easier with some tips and tricks..............150
Sample Pregnancy Meal Plans ...........................................151
2,000-calorie sample meal plans for the first trimester ................151
2,300-calorie sample meal plans for the second trimester..........153
2,450-calorie sample meal plans for the third trimester..............155

**Part III: Cooking for Pregnancy ..................................157**

**Chapter 12: Rise and Shine: Breakfast and Smoothie Recipes .....159**
Glorious Grains ................................................................160
Incredibly Edible Eggs......................................................166
On-the-Go Breakfasts — Smoothie Style...........................172

**Chapter 13: Adding Fuel to Your Day: Snack, Appetizer, and Salad Recipes** . . . . . . . . . . . . . . . . . . . . . . . . . . . . . . **175**

Preparing Healthy Snacks.....................................................................175
Small Bites for Your Growing Belly: Tapas-Style Meals......................182
Adding Color (And Nutrients) to Your Plate with Salads.....................191

**Chapter 14: The Land, Sea, and Air: Main Dish Recipes** . . . . . . . . **201**

Beef, It's What's for Pregnancy..............................................................202
Fishing for Something Different for Dinner: Seafood Dishes...............210
Embracing the Many White Meats ........................................................216

**Chapter 15: Plants, Please! Meatless Side and Main Dishes** . . . . . . . . . . . . . . . . . . . . . . . . . . . . . . . . . . . . . . **227**

Filling Up on Soups and Chilis ..............................................................228
Creative and Tasty Bean- and Soy-Based Alternatives to Meat...........233
Embracing Vegetables ...........................................................................242
Serving Up Pasta and Pizza ...................................................................247

**Chapter 16: How Sweet It Is: Dessert Recipes** . . . . . . . . . . . . . . . . **253**

Whipping Up Smooth and Creamy Treats..............................................254
Pregnancy Must-Have: Chocolate! .......................................................259
Diving into the Refreshing, Sweet Taste of Fruit .................................265

**Chapter 17: Cook It Fast: Speedy Recipes Ready in 10 Minutes or Less** . . . . . . . . . . . . . . . . . . . . . . . . . . . . . . . . **271**

Relying on Convenience Foods ..............................................................272
Letting Flavor Stand Out in Quick Dishes.............................................279

**Part IV: What You May Not Be Thinking about but Should** . . . . . . . . . . . . . . . . . . . . . . . . . . . . . . . . . **285**

**Chapter 18: Help Me, Doc! Situations That Require Medical Attention** . . . . . . . . . . . . . . . . . . . . . . . . . . . . . . . . . . . . **287**

Using Diet and Exercise to Help Control Certain Medical Conditions..287
Gestational diabetes.........................................................................288
Polycystic ovary syndrome ..............................................................290
High blood pressure and preeclampsia............................................291
Anemia...............................................................................................293
Nutrition Advice for Mothers with Special Considerations .................294
Nutritional concerns for teenage mothers .....................................294
Nutritional concerns for mothers who are cancer survivors ......295
Nutritional concerns for mothers of multiples ............................295

## Chapter 19: Mommy-and-Me Food Allergies . . . . . . . . . . . . . . . . . . 297

Identifying Common Food Allergens.................................................297
What to Do If You Suspect a Food Allergy......................................299
Preventing Food Allergies in Your Baby..........................................300
    Deciding whether you need to avoid
      certain foods while pregnant.......................................300
    Recognizing the role breast-feeding
      plays in allergy prevention ........................................301
    Introducing food allergens to your child.......................302

## Chapter 20: After the Arrival: Caring for You and Your Baby . . . . . . 303

Getting the Nutrients You Need to Fuel Your Recovery....................303
To Nurse, or Not to Nurse? ............................................................305
    Benefits of nursing for Mom .......................................305
    Benefits of breast milk for Baby..................................307
    Overcoming obstacles of breast-feeding .....................307
Practicing Good Nutrition When You're Nursing...............................308
    Focusing on carbohydrates, proteins, and fats ...........309
    Highlighting other important nutrients .......................309
    Staying hydrated........................................................310
    Sampling some meal plans for nursing moms..............311
    Being smart about alcohol and caffeine......................312
Feeding Baby................................................................................313
    With breast milk.........................................................314
    With formula..............................................................315

## Chapter 21: Losing Those Lingering Pounds . . . . . . . . . . . . . . . . . . . 317

Setting Yourself Up for Success with Realistic Expectations .............318
    Knowing how long your belly will stay .........................318
    Understanding proper rates of weight loss...................319
Fueling Your Body the Right Way......................................................319
    Focusing on nutrient-dense foods ..............................320
    Creating a calorie deficit............................................321
    Sampling some meal plans to help you lose weight......322
Incorporating Exercise into Your Post-Delivery Routine ...................324
    Getting started .........................................................324
    Fitting in all three types of exercise ...........................326
Preparing for the Next Baby Bump .................................................327
    Deciding how soon to start trying again......................327
    Restoring your nutritional status ................................328

*Part V: The Part of Tens* .............................................. **329**

**Chapter 22: More Than Ten Nourishing Foods
for Your Whole Pregnancy** ................................... **331**
    Asparagus ........................................................331
    Avocado ..........................................................332
    Beef.................................................................332
    Berries.............................................................332
    Edamame .........................................................333
    Eggs ...............................................................333
    Greek Yogurt ....................................................334
    Legumes ..........................................................334
    Milk ...............................................................335
    Quinoa.............................................................335
    Salmon............................................................336

**Chapter 23: Ten Tricks for Getting Back to
Your Pre-Pregnancy Weight** ................................ **337**
    Listen When Your Belly Says It's Full.......................337
    Don't Starve Yourself .........................................338
    Eat Small Portions and Eat Frequently ....................338
    Be Mindful of What You're Eating ..........................339
    Get Moving ......................................................339
    Increase Your Muscle Mass...................................340
    Breast-feed to Burn More Calories .........................341
    Get Enough Sleep...............................................341
    Make Time for Yourself........................................342
    Remember Why You're Trying to Lose Weight — For Baby................342

*Appendix: Metric Conversion Guide* ........................... **343**

*Index* .................................................................. **347**

# Introduction

· · · · · · · · · · · · · · · · · · · · · · · · · · · · · · · · · · · · · · · · · · · · · · · · · · ·

*I*f you're reading this book, I'm guessing you or someone you love is either pregnant or thinking about becoming pregnant. Either way, congratulations! Having children is one of the greatest joys (and challenges) in life. I applaud you for taking an interest in how and what you eat during pregnancy so that you can keep yourself healthy and, of course, deliver a bouncing, beautiful baby boy or girl.

While pregnancy is certainly a joyous time, it can also be a time full of stress and anxiety as you constantly wonder if you're doing everything right. Your diet may be one of the areas you're confused and panicked about. Never fear! You've now got a resource to help guide you through the ins and outs of pregnancy nutrition — from what food to buy to how to prepare and enjoy it.

My goal in writing this book is to present the scientifically factual information you need to know about pregnancy nutrition in a way that doesn't add any more stress to your life. I explain which foods to avoid and which ones to get plenty of so that both you and your baby get all the nutrients you need for healthy growth. As a bonus, I include six whole chapters of new recipes that will nourish your growing belly, and I explain what you need to consider as far as postpartum nutrition goes.

## About This Book

I wrote this book because as a registered dietitian who recently went through two pregnancies, I know what it's like to have lots of questions when you first become pregnant. I too wondered what can I eat, what can't I eat, and what can I do if I'm nauseous, constipated, or just plain tired? I've since discovered the answers, and it's my pleasure to share them with you. In fact, I hope this book helps you feel better about your food and beverage choices and puts your mind at ease regarding pregnancy nutrition.

In addition to nutrition advice, I also include advice on how to eat while pregnant, pointers on safe food preparation, and 100 delicious recipes for you to try out. After all, eating during your pregnancy should be an enjoyable experience.

In typical *For Dummies* style, all this information is organized in a way that allows you to pick up the book and head to the topic that interests you in that moment. You don't have to start at the beginning or go through the chapters in chronological order. Feel free to visit a chapter, or even sections of a chapter, as the subjects interest you or apply to you at various times in your pregnancy.

# Conventions Used in This Book

I use the following conventions throughout the book to make things consistent and easy to understand:

- ✔ Monofont indicates web addresses.

- ✔ *Italics* draw your attention to new terms that I'm defining. They also occasionally indicate words I want to emphasize.

- ✔ **Boldface** tells you you're looking at the keywords in bulleted lists and the action parts of numbered steps.

When you're reading through this book's recipes, keep in mind the following guidelines:

- ✔ Milk is lowfat or fat-free.

- ✔ All milk, cheese, juice, and honey are pasteurized.

- ✔ Butter is unsalted unless otherwise specified. Margarine isn't a suitable substitute for butter unless I state you can use either one.

- ✔ Eggs are large.

- ✔ All olive oil is extra-virgin.

- ✔ All lemon or lime juice can be either fresh squeezed or from a bottle unless otherwise specified. (If you go the fresh-squeezed route, just be sure to wash the outside of the lemon or lime before you cut into it.)

- ✔ Powdered sugar refers to confectioner's sugar.

- ✔ Salt refers to regular table salt unless otherwise noted.

- ✔ Pepper is freshly ground black pepper unless otherwise specified.

- ✔ Onions are yellow unless otherwise specified.

- ✔ Flour is all-purpose unless otherwise specified.

- ✔ Sugar is granulated unless otherwise specified.

- ✔ All herbs are fresh unless dried herbs are specified.

- ✔ All temperatures are Fahrenheit. (If you prefer working in the metric system, see the Appendix for help with converting temperatures to Celsius.)

Last but not least, when referring to your baby throughout the book, I take turns with gender, alternating between he or she and him or her.

# What You're Not to Read

Although I think absolutely every word in this book is worth reading, I realize that you may not have the time or energy to read it from cover to cover. To help you focus on the most important parts, I highlight the interesting but unessential info so that you can quickly skip over it:

✔ When you see text in a shaded box, you know it's a sidebar. Sidebar information is good to know and usually quite interesting, but it's not necessary to your understanding of the topic at hand.

✔ When you see a Technical Stuff icon, you know that I've delved a bit deeper into a subject and provided some information that you can live without — although you may be less likely to win trivia contests in the future if you don't read it! If you have the time and interest, dig in; if not, move on.

# Foolish Assumptions

Call me crazy, but I assume that most people reading this book are pregnant. In particular, I assume that you're pregnant with your first child and are feeling slightly overwhelmed with all the information out there about what you can and can't eat. That's why I talk directly to the pregnant woman throughout the book. If you're a partner or loved one of a pregnant woman and you're reading this book, please pass the information along to the momma-to-be.

Because this book also includes 100 very tasty recipes, I also assume you know a thing or two about cooking — as in you've at least boiled water and used a mixer in your somewhat recent past.

# How This Book Is Organized

This book contains five parts, and each part contains several chapters. I give you a rundown of what these parts cover in the following sections. Whenever I mention information that I discuss elsewhere in the book, I refer you to that particular chapter so you know where to go if you're interested in that topic.

## Part I: In the Beginning: Growing a Baby Bump

If you happen to be doing your homework on pregnancy nutrition before getting pregnant, then this is the part for you. It includes a chapter with advice that will prepare you to start growing your very own baby bump.

If you're already pregnant, then get ready to find out more about every one of the nutrients that are critical to your baby's development, from folate and fat to calcium and carbs. I also warn you about foods and beverages that can potentially cause harm to you or your baby so you can avoid or limit them in your diet. And because pregnancy comes with some obvious side effects (hello, weight gain!) and some potentially embarrassing ones (think vomiting and gas), I guide you in gaining the proper amount of weight and explain how to manipulate your diet to overcome nausea, gas, and the other unmentionables of pregnancy.

## Part II: Eating Right for Pregnancy

As you discover in this part, you basically have to develop a whole new eating routine when you become pregnant; that routine revolves around eating small amounts frequently. Also when you're pregnant, deciding what to eat takes a bit more thought. That's why this part also explains how to make good-for-baby (and you) choices while dining out, how to make smart grocery shopping decisions, and how to prepare your kitchen for optimal food safety. This part finishes up by providing you with some sample meal plans to follow for the various stages of your pregnancy.

## Part III: Cooking for Pregnancy

Whatever your taste preferences are, at least a few of the 100 recipes in this part have to appeal to you. Here you find a wide array of breakfast meals, appetizers, salads, main dishes, vegetarian dishes, and desserts. Each recipe contains at least one ingredient that has special nutritional value for you during your pregnancy.

Whichever recipe you choose to make, I recommend that you read it in its entirety before getting started. Then gather your ingredients and follow the directions carefully for the best possible outcome.

## Part IV: What You May Not Be Thinking about but Should

Every pregnancy is different because every woman brings with her a unique set of genetics and lifestyle habits. Of course you want to have a relatively normal pregnancy, but just in case certain medical complications, like gestational diabetes or high blood pressure, do crop up, I dedicate a chapter in this part to how to adjust your diet to manage these issues. I also cover how to deal with food allergies you may have and how to prevent them in your baby.

While you may not be thinking of it yet, I can almost guarantee that at some point you'll start considering what life will be like after your baby is born. So in this part, I also clue you into post-delivery nutrition and your options for feeding your little one. And just in case you're wondering how you're going to get back in shape after delivery, I offer some advice at the end of this part on how to do just that.

## Part V: The Part of Tens

If you're a regular *For Dummies* reader, you know that every *For Dummies* book features a Part of Tens that includes short lists of tidbits that are helpful for you to know about the subject in question. This book is no different. In this part, you find a list of ten nutrient-rich foods to eat during pregnancy and ten simple yet effective ways to lose lingering "baby weight" after you deliver. I also throw in an appendix of metric conversions in case you prefer cooking with milliliters rather than cups.

# Icons Used in This Book

To make this book easier to use, I include some icons that can help you find and grasp key information quickly. Here's what those icons look like and what they mean:

This icon is pretty self-explanatory. When you see it, be sure to follow up with your doctor for his or her expert opinion on the information in question.

This icon represents some of the most important information in the book. You may even want to read it a few times so that it really takes hold (especially if you have "pregnancy brain" and have a difficult time keeping things straight).

The tidbits marked by this icon may be really interesting (at least, to me), but you don't have to read them word for word to grasp the main concepts at hand. In fact, feel free to skip over paragraphs flagged with this icon.

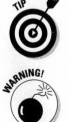

I'm all for saving a pregnant woman's time and making things easier for her, so know that you're in for some great tips that achieve just that every time you see this bull's-eye.

Watch out for any paragraphs bearing this ticking time bomb. Paying attention to the information they contain can help keep you and your baby safe.

# Where to Go from Here

Where you go from here is completely up to you and your needs. If you're not pregnant yet and you want to know how to eat to best prepare your body for pregnancy, start with Chapter 2. If morning sickness is getting you down, check out the tips in Chapter 6 for how to deal with this unpleasant side effect of pregnancy. If you're craving some dessert, turn to Chapter 16, which features some amazing recipes that are sure to satisfy any sweet tooth. You get the idea.

Wherever you decide to begin, my hope is that you enjoy eating all throughout your pregnancy. Focus on nourishing your body with nutritious foods while at the same time taking advantage of being able to eat a few extra calories!

# Part I

# In the Beginning: Growing a Baby Bump

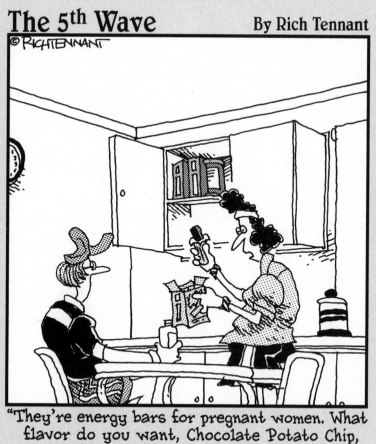

The 5th Wave                    By Rich Tennant

"They're energy bars for pregnant women. What flavor do you want, Chocolate Potato Chip, Ketchup & Pickles, or Sardine Blast?"

## In this part . . .

*E*ven starting with preconception, what you eat can have an impact on everything from your fertility to the development of your baby's vital organs. Certain foods, like those containing alcohol, caffeine at certain levels, or harmful bacteria, can hinder growth. The good news is that many of the nutritious foods you eat have a direct role in forming your baby's organs and systems as your belly grows.

In this part, you discover how to prepare your body for Baby. If you've already conceived, you can dive right into the information on which foods provide critical nutrients for you and your baby and the truth about how many calories it takes to gain the right amount of weight during each trimester of pregnancy. This part also tells you which foods and beverages to steer clear of, how to gain your pregnancy pounds the healthy way, and how to overcome some of the embarrassing side effects that can come along with pregnancy simply by modifying your dietary habits.

# Chapter 1

# Eating Right for You and Your Baby

. . . . . . . . . . . . . . . . . . . . . . . . . . . . . . . . . . . . . . . . . . . . . . . . . . .

## In This Chapter

▶ Recognizing the roles good nutrition and steady weight gain play in a healthy pregnancy

▶ Dealing with unpleasant pregnancy side effects by eating right

▶ Understanding why eating small, frequent meals is important

▶ Making the right food decisions throughout your pregnancy

▶ Looking ahead to your body's post-delivery needs

. . . . . . . . . . . . . . . . . . . . . . . . . . . . . . . . . . . . . . . . . . . . . . . . . . .

The role nutrition plays in your baby's development is critical. In fact, some researchers suggest that the nutrients a developing fetus receives in the womb (and that a newborn receives in the first few weeks of life) are more critical than the nutrients received at any other time in life. That may seem quite shocking, but more and more evidence is connecting a woman's nutritional status during pregnancy to the health of her child, not just at birth but throughout his or her life.

This chapter provides you with an overview of pregnancy nutrition. Prepare to discover the basics of what to eat and how to eat it over the course of the next nine months. (As an added bonus, reading this chapter arms you with fact-based answers for when your mother-in-law or that perfect stranger asks you whether eating XYZ food is safe.)

## Delving into Pregnancy Nutrition

Eating the right foods while you're pregnant may not be as difficult as you think. Depending on what you ate before you started trying to get pregnant or before you got that positive pregnancy test, you may not need to make many changes after all. If you already gravitate toward fruits, vegetables, lean proteins, whole grains, and lowfat dairy, the pregnancy diet will be really easy for you to follow. If, on the other hand, you survive on donuts, chips, and fast food, you may need to dig a bit deeper into changing those habits for the sake of your unborn child.

## Start eating right before you get pregnant

Eating right is important even when you're still trying to get pregnant. As I explain in Chapter 2, certain nutrients (such as folate) are essential for the development of critical organs within your baby before you realize you're pregnant. So even before you get a positive pregnancy test, focus on filling your body with nutrient-rich foods that will help you stock up your nutritional status so you can start your pregnancy on the right foot.

*Tip:* All women of childbearing age are encouraged to take a multivitamin that contains folic acid because of the important role folic acid plays in the early development of the neural tube that connects the brain and spinal cord. Switch to a prenatal vitamin when you start trying to get pregnant and keep taking it throughout your pregnancy.

Finding the right balance of calories is one of the many things that women wonder about when they get pregnant. You often hear people say, "Oh, you're pregnant. So now you can eat for two!" But that's not really the case. Just think about it for a minute. You're growing a little baby, not a full-sized adult. Yes, you do typically need to take in extra calories starting in your second trimester, but you certainly don't need to start eating double. Turn to Chapter 3 to find out exactly how many more calories you need.

The following sections give you a general idea of which foods you should steer clear of throughout your pregnancy and how you should aim to put on those pregnancy pounds.

## *Knowing which foods to avoid*

Before you got pregnant, you may have thought that all you needed to stay away from during your pregnancy was alcohol and possibly caffeine. I'm afraid the list of taboo foods is quite a bit longer than that and includes the following:

- **Raw and undercooked beef, chicken, fish, and pork:** A meat thermometer can tell you for sure whether a particular meat has reached a safe temperature. (I provide a list of the minimum safe temperatures in Chapter 10.) If you don't own a meat thermometer, I strongly suggest picking one up. It'll be your new best friend in the kitchen.

  When most people think of sushi, they think of raw fish. As a sushi fan, I was heartbroken by the thought of not having it while I was pregnant, but in reality you can have sushi — as long as it's not the raw tuna or salmon kind. Imitation crab (used in the California roll), real crab, shrimp, and eel are all cooked, so you can enjoy any of those in your sushi.

✔ **Runny eggs:** Eggs need to be cooked all the way through, whether they're in the skillet, a sauce, or a casserole. Cook (or order your eggs in a restaurant) scrambled well or over hard. If the white or yolk is still runny, send it back to the skillet to be cooked until firm. Egg casseroles should be cooked until they reach 160 degrees. Avoid sauces that contain raw eggs, such as hollandaise and béarnaise. And don't forget about raw cookie dough — no licking the spoon if there are raw eggs in the dough!

✔ **Unpasteurized milk and cheeses:** Avoid milk or cheese that claims to be *raw* or that doesn't say *pasteurized* on the label. You're free to eat any cheese (including soft cheeses) as long as it has been made with pasteurized milk.

For the full scoop on which foods to avoid completely and which to be cautious of during pregnancy, see Chapter 4.

## Gaining your baby weight slowly and steadily

Putting on those pregnancy pounds gradually as your baby puts on weight is really the best approach to weight gain during pregnancy. The pounds you gain will distribute themselves in various tissues of your body, including fat and fluid, as well as your developing baby. (***Remember:*** Gaining some fat deposits when you're pregnant is normal and actually necessary!)

Try not to step on the scale every day during your pregnancy. Because of the variation in weight due to fluid balance, you may find that you gain 3 pounds in one day and then lose 1 pound the next day. As long as the overall trend is that you're gaining weight (slowly and steadily, of course) and your doctor determines that your baby is also growing and gaining weight, don't stress out about the exact number on the scale.

To prevent excess weight gain and to keep your heart, lungs, and muscles strong, exercise throughout your pregnancy. In particular, aim for a mix of aerobic exercise, strength training, and yoga (see Chapter 5 for details).

## Overcoming Pregnancy's Not-So-Fun Side Effects with Simple Food Tricks

As you may already know, pregnancy brings with it a variety of unpleasant side effects, like constipation, gas, hemorrhoids, heartburn, fatigue, and, of course, that first trimester nausea that can be unbearable. If this is the first time you're hearing about these side effects, I'm sorry that I'm the one breaking the news to you! But you need to be prepared because you may soon find yourself throwing up, farting, or just feeling really tired all because of that little bundle of joy growing in your belly.

The good news is that not all of these side effects happen to every woman. In fact, you may experience none of them! Additionally, they all have nutritional solutions that can make them tolerable. For example, if nausea is ruling your world, the key is to not let your stomach get too empty. I know this is the last thing you want to hear because you don't feel like eating, but even munching on dry cereal or crackers gives your stomach acid something else to focus on besides making you feel sick.

The caveat regarding food-related tricks for overcoming pregnancy's not-so-pleasant side effects is that there's lots of advice out there. Don't try to follow every tip you hear. Instead, focus on the tip that helps you manage the problem you're experiencing at the time. For instance, eating before bed is a good way to combat nausea in the first trimester, but this routine can be a problem in the second trimester if you start experiencing heartburn. In that case, stop eating a little before bedtime.

Want more tips and tricks for your pregnancy side effect arsenal? Head to Chapter 6.

## Discovering How to Eat

People tend to focus most of their nutrition attention on what to eat or what not to eat. Not nearly enough attention goes toward *how* to eat. I'm a believer in eating small quantities frequently throughout the day all the time, but this eating strategy becomes especially important as your belly grows.

In the first trimester, the end goal of eating small amounts frequently is to prevent nausea by having a little bit of food in your stomach at all times (that way, your stomach doesn't have to go into acid overload). As your baby bump grows and you progress into your second and third trimesters, you'll find that your body literally has less room for your stomach! As a result, the baby may press on your stomach and the area where your esophagus meets your stomach, causing heartburn. If you have small amounts of food in your stomach, you're less likely to experience this reflux.

The key to eating small amounts frequently is to enjoy a mix of smaller meals and regular snacks throughout the day. Now before you start envisioning bags of chips and pints of ice cream in your snacking future, remember that the majority of your snacks need to contain the nutrients you and your little one need. Otherwise, you're just eating empty calories. I provide a list of tasty nutritious snacks, as well as advice on how many snacks you may need throughout the day and how big they should be, in Chapter 7.

Another trick for keeping your eating in check is to avoid overindulging in cravings. You'll no doubt hear other women talk about cravings they had in pregnancy, and maybe you've already been experiencing them yourself. I like to blame everything in pregnancy on hormones, but cravings are truly a case of hormones gone wild! Sometimes those hormones cause food aversions (I actually didn't want chocolate during my first trimester with both kids!), and sometimes those hormones make it impossible to imagine living through another moment without one particular food. Don't worry; I show you how to get through this crazy part of pregnancy in Chapter 7.

# Making Healthy Choices

If only deciding what to eat every day during pregnancy were simple. First, you have to think about what you *want* to eat; then you have to consider what you *should* eat. Finally, you have to narrow down your choices to what's *available* to eat. To make the decision even harder, these three things are often on completely opposite ends of the healthy-tasty spectrum.

You can make the best decisions for you and your growing belly by arming yourself with some basic information before you head to your favorite restaurant, visit your local grocery store, or prepare your daily meals.

## Picking the nutritious options at restaurants and grocery stores

If you're dining out, those wonderful adjectives like *smothered* and *golden* can really take you into a place of love at first description. You may even be getting hungry right now! Making the healthy choice at a restaurant isn't easy, and eating the right portion is even more challenging.

Even though you're entitled to consume more calories during most of your pregnancy, you'd likely wind up consuming far more than your daily recommended amount if you finished off all the huge dinner portions so common in restaurants today. Fortunately, you can combat these oversized portions by asking for half of your meal to go before you even get it or by splitting a dish with a friend or partner. For additional pointers on dining out the healthy way while pregnant, flip to Chapter 8.

Grocery shopping may be last on the totem pole of things that excite you. But it's one of those chores that you have to do — if you want to eat from something other than a take-out box, that is. Pregnancy brings with it many decisions that you have to make at the supermarket, like whether to buy organically grown produce or the conventionally grown kind, which fish to choose, and whether to buy foods containing artificial sweeteners (and if so, which sweeteners you're comfortable consuming). Fortunately, one way to avoid getting hung up in the decision-making process at the store — and avoid impulse purchases — is by preparing a grocery list ahead of time. See Chapter 9 for a pregnancy-friendly grocery list that you can modify based on your preferences.

## Preparing good-for-you-both meals

Your kitchen can be a haven away from the uncertainty of how something was cooked (or who touched it) at a restaurant — not to mention you have more control over the ingredients when you prepare a meal yourself. As I explain in Chapter 10, all you have to do to make your kitchen a safe and healthy place for you to cook and eat during your pregnancy is check the refrigerator, freezer, and pantry for expired items and practice some basic food safety steps, such as:

✔ Always wash your hands before you start preparing food.

✔ Prepare vegetables away from raw meats.

✔ Cook (or reheat) food to the proper temperature.

✔ Store food promptly in the fridge or freezer.

Of course, a well-stocked and safe kitchen does you little good if you're not whipping up some tasty meals. For me, half the battle when eating right is simply knowing what to cook for myself and my family. To help you avoid that problem, I've filled Part III of this book with 100 recipes designed to nourish your belly with foods that taste yummy and contain the essential nutrients you and your developing baby need. Whether you're looking for breakfast, snack, salad, main dish, side dish, or dessert options, you'll find a delicious mix of traditional and more adventurous recipes.

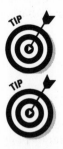

To make eating right during pregnancy a little easier (and less stressful), plan out your meals ahead of time. I show you how in Chapter 11.

As you cook, particularly as you get further along in your pregnancy, take frequent breaks. Sit down in a chair or stool and give your feet a rest for a few minutes if you notice you've been standing for a while.

# Sticking to Good Nutrition When Faced with Unique Circumstances

Every woman brings with her a unique set of genetics and lifestyle habits that guides how her pregnancy will progress. My hope is that you don't have any complications or unusual circumstances, but I want to prepare you just in case.

Various nutrition-related medical complications may creep up on you. For example, if you find out you have gestational diabetes, your best bet is to seek out the counsel of a registered dietitian to guide you in exactly how many and what kind of carbohydrates to eat. If you're faced with preeclampsia or high blood pressure, you'll have to watch your sodium intake very carefully. If you develop anemia, you'll need to focus on getting plenty of iron-rich foods and making sure your body absorbs as much of it as possible. (For additional guidance on maintaining proper nutrition in the face of pregnancy complications, head to Chapter 18.)

If you're allergic to milk or wheat and worried about whether your allergy is causing you to miss out on important nutrients, never fear. Just make the simple food substitutions I recommend in Chapter 19 to ensure you're eating a diet that's filled with all the nutrients you and your baby need. *Note:* Allergies can run in the family, so Chapter 19 also includes tips on when to introduce highly allergenic foods during your pregnancy and while you're nursing.

# Thinking Ahead to Life Post-Delivery

Right now you're probably smiling as you imagine holding your precious baby in your arms for the first time. I encourage those thoughts wholeheartedly, but don't forget to also think about how your life is going to change after your little one arrives.

For one thing, your body is going to need to recover, and it's going to need your help to do so. Also, eventually you'll need to think about shedding any lingering pregnancy pounds so that your body is in good shape — particularly if you want to have more kids. The following sections clue you in to the basics of post-delivery nutrition and the tricks to getting your pre-pregnancy body back.

## Figuring out your body's post-pregnancy nutrition needs

Being pregnant obviously comes with specific nutrition requirements, but so does giving birth to your child and recovering from that birth. No matter how you end up delivering, your body will require energy and specific nutrients to heal itself. Eat protein foods (think meats, eggs, dairy, and beans) because they're essential for repairing your body. Include carbohydrates (especially whole grains that are high in fiber) because they're necessary for energy. Also incorporate some healthy fats (such as olive oil, nuts, and seeds) to provide important nutrients and additional energy for your body. (I share more specifics on nutrition strategies for childbirth recovery in Chapter 20).

If you decide to breast-feed your baby, plan on eating pretty much the same foods you ate while pregnant throughout the length of time you choose to nurse. Of course, you may find that you need more calories while you're nursing than you did while you were pregnant; whether you do depends on how much milk you produce. *Note:* Nursing moms may lose some of their lingering pregnancy pounds fairly quickly due to their bodies' increased calorie needs and ability to use stored fat as energy to produce milk.

If you're breast-feeding, drink plenty of fluids, get rest, and continue to take your prenatal vitamin because you can use the extra vitamins and minerals while nursing.

## Getting back in shape

The key to post-pregnancy weight loss is to take it slow and steady, just as you did when gaining weight while you were pregnant. After all, you didn't gain all those pounds overnight, and they certainly won't come off that fast! As you get started, focus on eating smaller portions and leaving a few bites behind on your plate. Listen to your stomach when it tells your brain that it's satisfied and stop eating before you get overfull.

Don't give into the temptation of starving yourself after pregnancy. I know you're tired of carrying those extra pounds, but eating too little isn't good for you or your baby. Remember that your body is still recovering. If you're nursing, keep in mind that you need a good deal of calories to fuel milk production. Turn to Chapter 21 for more specific advice on how to eat for weight loss after your babe is born.

You may be surprised to find out that your pregnancy belly stays for a little while after delivery. The truth is much of your expanded stomach is actually your uterus, and it takes several weeks to shrink back to its normal size. Ignore anyone who tells you she wore her pre-pregnancy clothes home from the hospital and make sure you hang on to your elastic-banded pregnancy pants for a little while longer (or live in comfy dresses like I did for the first month).

As soon as you receive clearance from your doctor, which may take eight weeks or more if you have a cesarean (C-section) delivery, start adding exercise to your routine. Put your baby in the stroller and go for a walk, swim, pop in a yoga DVD, or attend a postnatal exercise class. Doing so will not only help you burn calories but also provide you with some much-needed stress relief and give you a nice boost of mood-elevating hormones.

# Chapter 2

# Expecting to Expect: Good Nutrition before Pregnancy

## In This Chapter

▶ Getting your nutrition and health in order before you start trying to have a little one

▶ Understanding how what you eat or don't eat affects fertility

▶ Finding out what your weight has to do with how quickly you can conceive

Congratulations! You've made one of the most important decisions of your life: the choice to have children. Even if you aren't pregnant yet, just deciding that you want to join the millions of people who've found joy in reproducing is a big step!

In this chapter, I tell you exactly what you need to consider before you get pregnant. (If you're already pregnant, stick around because you'll still pick up some good stuff.) First, I delve into the true importance of eating well during pregnancy and preparing your body before you even get pregnant. Then I help you understand two big factors that can affect your fertility: what you eat and how much you weigh.

## Preparing for the Baby Bump

If you and your partner are thinking about trying to conceive, then you know it's not just about you anymore. Mentally, you're readying yourself to get used to the idea of having a child, but you have to do some physical preparation, too. Specifically, you need to start watching what you eat and getting your health in order, no matter what your current health status or shape may be.

## *Understanding why you should eat right (and exercise) now*

Gone are the days of waiting for the positive sign on the pregnancy stick to get serious about getting healthy. Why? Because your body needs certain nutrients in reserve even before you get pregnant. If you're properly nourished when you get pregnant, you'll start off with the right building blocks to nourish your baby, too. Planning several months in advance can give you a jump-start in preparing yourself for pregnancy. Plus, if you clean up your diet now, you won't have to make major changes when you do find out you're pregnant. (So even if you aren't pregnant yet, go ahead and start following the advice in Chapters 3 and 4 and Part II, and don't miss out on the yummy — and healthy — recipes in Part III.)

Your body's reserves and the food you eat are the only meal service for your developing baby. From the minute the sperm and egg collide to make new life, certain nutrients are necessary to make everything else possible. For example, your baby's neural tube, which covers the spinal cord, forms in the first few weeks to one month following conception. At that point, some women don't even know they're pregnant yet. Having enough of the B vitamin folic acid in your body in those first few weeks is necessary to form a healthy spinal cord for your baby and can prevent certain neural tube birth defects, such as spina bifida. (For details on exactly how much folic acid you need, see the next section, and for information on other important nutrients your growing baby needs, see Chapter 3.)

Before you even start trying to have a baby, stop eating high-mercury fish, like king mackerel, shark, swordfish, and tilefish. If mercury passes to the fetus after you become pregnant, it can have a negative effect on the baby's developing nervous system. Because mercury can build up in the bloodstream and take years to remove naturally, experts recommend that women who are thinking of becoming pregnant limit their consumption of high-mercury fish for several months to a year prior to becoming pregnant. (See Chapter 9 for more details on which fish to eat and which fish to avoid during pregnancy.)

*Note:* If you're a vegetarian, you can continue living your vegetarian lifestyle throughout pregnancy and nursing. You simply need to make sure you're getting all the essential nutrients that you and your baby need. Focus on iron, zinc, omega-3 fatty acids, and protein. I cover vegetarian diets in greater detail in Chapter 3.

Of course, eating right isn't the only way to physically prepare for a baby bump. Exercise helps, too. Even though trying to get pregnant should be nothing but fun, the whole process can be stressful at times. Exercise is a natural way to relieve stress. So take your aggressions out physically with moderate and even vigorous exercise. Exercise also elevates your mood by boosting endorphins that make you feel better, and a better mood means better sex.

On a cellular level, exercise helps your body process *glucose* (blood sugar) and use *insulin* (the hormone that takes glucose to your cells). Better glucose control means better chances of getting pregnant. Finally, exercise helps strengthen your heart, muscles, and bones — preparing them for the extra physical demand that pregnancy puts on your body.

## Getting your body ready

If you were planning to take your car on a cross-country road trip, you'd take it in for a tune-up before you left to make sure all the hoses and spark plugs were in good working order. Just like a tune-up for a car, getting a full-system checkup on your body is key for getting pregnant and delivering a healthy baby. Consider this your pre-pregnancy checklist:

- ✔ **Visit your family doctor.** A visit with your family doctor (or internal medicine doctor) is a good idea every year anyway, but a pre-pregnancy checkup will either give you a medical green light to get pregnant or provide information about aspects of your health that you need to improve before you conceive. Go through your family and personal health history to see whether your doctor has any concerns about your trying to become pregnant. He or she may also have some good advice for lifestyle changes to ensure a healthy pregnancy that you may not have considered.

- ✔ **Establish a relationship with an OB/GYN.** If you don't already have an obstetrician/gynecologist (OB/GYN), search around until you find one you're comfortable with. Pregnancy requires numerous office visits throughout the journey, so find someone you can build a rapport with. You need to feel comfortable asking all the silly and not-so-silly questions about pregnancy and delivery as you go through the process.

- ✔ **Visit the dentist.** Your mouth is the gateway for nutrition. Even if you think your teeth and gums are healthy, get a checkup and cleaning prior to pregnancy. Take care of any dental work (including treating bleeding gums or any other signs of periodontal disease) that needs to be done before you get pregnant, if at all possible. Studies show that pregnant women with periodontal disease give birth more often to low-birth-weight babies and have more babies born preterm.

  When you do get pregnant, you may experience bleeding gums due to more blood volume and more blood flow to the gums. With both of my pregnancies, my gums bled more than usual every time I flossed. I wanted to skip my six-month cleaning when I was pregnant, but my dentist insisted that I come in and promised to go easy on me. I went and was glad I took that step to keep my mouth healthy.

✔ **Manage your weight.** Many women go into pregnancy fearing that they'll gain too much weight and not be able to lose it. If you're overweight, try to lose weight prior to pregnancy. It's safe to lose weight and try to get pregnant at the same time. Plus, losing those excess pounds helps increase your chances of getting pregnant (see more details in the later section "Discovering Why Your Weight Matters") and improves your health.

As soon as you become pregnant, talk to your doctor or registered dietitian about weight-management strategies because weight loss isn't recommended during pregnancy.

✔ **Get plenty of folic acid.** Folic acid is the synthetic form of folate, which is found naturally in certain plant foods. Women in their childbearing years should take 400 to 800 micrograms (mcg) of folic acid every day, but especially for the three or more months before they start trying to get pregnant. The first 28 days following conception are the most critical for folic acid and prevention of neural tube birth defects. If you're already pregnant, start taking folic acid right away. A prenatal vitamin or even a regular multivitamin should have what you need, but check the label for a minimum of 400 mcg.

✔ **Cut back on alcohol.** If you think you have an alcohol problem, seek help before trying to get pregnant. If you drink daily but moderately (one drink per day), consider cutting back while you're trying to get pregnant. When you get pregnant, cut out alcohol completely. (Cutting back pre-pregnancy may make eliminating alcohol from your diet easier to do when you actually get pregnant.)

Jump ahead to the section "The controversies surrounding alcohol and caffeine" for details on the relationship between alcohol and conception.

✔ **Limit caffeine.** If you have to have three or more fully caffeinated cups of coffee per day (8 ounces each), consider cutting back. Because caffeine is physically addicting and withdrawal symptoms can occur (mainly headaches and irritability), cutting back slowly is a better approach than going cold turkey. Take this time while you're trying to become pregnant to pour fewer daily cups to physically (and mentally) get used to consuming less caffeine because after you conceive, it's best to limit your caffeine intake to just 200 milligrams (mg) per day.

For more information on the relationship between caffeine and conception, check out the section "The controversies surrounding alcohol and caffeine."

✔ **Quit smoking.** Quit smoking well before you plan on getting pregnant. Smoking during pregnancy compromises blood flow and oxygen to the baby. Plus, pregnant women who smoke have a higher risk of giving birth to low-birth-weight babies, and their babies have a higher risk of developing asthma and other breathing lung problems.

Also eliminate secondhand smoke during pregnancy. Don't be afraid to ask someone to take it outside for the health of your baby.

✔ **Make over your medicine cabinet.** If you're taking prescription medications and you're thinking about becoming (or already are) pregnant, review them with the prescribing physician as well as your obstetric physician. Many medications carry a warning not to take them during pregnancy, and chatting with your doctor can help you decide whether it's medically necessary for you to continue taking your meds if they fall into this category. Be sure to review over-the-counter medications and dietary supplements, such as cold medicines, pain relievers, and vitamin or herbal supplements, with your doctor, too, so that you can make sure you have the right stuff on hand in case you become ill before you realize that you're pregnant.

## *Managing current health conditions*

If you have a particular health condition, such as one from the following list, discuss your condition with your doctor before trying to get pregnant so that together you can form a plan for the best possible outcome.

✔ **Diabetes:** When you have diabetes, maintaining the right range of blood sugar prior to conception is key to getting pregnant and preventing miscarriage. Studies have linked diabetes during pregnancy to large babies and difficult deliveries with increased risk of C-section deliveries. If you have diabetes, focus on eating right before and while you're pregnant and including the right kinds of carbs in the right amounts. Limit refined grains and added sugars while focusing on getting the right mix of nutrients such as fiber and protein. (Note that some pregnant women wind up with *gestational diabetes,* a type of diabetes that develops only after a woman is pregnant. I explain how to deal with this condition in Chapter 18.)

If you have a family history of diabetes or suspect you have diabetes, make an appointment with your doctor to see if you are diabetic.

✔ **Polycystic ovary syndrome (PCOS):** PCOS reduces fertility in women because it compromises their body's use of insulin, leaving them with high glucose and insulin levels that lead to hormone disruption and weight gain. Losing weight by managing portions and exercising regularly helps control glucose and regulate hormones. But some women with PCOS may also need to use medications for glucose control and ovulation regulation. (See Chapter 18 for more details.)

✔ **High blood pressure (hypertension):** Blood flow to the baby is critical during pregnancy, and women with high blood pressure may have reduced blood flow. If you're on a medication for blood pressure, consult your doctor about continuing the medication during pregnancy; many high blood pressure meds are safe. Strict sodium restriction may also be necessary to control blood pressure. (I cover hypertension during pregnancy in more detail in Chapter 18.)

✔ **High cholesterol:** If you're on cholesterol-lowering medications, your doctor will very likely want you to stop taking them during pregnancy because they aren't considered safe for pregnant women. As a result, you have to rely on your diet to control your cholesterol during the period of time you're off the medications. Read labels carefully to limit your saturated and trans fat intake as much as possible. Increase soluble fiber, soy protein, and plant sterols to help keep your cholesterol under control. You may also take omega-3 fish oil supplements, especially if your triglycerides are elevated.

If you have a health condition that involves dietary considerations, or if you want a healthy preconception and pregnancy eating plan, make an appointment with a registered dietitian (RD) before you get pregnant, if possible. Dietitians are trained to teach you exactly what, how much, and when to eat to get the best outcome for you and your baby. Plan on meeting with your dietitian periodically throughout your pregnancy so that you can get help along the way. To find an RD in your area, visit the American Dietetic Association's website, www.eatright.org.

# Conception Troubles: Recognizing How Diet Affects Fertility

An estimated one in seven couples has trouble getting pregnant. Millions of dollars have been spent on reproductive technologies to assist couples in getting pregnant, but comparatively little attention has been paid to the role of diet in fertility even though a woman's diet affects numerous systems within her body — including her reproductive system.

Let me point out right away that no magic bullet food will make you a fertile goddess if you eat it. That being said, the field of diet and fertility has been growing, and new research is emerging on a regular basis. The following sections outline some of the nutrients that affect fertility and explain why your daily vice of choice (like that cup o' joe or glass of Merlot) may be hurting your chances of conceiving.

If you've been trying to get pregnant for 6 to 12 months and have been unsuccessful, you may want to call your doctor. If you're older than 35 or have any other reason to think you may have trouble getting pregnant, see your doctor earlier than 6 months into the trying process.

## Nutrients that may influence your fertility

The reason you (and I and everyone else out there) need food is to provide nutrients for your body to have energy and to keep your organs functioning. Your reproductive system is just one of the many systems of the body that requires good nutrition to run effectively.

# Good sources of plant proteins

Not yet pregnant but wanting to eat a healthier diet to improve your odds of conceiving? Adding just one serving a day of any of the following plant-protein sources can protect against infertility that results from not ovulating properly:

✔ **Soy-based foods:** Soymilk, tofu, tempeh, and vegetarian alternatives (like veggie bacon, burgers, sausage, and so on)

✔ **Legumes:** Black beans, garbanzo beans (chickpeas), pinto beans, lentils, kidney beans, black-eyed peas, and so on

✔ **Nuts:** Peanuts, almonds, pistachios, walnuts, soy nuts, pecans, and so on

Unfortunately, not a lot of research has been done on the direct effect of diet and fertility. But researchers at Harvard Medical School have found a few connections between diet and ovulation. If you're trying to get pregnant, pay special attention to the following nutrients, which I list in order of importance regarding how they affect the most common female fertility problem — not ovulating properly:

✔ **Carbohydrates:** Carbs, your body's preferred source of energy, can send your glucose and insulin levels sky-high if you eat too many of the refined carbs out there (like sugary and white-flour-based foods). In turn, spiking glucose and insulin levels may negatively affect the hormones needed for ovulation and can decrease fertility. Choose carb-containing foods that are full of nutritional value and that provide a slow release of glucose (blood sugar). Try the whole-grain variety whenever possible and fill up on whole fruits and vegetables.

✔ **Protein:** Women with high intakes of animal protein are more likely to have ovulation-disruption fertility problems than women who eat more plant-based proteins. Red meat, chicken, and turkey seem to have a negative impact on fertility, while fish and eggs have no effect. Now I'm not saying you need to become a vegetarian. Simply consider substituting 25 grams (g) of plant protein for 25 g of animal protein each day. Doing so can reduce your risk of infertility due to not ovulating properly by 50 percent.

✔ **Fats:** Recent evidence has connected the types of fat that people eat to fertility. The more trans fats in your diet, the higher your risk of infertility related to ovulation problems. So minimize your intake of trans fats as much as possible and limit your saturated fat intake. Boost your intake of monounsaturated fats and polyunsaturated fats as these fats can have a positive effect on fertility. I explain these fats in more detail in Chapter 3.

✔ **Dairy:** If you're choosing the skim or fat-free dairy products currently, you may want to switch to the higher-fat versions, at least for a few months while you're trying to get pregnant. Information from the 2007 Nurses' Health Study showed that women who had lowfat dairy in their diets were more likely to have trouble getting pregnant than women who had high-fat dairy. Why? High-fat dairy has greater hormone content, which may help fertility. Before you start downing a pint of regular ice cream in one sitting, consider having just one to two servings of higher-fat dairy each day.

✔ **Folate/folic acid:** Extra *folate* (the food form) or *folic acid* (the form found in dietary supplements and fortified foods) can improve a woman's chances of getting pregnant and staying pregnant. Folate helps build DNA, a process that happens at a high rate during reproduction. Which form you get doesn't matter; just make sure you get one of them. Eat food or take a supplement that provides 400 to 800 mcg per day prior to and during pregnancy.

✔ **Iron:** Recent research has suggested that even mild iron deficiency may affect ovulation. Iron also has a role in DNA production and in carrying oxygen as part of hemoglobin inside red blood cells. Estimates show that one in seven women have below-normal iron levels. Get your iron tested and take 40 to 80 mg of supplemental iron if you're diagnosed with low iron levels to improve your chances of getting pregnant.

If you make the dietary changes recommended in the preceding list, your fertility may improve — or it may not. Work with your doctor to put together a comprehensive, individualized fertility improvement plan.

## *The controversies surrounding alcohol and caffeine*

The relationship between alcohol and fertility is quite controversial. Heavy drinking isn't good at any stage of life, but what about having an occasional (or even daily) drink while trying to get pregnant? The research is split. Some studies show that moderate drinkers take longer to get pregnant; other studies show no connection between drinking and length of time it takes to conceive. Even so, the March of Dimes and Centers for Disease Control and Prevention recommend avoiding alcohol completely while trying to conceive. (As far as pregnancy and alcohol go, the research is very clear that you shouldn't drink any alcohol when you actually do get pregnant.)

If you think the research on the effects of alcohol on fertility is controversial, consider the same research on caffeine. Part of the problem with getting a straight answer is the fact that women metabolize caffeine differently based on genetics and the phase of the menstrual cycle they're in at the time. Consequently, caffeine may have more of an impact in some women than others. To be safe, limit your caffeine consumption to 200 mg or less per day, both when you're trying to conceive and during pregnancy. To see how much caffeine is in common foods and beverages, take a look at Table 2-1, which features data from the Center for Science in the Public Interest.

| Table 2-1 | Caffeine Content of Common Foods |
|---|---|
| *Food* | *Caffeine Content (mg)* |
| *Coffee* | |
| Starbucks, brewed (16 oz, grande) | 320 |
| Dunkin Donuts, brewed (16 oz) | 206 |
| Coffee, generic brewed (8 oz) | 133 (Range 102–200)* |
| Coffee, generic instant (8 oz) | 93 (Range 27–173) |
| Espresso, generic (1 oz) | 40 (Range 30–90) |
| Coffee, generic decaf (8 oz) | 5 |
| *Tea* | |
| Tea, brewed (8 oz) | 53 (Range 40–120) |
| Snapple, Lemon (16 oz) | 42 |
| Nestea (12 oz) | 26 |
| *Soda* | |
| Mountain Dew, regular or diet (12 oz) | 54 |
| Diet Coke (12 oz) | 47 |
| Pepsi (12 oz) | 38 |
| Diet Pepsi (12 oz) | 36 |
| Coke (12 oz) | 35 |
| Barq's Root Beer (12 oz) | 23 |
| Sprite, 7-Up, Fresca, Sierra Mist (12 oz) | 0 |
| *Energy Drink* | |
| Monster Energy (16 oz) | 160 |
| Red Bull (8.3 oz) | 80 |
| AMP (8.4 oz) | 74 |
| *Chocolate* | |
| Dark chocolate (1.45-oz bar) | 31 |
| Milk chocolate (1.55-oz bar) | 9 |

*The exact amount of caffeine in coffee and tea depends on the brand and how strongly it's brewed. I include the average caffeine content of generic brands for comparison purposes, but note that the actual amount can be anywhere within the range I provide in parentheses.*

# Discovering Why Your Weight Matters

Your weight may have an impact on your fertility. If you weigh too little (and have a body mass index, or BMI, of less than 18.5), your body fat reserves are likely low. When your body fat reserves are low, ovulation and menstruation become irregular or stop completely. If the body doesn't have any reserves of energy (fat), it naturally prevents the body from being able to reproduce. The body needs energy to keep the brain sending signals, to keep the heart pumping, and to keep the muscles and organs moving. If the body doesn't have enough energy to keep its own systems going, it definitely doesn't have enough to create and grow a new life.

On the other hand, weighing too much (having a BMI of greater than 25) can also have a detrimental effect on fertility. You may think that an excess of energy (fat) would keep the body happy, since it knows it has plenty of energy stored up to grow a baby. However, as weight increases above the desired range, it puts stress on the body. Specifically, the excess weight gain affects the numerous hormones being secreted by fat cells; those hormones, in turn, affect fertility by interfering with ovulation.

Women who weigh too much are at risk for the following reproductive issues:

- ✔ Irregular periods/disrupted ovulation
- ✔ Disruption of hormones affecting fertility
- ✔ Polycystic ovary syndrome (PCOS)
- ✔ Increased risk of ovarian, cervical, and breast cancers

To ensure optimal fertility, keep your BMI between 20 and 24. To figure out your BMI, refer to Figure 2-1. Locate your height in the left-hand column and follow that row until you find the number that's closest to your weight. Then look at the top of the table to find your BMI.

If you're overweight, losing between 5 and 10 percent of your weight can get your ovulation back on track. For example, if you weigh 160 pounds, focus on losing at least 8 to 16 pounds. Even though losing 5 percent of your weight may not put you in the "ideal" range for fertility, that little loss can still help increase your chances of getting pregnant.

Understanding weight loss is simple: You need to eat fewer calories than you burn. Unfortunately, putting that equation into action isn't so simple! Here are the keys to losing weight the healthy way:

- ✔ Focus on portion control at all meals.
- ✔ Stop eating when you're satisfied but not completely full or stuffed.

✔ Add healthy snacks of 100 to 150 calories throughout the day to bridge your hunger in between meals, making sure these calories fit into your daily calorie budget for weight loss.

✔ Choose foods that are lower in calories, such as lowfat or reduced-sugar options.

✔ Start doing some daily exercise, like walking 20 to 25 minutes each day, if you aren't active. If you already exercise on a regular basis, increase the intensity or duration of your workouts.

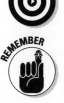

For more ideas on exercise, check out the latest edition of *Fitness For Dummies* by Suzanne Schlosberg and Liz Neporent or *Fit Pregnancy For Dummies* by Catherine Cram and Tere Stouffer Drenth (John Wiley & Sons, Inc.).

✔ Keep your eye on the prize: a beautiful, bouncing, baby boy or girl.

Of course, talk to your doctor before beginning any weight-loss or exercise plan.

| | Normal | | | | | | Overweight | | | | | Obese | | | | | |
|---|---|---|---|---|---|---|---|---|---|---|---|---|---|---|---|---|---|
| BMI | 19 | 20 | 21 | 22 | 23 | 24 | 25 | 26 | 27 | 28 | 29 | 30 | 31 | 32 | 33 | 34 | 35 |
| Height (Inches) | | | | | | | Body Weight (Pounds) | | | | | | | | | | |
| 58 | 91 | 96 | 100 | 105 | 110 | 115 | 119 | 124 | 129 | 134 | 138 | 143 | 148 | 153 | 158 | 162 | 167 |
| 59 | 94 | 99 | 104 | 109 | 114 | 119 | 124 | 128 | 133 | 138 | 143 | 148 | 153 | 158 | 163 | 168 | 173 |
| 60 | 97 | 102 | 107 | 112 | 118 | 123 | 128 | 133 | 138 | 143 | 148 | 153 | 158 | 163 | 168 | 174 | 179 |
| 61 | 100 | 106 | 111 | 116 | 122 | 127 | 132 | 137 | 143 | 148 | 153 | 158 | 164 | 169 | 174 | 180 | 185 |
| 62 | 104 | 109 | 115 | 120 | 126 | 131 | 136 | 142 | 147 | 153 | 158 | 164 | 169 | 175 | 180 | 186 | 191 |
| 63 | 107 | 113 | 118 | 124 | 130 | 135 | 141 | 146 | 152 | 158 | 163 | 169 | 175 | 180 | 186 | 191 | 197 |
| 64 | 110 | 116 | 122 | 128 | 134 | 140 | 145 | 151 | 157 | 163 | 169 | 174 | 180 | 186 | 192 | 197 | 204 |
| 65 | 114 | 120 | 126 | 132 | 138 | 144 | 150 | 156 | 162 | 168 | 174 | 180 | 186 | 192 | 198 | 204 | 210 |
| 66 | 118 | 124 | 130 | 136 | 142 | 148 | 155 | 161 | 167 | 173 | 179 | 186 | 192 | 198 | 204 | 210 | 216 |
| 67 | 121 | 127 | 134 | 140 | 146 | 153 | 159 | 166 | 172 | 178 | 185 | 191 | 198 | 204 | 211 | 217 | 223 |
| 68 | 125 | 131 | 138 | 144 | 151 | 158 | 164 | 171 | 177 | 184 | 190 | 197 | 203 | 210 | 216 | 223 | 230 |
| 69 | 128 | 135 | 142 | 149 | 155 | 162 | 169 | 176 | 182 | 189 | 196 | 203 | 209 | 216 | 223 | 230 | 236 |
| 70 | 132 | 139 | 146 | 153 | 160 | 167 | 174 | 181 | 188 | 195 | 202 | 209 | 216 | 222 | 229 | 236 | 243 |
| 71 | 136 | 143 | 150 | 157 | 165 | 172 | 179 | 186 | 193 | 200 | 208 | 215 | 222 | 229 | 236 | 243 | 250 |
| 72 | 140 | 147 | 154 | 162 | 169 | 177 | 184 | 191 | 199 | 206 | 213 | 228 | 221 | 235 | 242 | 250 | 258 |

**Figure 2-1:** Calculating your BMI.

# Fertility nutrition for the dad-to-be

What you eat isn't the only thing that affects your chances of conceiving a child. What your partner eats matters, too. Specifically, his dietary choices affect the development of his sperm, so eating right while trying to get pregnant isn't just the woman's job!

Following are some tips to share with your desired baby-daddy so he can make sure he's doing his part to contribute to Operation Fertility:

- **Lose weight.** Excess weight can decrease sperm production. Refer to the section "Discovering Why Your Weight Matters" for help calculating your BMI and determining whether it falls in the healthy or overweight range.

- **Pop a daily multivitamin.** Future dads need adequate folic acid and zinc for sperm production. Taking a daily multivitamin can fill in small gaps in these and other nutrients.

- **Eat your veggies.** On average, men don't eat as many fruits and vegetables as women do. An estimated 80 percent of men don't get the recommended five fruit and vegetable servings per day, which means they may not be getting the nutrients needed for optimal sperm production. Even more reason to also take that multivitamin!

- **Eat a nutrient-rich diet.** Nutrients such as folate, iron, and zinc are vital in creating new sperm cells, and vitamins A and E play a role in the secretion of prostate proteins. Bottom line: Eat healthy not only to support your partner but also to help do your job in the creation of a healthy baby.

- **Go easy on the alcohol.** Heavy drinkers are more likely to produce defective sperm that are unable to fertilize an egg. You don't have to cut out alcohol completely; just make sure you enjoy it in moderation. Limit yourself to no more than two alcoholic drinks per day.

# Chapter 3

# Nourishing Your Bump: Proper Nutrition while Pregnant

• • • • • • • • • • • • • • • • • • • • • • • • • • • • • • • • • • • • • • • • • • • • • • •

*In This Chapter*

▶ Balancing the food you eat with the energy you burn every day of your pregnancy

▶ Knowing how to get more calories from nutritious foods

▶ Understanding why carbs, proteins, fats, fiber, and water are all essential nutrients

▶ Recognizing special nutrient needs you may have if you're a vegetarian

• • • • • • • • • • • • • • • • • • • • • • • • • • • • • • • • • • • • • • • • • • • • • • •

*I*f there's ever a time to eat right, it's during pregnancy. Why? Because the right mix of nutrients (everything that's nourishing your body, from protein and iron to fiber and water) helps keep you going strong and your baby growing steadily. This chapter gives you the nitty-gritty details of pregnancy nutrition. If you're a numbers person, you'll love it because I specify how many more calories you really need during pregnancy and show you how to distribute those calories into the three major nutrients that make up your diet: carbohydrates, protein, and fat. If you're not a numbers person, just gloss over the numbers and pay attention to the foods I recommend that you focus on.

Either way, you need to be aware that certain vitamin and mineral needs change when you're pregnant, whereas others don't change at all. Don't worry, though. I tell you exactly which nutrients require your attention and which foods can provide you with them. I also cover fiber and hydration — the keys to smooth digestion — and reveal how to get the proper nutrients in your pregnancy diet if you're a vegetarian.

## Eating for Baby and You: Balancing Calories Eaten and Calories Burned

Rule number one of pregnancy nutrition: Don't let anyone tell you (and don't tell yourself either!) that you're eating for two. Thankfully, your baby will never be as big as you while inhabiting your uterus. To think that you need to eat as many calories to support your baby as you need to support yourself is misguided. Eating for two may be a cute saying, but, in reality, eating for two won't make you look or feel cute!

You do need to consume some extra calories during the course of your pregnancy, but how many you consume varies according to the trimester you're in. (Also, depending on your size pre-pregnancy — whether you're petite or tall — you may need slightly more or less than the recommended numbers.) The following sections give you the specifics.

Your weight status prior to pregnancy can dictate the number of calories you need. If you were overweight before you got pregnant, you may need fewer calories. If you were underweight, you may need to supplement the calorie numbers I provide in this chapter with more calories to gain the proper amount of weight. Talk to your obstetrician (OB) to determine the approximate total amount of weight you can gain for a healthy pregnancy and the number of additional (or fewer) calories you need to consume to get there.

## First trimester (weeks 1–13): Don't purposely take in extra calories

Even though the first trimester (weeks 1 through 13) is a time of incredible growth for your baby, she's still so small that her growth doesn't require any significant energy. So during these first few months, don't worry about purposely eating any more calories than you ate pre-pregnancy. If you happen to eat a few more bites of food or an extra piece of fruit or glass of milk, you're likely getting everything you need.

If food is the last thing on your mind because of nausea, take a deep breath and relax. Your pre-pregnancy nutrient stores will get you through this first trimester even if you aren't able to hold down much food. Just be sure to take your prenatal vitamin every day so you know you're getting enough folic acid. (For advice on dealing with nausea, see Chapter 6.)

If you're not experiencing nausea, you may have the opposite problem — ravenous hunger! When hunger strikes, go with your instincts and eat, but eat foods that will fill you up and provide good nutrients. Avoid foods high in sugar and fat and focus instead on healthy foods. While you're at it, why not venture into the kitchen and whip up some of the delicious recipes I present in Part III?

## Trust your gut

When I was pregnant with my first child, I went in for my first OB appointment at eight weeks, excited for all the pregnancy advice he was about to dole out. When he got to the nutritional advice, he told me not to purposely start eating extra calories right away but instead to follow my body's natural hunger cues.

What? As a dietitian, I was horrified. Based on my nutritional knowledge, I knew that women need more calories while they're pregnant and I couldn't believe that for 20 plus years this doctor had been telling all his pregnant patients not to eat more calories. How irresponsible! How would his patients know to get the nutrition they need to support their pregnancy if he was telling them not to eat more?

After living as a pregnant woman for another month or so, I started to realize that Dr. Kyle Crofoot (my OB) was simply brilliant. I noticed that if I truly listened to my hormone-raging pregnant body, I would eat more when I needed to eat more to support my pregnancy. Some days I was nauseous and didn't eat much, but other days my appetite was ravenous and I would eat more. I'm so glad that I didn't start at week eight with purposely trying to eat more calories every day. I likely would have gained too much in the first trimester, setting the stage for excess weight gain for the entire pregnancy.

## *Second trimester (weeks 14–27): Take in an extra 300–350 calories*

The second trimester (weeks 14 through 27) is a time of incredible growth for your baby, as you can see in Figure 3-1. She goes from weighing only about an ounce at the end of week 13 to weighing more than 2 pounds by the end of week 26. To support your little one's growth during this phase of pregnancy, you need to consume about 300 to 350 extra calories per day.

You don't have to eat all 300 to 350 calories at one time. You can spread them out over the course of the day. Check out the following list for some great meal and snack ideas that'll give you the calories you need during your second trimester (the number of calories is in parentheses). Feel free to mix and match to make your own yummy combinations.

- 1 large banana (120) + 1 large apple (95) + 30 pistachios (100)
- 1 ounce whole-grain crackers (120) + 1 string cheese (85) + ½ cup frozen yogurt (140)

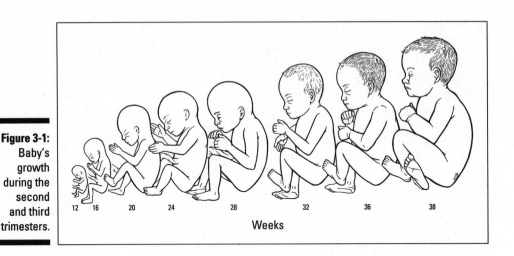

**Figure 3-1:**
Baby's growth during the second and third trimesters.

Weeks

12   16   20   24   28   32   36   38

- 1 cup 1% cottage cheese (160) + 1 cup fresh sliced strawberries (50) + ½ cup edamame (95)

- 1 cup fat-free milk (90) + 1 cup whole-grain cereal (175) + ½ cup blueberries (45)

- Two slices whole-wheat toast (160) + 1 tablespoon almond butter (100) + 1 tablespoon raspberry preserves (55)

- 1 ounce tortilla chips (140) + ¼ cup salsa (20) + ½ cup black beans (110) + 1 cup fresh pineapple chunks (80)

- 6 ounces Concord grape juice (130) + ½ ounce dark chocolate (85) + 6 ounces nonfat fruited Greek yogurt (130)

- 1 smoothie (310) made with ½ banana + ½ cup strawberries + ½ cup nonfat milk + 1 scoop protein powder + 1 tablespoon wheat germ

- 1 frozen meal of your choice (about 300)

Some days you'll be hungrier than others. Follow your hunger cues and eat more on the days when your hungrier, but don't force yourself to eat on the days when you aren't. It'll all even out for most women. Besides, your doctor will let you know whether you're gaining too little or too much weight, so you can adjust your calories up or down as appropriate.

If you're so inclined, you can rely on the scale to tell you whether you're getting enough to eat (or too much, for that matter). Look at your average weight gain over the course of a few weeks to assess your progress. Turn to Chapter 5 to see how much weight you should be gaining throughout your pregnancy.

## The science behind those extra calories

Women need about 85,000 calories for the entire 40 weeks of pregnancy. If you do the math, those 85,000 calories break down to about 300 extra calories per day. However, studies vary, some estimating pregnant women need more calories and others estimating they need fewer calories.

One reason why you need more calories when you're pregnant (at least in the second and third trimesters) is that your *resting metabolic rate* (RMR) increases. Your RMR is the number of calories you burn each day at rest. Your RMR increases with pregnancy because you burn more calories to grow another life. The other reason you need more calories is that you have to store fat and protein in your body throughout pregnancy. (I explain more about how much weight to gain during pregnancy in Chapter 5.)

While your RMR plays a large part in determining the number of calories you burn in a day, you can't forget about your daily physical activities. Some studies suggest that pregnant women don't need as many calories as many experts estimate because many women end up decreasing their physical activity during pregnancy. Whether that means exercising less intensely or simply sitting with your feet up more often, you may find yourself moving less than your pre-pregnancy self who never sat down and kick-boxed her way to fitness. As you work with your doctor to determine how many more calories you need, be sure to think about how much more or less you're moving during your pregnancy.

## *Third trimester (weeks 28–40): Take in an extra 450–500 calories*

During the third trimester, your baby gains about 4 more pounds (refer to Figure 3-1 to see the baby's size difference between the end of the second trimester and the end of the third). Because you're now carrying around even more weight than you were in the second trimester, you need to consume more calories so you have the energy to cart that extra weight around. Aim to eat about 450 to 500 more calories than you did pre-pregnancy.

Follow your hunger. Some days you'll be ravenous and other days your appetite will subside. As long as you're gaining the proper weight, don't stress about eating exactly 450 to 500 extra calories per day.

Here are some ideas for how to get those extra 450 to 500 calories each day (the number of calories is in parentheses). Keep in mind that you can spread out the extra calories throughout the day. Mix and match foods from this list to create your own meals and snacks.

- ✔ ¼ cup hummus (100) + 1 cup fresh raw veggies (50) + 1 whole-grain pita pocket (120) + 1 ounce pasteurized feta cheese (75) + 1 cup chocolate soymilk (140)

- ✔ 2 Medjool dates (130) + 1 ounce (or 19 halves) pecans (195) + 1 ounce cheddar cheese (115) + 1 plum (30)

- ✔ 1 hard-boiled egg (75) + one 4-inch cinnamon raisin bagel (230) + 1 table-spoon peanut butter (95) + 4 ounces 100% pomegranate juice (80)

- ✔ 3 ounces salmon (175) + ½ cup quinoa (115) + 1 cup asparagus (40) + 1 tablespoon olive oil (120)

- ✔ 3 ounces lean strip steak (165) + 2 cups raw spinach (15) + 20 pine nuts (25) + 2 tablespoons Italian salad dressing (100) + 1 KIND or other fruit and nut nutrition bar (190)

- ✔ ½ cup garbanzo beans (130) + 1 mango (135) + 1 cup chocolate pudding (210)

- ✔ 6 ounces nonfat fruited Greek yogurt (130) + ½ cup granola (200) + 1 tablespoon honey (65) + 1 cup raspberries (65)

- ✔ ⅓ cup dry rolled oats (150) + 1 cup skim milk (90) + 1 ounce (or 14 halves) walnuts (185) + 1 large peach (70)

- ✔ ½ cup homemade tuna or chicken salad (200) + 1 cup grapes (65) + 15 almonds (105) + 1 SOYJOY or other soy protein nutrition bar (130)

- ✔ 2 mini Babybel or other round cheeses (140) + ½ cup barley (100) + 6 dried apricot halves (50) + 2 small chocolate chip cookies (160)

You can also get your extra 450 to 500 calories by eating larger portions at your meals, but adding some nutritious snacks in between meals is probably a better idea. Why? Because as the third trimester goes on, the sheer size of your belly may suppress your appetite or cause gastric reflux by pressing on your stomach. Limiting portions at meals and relying on snacks for added nutrients and energy can help you feel better overall.

# Figuring Out Where Your Calories Should Come from

Variety is the spice of life, and it should definitely be a part of your diet, whether you're pregnant or not. If you eat the same foods all the time, you get the same nutrients all the time. But if you vary your food choices, you get different nutrients in the foods you consume. But what should those foods be?

The United States Department of Agriculture (USDA) provides a guideline for the average person to follow for good nutrition. This guideline is called *MyPlate,* and it shows the proportion of calories that should come from each of the five food groups (grains, protein, vegetables, fruits, and dairy). Figure 3-2 shows what the MyPlate guideline looks like. You can get specific recommendations for calories and portions based on your height, weight, age, and activity level by going to www.choosemyplate.gov.

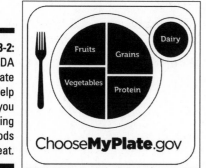

**Figure 3-2:**
The USDA
MyPlate
can help
guide you
in knowing
which foods
to eat.

The majority of the extra calories you get while you're pregnant should come from three sources: carbohydrates, protein, and fat. The following sections explain why each of these nutrients is so important during pregnancy.

## Carbohydrates: Energy for the body

*Carbohydrates* (or *carbs,* as they're often called) are your body's (and your baby's) preferred source of energy, providing you with the glucose you need to keep your brain functioning. Some examples of carb-containing foods include grains (bread, cereal, oatmeal, and tortillas, just to name a few), fruits, vegetables, milk, desserts, and anything that contains sugar.

Without enough carbohydrates, your body has to break down other nutrients, like proteins and fats, for energy instead of letting them do what they're supposed to do in the body (see the next two sections for details). You can avoid this situation by making sure that anywhere from 45 to 65 percent of your daily calories come from carbs. A single gram of carbs contains 4 calories, so just multiply the grams of carbs in a food by 4 to figure out how many carb calories that food contains. (You can see how many carbs are in the foods you eat by looking for the phrase *Total carbohydrates* on the food label. Under the total carbohydrates, you usually also see the amount of fiber and sugar, in grams, that the food contains. Both fiber and sugar are part of the total carbohydrate number.)

An easier option is to keep track of the total grams of carbs you consume. If you take this approach, aim to eat between 225 and 325 grams (g) of carbs per day for an average 2,000-calorie intake.

The two categories of carbs are simple and complex. *Simple carbs* are sugars — not just table sugar but also the sugar found naturally in food, like fructose in fruit and lactose in milk. *Complex carbs,* also called *starches,* are long chains of sugars; they're found in foods like grains, rice, pasta, potatoes, and beans. Your body has to break down complex carbs into simple sugars for them to be absorbed from the digestive tract into the bloodstream. Focus on getting the majority of your carbohydrates as complex carbs.

Plan on having carbohydrates in the form of grains, fruits, and vegetables at every meal. Maintaining good energy means keeping your body fueled with its preferred energy source (you guessed it, carbs!) all day long.

## Protein: Cell building and repair

Protein is made up of *amino acids,* which are basically the building blocks of every cell in your body and in your developing baby's body. Aim to get 20 percent of your daily calories from protein (that's about 100 grams per day if you're eating a 2,000-calorie diet). A single gram of protein contains 4 calories. To figure out how many protein calories a food contains, simply multiply the grams-of-protein-per-serving info by 4. Of course, you can always eat more protein if you want, up to 35 percent of your daily calories (which amounts to 175 g if you're eating a 2,000-calorie diet).

Because a lot of protein-containing foods are fresh (think raw meat), they don't require a food label. That's nice for manufacturers but challenging for you when you're trying to keep track of your protein intake. Let Table 3-1 be your guide to how many grams of protein are in some common foods.

| Table 3-1 | Amount of Protein in Some Common Foods |
|---|---|
| *Food* | *Amount of Protein* |
| 3 ounces lean cooked meat (poultry, pork, beef, and fish) | About 21 g (7 g/ounce) |
| 6 ounces Greek yogurt | 12–16 g |
| 3 ounces firm tofu | 9 g |
| 1 cup lowfat milk | 8 g |
| 2 tablespoons peanut butter | 8 g |
| ½ cup black beans | 7 g |
| 6 ounces lowfat yogurt | 5–7 g |
| 1 large egg | 6 g |
| 1 ounce (or about 23) almonds | 6 g |
| Most grain products (for example, a slice of bread, 1 ounce of cereal, or 2 ounces of dry pasta) | 1–4 g per serving |

Protein takes longer to digest than carbs, so eating protein keeps you full for a longer period of time than eating carbs. Always try to include protein at every meal. At breakfast, your protein source can be milk, eggs, or yogurt, and, at lunch and dinner, it can be meat or meat alternatives. You can also get protein from your snacks by eating nuts and nut butters.

## Fat: Nervous system development and function

Even though you may be nervous about the weight you'll gain, pregnancy is *not* the time to go on a fat-free diet! Fat plays a key role in developing your baby's brain and keeping your brain and nervous system running smoothly. It's also an energy source for your body and helps keep you feeling fuller longer. Aim to get 20 to 35 percent of your calories from fat. Fat is more calorically dense than carbs and protein; a single fat gram contains 9 calories. Multiply the grams of fat in a food by 9 to figure out how many fat calories a food contains.

An easier way to track how many of your daily calories come from fat is to look for the *Fat Cal per serving* info on the Nutrition Facts panel. Another alternative is to track grams of fat. If you're eating a 2,000-calorie diet, you need to consume 45 to 78 g of fat per day.

Different fats have very different reactions in your body. So you need to be aware of what types of fats you're eating. Research has proven that certain fats are better for you than others. For example, saturated fat (butter, whole-fat dairy, and fatty meats) and trans fat (hydrogenated oils) have been shown to raise "bad" LDL cholesterol levels, leading to clogging of arteries and increased risk of heart disease. On the flip side, monounsaturated fats, like those found in olive oil and avocados, trigger less LDL cholesterol and more of the "good" HDL cholesterol. Polyunsaturated fats, like those found in vegetable oils and fish, are also beneficial. In fact, two specific types of polyunsaturated fats have a significant impact on brain development; I introduce you to these fats in the later section "Omega-3 fatty acids."

Limit your consumption of saturated fat to less than 22 g per day (that's 10 percent if you're consuming 2,000 calories a day) and try to avoid artificial trans fat (like the kind found in hydrogenated oils and fried foods).

Not sure how to figure out how much fat you're getting? Just look for the *Total Fat* listing on the food label. The amounts of saturated fat and trans fat appear underneath that listing. Sometimes you also find the amounts of monounsaturated fat and polyunsaturated fat listed, but they don't have to be there.

# Getting the Nutrients You Need

During pregnancy, you're literally forming a new life within your body – an act that requires more than just carbs, protein, and fat. Vitamins and minerals are also important members of the nutrition team, playing many different roles in the growth and development of your baby.

A supplement is one way to ensure you're getting the vitamins and minerals you and your little one need throughout your pregnancy. You find most, if not all, of the nutrients you need to supplement in a basic prenatal vitamin. Several brands of prenatal vitamins exist, including both over-the-counter and prescription varieties. A prescription prenatal isn't necessarily better, but your doctor may prescribe one for two reasons:

- ✔ Women take pills better when they're prescribed rather than just recommended.

- ✔ Some health insurance companies cover prescription prenatal vitamins, meaning that they may cost you less than the over-the-counter varieties.

In addition to a balanced diet, a regular multivitamin made with a women's formula (so it has extra folic acid and iron) may also get the job done. Women's multivitamins usually have all the essential nutrients for pregnancy, although they may not have as high of doses as the prenatal varieties. Prenatal vitamins also tend to have more iron and sometimes even the DHA omega-3 all in one place (see the later sections "Iron" and "Omega-3 fatty acids" for details).

Iron can cause nausea and constipation in some women. If you're one of them, skip the prenatal vitamin and at least take a separate folic acid supplement (with between 600 and 800 micrograms) or a general multivitamin with less iron.

Depending on your diet, you may also want to take extra calcium, iron, vitamin D, or DHA omega-3. Estimate how much of each nutrient you're getting in your diet and talk to your doctor about getting your blood values checked for certain nutrients, such as iron and vitamin D. Then supplement your diet with additional nutrients as needed.

A supplement is just that — a *supplement* to your diet. In other words, don't eat junk and think the vitamins you're taking will be enough to keep you and your baby healthy. Nutritious, healthy food is still important!

Of course, because some nutrients are of special concern during pregnancy, you may want to take a closer look at them so you can really understand what they do for your growing baby, how much of them you need, and what you can eat to get them. I provide these details in the next sections.

# *Folate (folic acid)*

*Folate* (the food form), also called *folic acid* (the supplement form), plays a key role in developing your baby's spinal cord early in pregnancy, but it's also an important nutrient to get later in pregnancy. Aim to get 600 micrograms (mcg) per day throughout your pregnancy. Your prenatal vitamin probably contains about this amount (check the label to make sure), but because vitamins are generally absorbed and utilized better through food than supplements, try to get it naturally in food, too.

You find folate in oranges (and orange juice), strawberries, avocados, beans (specifically black, garbanzo, kidney, navy, and pinto), black-eyed peas, lentils, nuts, dark-green leafy vegetables (like spinach, kale, and collards), asparagus, broccoli, and Brussels sprouts. You can also find folate-fortified grain products, such as flour and cereal.

# *Iron*

Your daily iron needs practically double during pregnancy, from 18 to 27 milligrams (mg). This increase is due in large part to the increase in blood volume you're experiencing. Iron helps your body form hemoglobin, the protein that carries oxygen to the blood. You need this oxygen to get to your placenta to help your baby develop.

Aside from your prenatal vitamin, you find iron in animal foods like beef, poultry (higher in dark meat), pork, fish, and egg yolks, although you can also get iron in seeds, beans, lentils, dark-green leafy vegetables, dried fruit (like prunes, raisins, and apricots), and whole grains. Manufacturers often add iron into other grains such as rice and cereals as well. In packaged food products, you can find the amount of iron per serving listed on the food label, but be aware that the percentage listed is based on the average 18 mg daily requirement and you now need 27 mg.

Iron, especially the form found in vegetable sources, is often not absorbed in high quantities by your body. To help improve absorption, eat foods that are high in vitamin C along with your iron-rich foods. For example, include oranges, tomatoes, cantaloupe, strawberries, kiwi, peppers, or broccoli in the same meal as your iron-rich foods. The vitamin C in these foods helps your body absorb more iron. Cooking iron-rich foods in an iron skillet may also help boost your iron intake because some of the iron actually gets into the foods.

Your doctor will probably check your iron levels periodically throughout your pregnancy to make sure they're within the normal range. One symptom of iron deficiency is fatigue, but you may have a hard time figuring out whether you're tired because you're iron deficient (called *anemic*) or because you're just plain exhausted from pregnancy! A blood test is the only real way to know for sure. If you find out that you're iron deficient, your doctor may recommend that you take a higher dose of supplemental iron. Iron supplements can cause nausea, loss of appetite, and constipation, though, so if you're suffering, talk to your doctor about taking a lower dose and focus on getting as much iron as possible from food.

# Calcium

Calcium helps with blood pressure control, but it's best known for its role in bone health — both maintaining yours and building your baby's. If you don't get enough calcium in your diet, 1,000 mg to be exact, your body will take it from your bones, leaving you at higher risk of osteoporosis. The good news is that your body actually absorbs calcium better when you're pregnant.

Most prenatal vitamins contain only about 250 mg of calcium, so plan to supplement that amount by eating dairy foods (like milk, cheese, and yogurt) daily. You can also find calcium-fortified soymilk, orange juice, breads, cereals, and nutrition bars. Some vegetables and fruits, like dark-green leafy vegetables, broccoli, okra, and figs, also contain calcium. For packaged foods, calcium has to appear on food labels, so you can easily find out how much calcium the food you're eating contains. Fortunately, the daily recommendation is the same for pregnant and nonpregnant people, so looking at the percent on food labels is a good way to see whether you're getting enough calcium.

# Choline

Although you may not have heard of it, choline is pretty important to your little one. Preliminary evidence suggests that it works along with folate to ensure the proper development of the neural tube and central nervous system. In addition, choline also plays a key role in developing the *hippocampus,* which is the memory center of the brain. So if you want your child to remember Mother's Day, get plenty of choline, specifically 450 mg of it.

Choline isn't difficult to get in your diet, but purposely include some of the best food sources daily so you get your fill. Eggs are the best source of choline, with 125 mg; just make sure you eat the yolk because all the choline is in the yolk, not in the white part. You also find choline in meats such as beef, poultry, pork, and fish. If you're looking for vegetarian sources, try wheat germ, cauliflower, broccoli, potatoes, and nuts (especially pistachios). Check the label of your prenatal vitamin to see if it includes choline; most prenatal vitamins have it but some may not.

# Omega-3 fatty acids

Omega-3 fatty acids have been shown to help reduce the risk of preterm births, preeclampsia, and hypertension in pregnancy. Two specific omega-3 fatty acids found mainly in fish and seafood are essential during pregnancy:

- **Docosahexaenoic acid (DHA):** Most research emphasizes getting plenty of DHA in pregnancy because the brain is made up primarily of DHA. I was so convinced of the research that I made sure I took omega-3 supplements while pregnant and nursing to ensure I would have brilliant children. It worked because so far they're too smart for their own good! All joking aside, aim to get a minimum of 300 mg of DHA a day while pregnant.

- **Eicosapentaenoic acid (EPA):** EPA is essential to building every structural cell in the body. Aim to get a minimum of 220 mg per day (which is actually the same amount you need when you're not pregnant).

The key to getting plenty of omega-3s in pregnancy is focusing on the best sources of omega-3s while avoiding the sources with higher mercury contents. How do you know which sources are best? Take a look at Table 3-2. It shows a list of high-omega-3 fish that are also low in mercury (and, thus, safe to eat during pregnancy).

| Table 3-2 | Low-Mercury Sources of DHA and EPA Omega-3s |
|---|---|
| *Fish* | *DHA + EPA Content* |
| Atlantic salmon, farmed, 3 ounces cooked | 1,835 mg |
| Coho salmon, farmed, 3 ounces cooked | 1,087 mg |
| Anchovies, 2 ounces canned | 924 mg |
| Sardines, 3 ounces canned | 835 mg |
| Crab, 3 ounces cooked | 335 mg |
| Flounder, 3 ounces cooked | 255 mg |
| Clams, 3 ounces cooked | 241 mg |
| Light tuna, 3 ounces canned | 230 mg |
| Scallops, 3 ounces cooked | 80 mg |
| Shrimp, 3 ounces cooked | 80 mg |
| Catfish, 3 ounces cooked | 77 mg |

*Source: USDA nutrient database (www.nal.usda.gov)*

If you're not a fan of fish, look for sources of algae because the algae the fish eat produce their high omega-3 content. But before you start scraping the sides of your fish tank, look for food products on store shelves that boast high DHA contents. Most of these products are fortified with algal oil and contain between 30 and 50 mg of DHA per serving.

One of my favorite nonfish sources of omega-3s is a DHA-enhanced egg. Eggland's Best farms feed their hens sea kelp, which results in each egg having about 57 mg of DHA per large egg. Regular eggs have 29 mg on average.

If you can't fathom eating a ton of fish or omega-3-fortified food, consider taking an omega-3 supplement. Your prenatal vitamin may already have some omega-3s in it, so look at the label for DHA and EPA. Aim to get a minimum of 300 mg of DHA but ideally more like a total of 1,000 mg of DHA and EPA combined. If your prenatal vitamin doesn't have enough omega-3s, consider a fish-oil supplement. Just be sure to read the label carefully to see how many pills you need to take to get to the 1,000 mg amount.

Fish oil supplements can cause a nasty case of fish burps. If you don't think you can handle tasting fish for a while after taking a supplement, look for a supplement that's made from high-quality, highly purified fish oil, like Nordic Naturals. Alternatively, choose one that's enteric coated, like Vital Remedy MD's VitalOils1000 or a store-shelf brand like Nature Made's Ultra Omega-3 Minis, which give you 1,000 mg of combined DHA and EPA in three small pills that are easier to swallow. If you're a vegan, look for Ascenta brand NutraVege, which has 400 mg of DHA in two teaspoons.

## *The rest of the essential pregnancy nutrients*

The previous five sections describe specific nutrients that have a direct relationship to various key areas of your baby's development, but they're not the only nutrients worth knowing about. In the following list, I highlight four additional nutrients that are important for keeping you and your baby properly nourished:

- **Vitamin D:** Vitamin D helps build bones and protect the immune system of both you and your baby. Low levels of vitamin D have been linked to increased risk of cesarean (C-section) delivery, preeclampsia, and gestational diabetes for pregnant moms and weak bones, seizures, respiratory infections, and brain disorders in babies. Vitamin D is difficult to get in the diet, so make sure your prenatal vitamin contains at least 600 international units (IU). If you want to do even better by you and your baby, try to get at least 1,000 IU of vitamin D per day. (You can take an extra vitamin D supplement to reach this amount.)

  The American Academy of Pediatrics recommends that every pregnant woman get her vitamin D level checked and aim for a blood level above 32 nanograms/milliliter (ng/mL). It takes about 1,000 IU of vitamin D to raise blood levels 10 ng/mL. Many researchers now recommend that all pregnant and nursing women take 5,000 IU of vitamin D daily, but check with your doctor for his or her recommendation.

✔ **Vitamin A:** This nutrient is necessary in pregnancy because of its key role in building healthy cells and developing vision in your baby. Do your best to get 2,566 IU (770 mcg) of vitamin A per day.

Getting enough vitamin A isn't typically a problem. The concern is consuming too much of this particular nutrient. Some studies have connected high levels of vitamin A to birth defects. Getting too much vitamin A in your diet is pretty hard to do unless you eat liver several times per week (liver is really high in vitamin A), but getting too much from supplements is much easier. Check all the supplements you're taking and make sure that you're not getting more than 10,000 IU total of preformed vitamin A daily. Also make sure your supplement uses beta carotene as its source of vitamin A rather than the potentially problematic form called retinol.

✔ **Zinc:** This mineral is essential for keeping your immune system strong and for cell growth in your baby. During your pregnancy, aim to get a minimum of 11 mg of zinc per day; it's okay to get more than that. Good sources of zinc include animal proteins as well as fortified grains, sunflower seeds, wheat germ, tofu, and peanuts. You may also be able to meet your daily zinc requirement just by taking your prenatal vitamin; check the label to be sure.

✔ **Iodine:** In pregnancy, iodine helps with brain development and hormone production in your baby, so be sure to get 220 mcg of it daily. You can find iodine in iodized salt, a common staple in many people's homes, as well as in fish (especially saltwater fish), dairy foods, and some vegetables, like potatoes and beans. Some prenatal vitamins contain iodine but some don't, so don't rely on your vitamin to get your iodine.

## Researching the link between Mom's nutrition and Baby's development

A recent study found that a mother's nutrition while pregnant can actually alter the function of her child's DNA, predisposing the child to conditions and diseases such as obesity, diabetes, and heart disease. Eating a poor diet during the times that are most critical in the development of your baby may even cause certain organs to not function correctly and may lead to complications in your baby. For example, one study on baboons (hey, they're not so different from humans!) found that poor nutrition during fetal and early life damaged the pancreas and predisposed the offspring to type 2 diabetes later on in life.

Another interesting study looked at survivors of the Dutch Famine in the 1940s. The women who were pregnant during the famine had children who were more likely to develop a preference for fatty foods and to be less active. They also had increased risk of type 2 diabetes, obesity, hypertension, and cardiovascular disease. Although a famine probably isn't on the horizon in your life, this study is a great example of the impact a lack of nutrition during pregnancy can have on your child's lifelong health.

# Discovering the Numerous Benefits of Fiber

Fiber offers your body several different health benefits. Probably the most well-known benefit is its broom-like quality. That is, fiber keeps things moving through your digestive tract, cleaning out the colon. Fiber is the part of complex carbohydrates that literally doesn't get digested. Because your body can't digest it, fiber creates bulk in the stool, leaving you with a softer stool that passes with regularity.

Fiber also keeps you feeling fuller longer and keeps your blood sugar under control while your body tries to digest it. In addition, fiber can help you control your blood pressure, decrease your risk of preeclampsia, and reduce your cholesterol levels. The following sections tell you everything you need to know about how much fiber to get during pregnancy and where to go to get it.

## Knowing how much fiber you need

During pregnancy, you need to get 28 g of fiber per day (that's 3 g more than the recommended pre-pregnancy amount). Pregnant women need more fiber in their diets to combat their increased risk of constipation, which is a common occurrence for many expectant mothers due to hormonal changes in the body. Turn to Chapter 6 for additional constipation-prevention tips.

Eating fiber can leave you feeling a bit gassy. To avoid this experience, increase your fiber intake slowly. Eat a bit more fiber every day for several weeks to get up to the full 28 g per day. Doing so allows your digestive tract to get used to the added fiber.

## Filling up on fiber-rich foods

The only place you find fiber is in plant foods. So look to whole grains, beans, fruits, vegetables, nuts, and seeds to get your fill of fiber. Table 3-3 provides you with a list of common plant foods along with their fiber content. (For any foods with a range of fiber contents, just check the label on the food you're about to eat to find out exactly how much fiber it contains.)

| Table 3-3 | Common High-Fiber Foods |
| --- | --- |
| **Food** | **Fiber Content** |
| High-fiber cereals (like All-Bran, Fiber One, Kashi, Raisin Bran, and Shredded Wheat) | 6–14 g |
| Beans (like black, kidney, garbanzo, pinto, lima, and baked beans), ½ cup cooked | 5–9 g |
| Lentils, ½ cup cooked | 8 g |
| Blackberries, 1 cup raw | 8 g |
| Pear, medium with skin | 5 g |
| Apple, medium with skin | 4 g |
| Russet potato, medium with skin | 4 g |
| Whole-wheat bread, pasta, and brown rice, serving size | 2–4 g |
| Popcorn, 3 cups popped | 3.5 g |
| Banana, medium | 3 g |
| Strawberries, 1 cup raw | 3 g |
| Broccoli, ½ cup cooked | 2.5 g |
| Spinach, ½ cup cooked | 2 g |
| Oatmeal, ½ cup cooked | 2 g |
| Flaxseed, 1 tablespoon ground | 2 g |
| Wheat germ, 2 tablespoons | 2 g |
| Hummus, 2 tablespoons | 1.5 g |

Fiber is listed as *Dietary Fiber* on the Nutrition Facts panel on food labels (under the *Total Carbohydrates* line). Looking for this entry is the best way to find the exact amount of fiber in a packaged food.

## Sneaking more fiber into your day

Look for opportunities throughout the day to add more fiber to your diet. Start with a high-fiber cereal or a piece of whole-grain toast and be amazed at how easily you can get your required 28 g every day. Here are some additional creative ways of adding fiber to your diet:

- Use whole-wheat flour in place of part or all of the white flour in recipes.
- Leave the skin on fruits and vegetables (if it's edible!).

✔ Sneak more vegetables into foods by shredding and pureeing them and adding them to casseroles, sauces, and soups.

✔ Use fresh or frozen fruits and vegetables to make smoothies.

✔ Add canned beans to salads, soups, and pasta dishes — basically anywhere and everywhere you can think to add them. (Just remember to drain and rinse the beans to cut back on sodium and potentially reduce gas.)

✔ Use snacks like popcorn, fresh fruit, raw veggies, canned beans, and high-fiber cereal or crackers as midday fiber opportunities.

# Realizing Why Proper Hydration Matters

Whether you're pregnant or not, fluid is absolutely critical. You could survive for a long time on your body's stores of nutrients, but without fluid you may not even last a week. Fluid transports nutrients to your cells and waste material away from them, keeps your body at the proper temperature (something that's especially important when you're pregnant), and moves fiber through your digestive system. Read on to find out how much fluid you need to stay *hydrated* (having proper fluid balance in your cells) and where to get it.

## How much fluid do I need?

You need 102 ounces (that's 3 liters or 12.7 cups) of fluid per day throughout your pregnancy. Why so much? Well, blood is about 83 percent water, and your blood volume increases when you're pregnant. Also, what do you think your baby is floating around in? You guessed it — fluid! Without that extra fluid, your baby wouldn't have the proper cushioning he needs to protect his delicate, developing body.

To determine whether you're properly hydrated, look at the color of your urine. You don't need to examine it for hours; just taking a quick peek to see whether your urine is barely yellow can leave you feeling assured that you're hydrated. If it's bright yellow or dark in color, reach for a beverage after you wash your hands. If you're having trouble with vomiting during your pregnancy, you may have a hard time staying hydrated. Check with your doctor about monitoring and improving your hydration.

## Where should my fluid come from?

Water should be your primary source for hydration (it's calorie-free and easily available), but the 102-ounce recommendation also includes the water you get from food and other fluids. Food (including fruits, vegetables, rice, pasta, and even bread) typically contributes about 20 ounces of your fluid for the day. The remaining 90 plus ounces come from everything — and I mean everything — you drink.

Coffee, tea, soft drinks, sparkling water, juice, and milk all earn you hydration points. Since you're not drinking alcohol and limiting your caffeine (see Chapter 4 for details), you won't be getting any major diuretic effects from those beverages. Decaffeinated beverages hydrate essentially the same as water.

*Note:* Tap water is safe in the United States, so don't feel like you have to drink bottled water throughout your pregnancy. If you're concerned about the safety of your tap water, use a reverse osmosis filter to be sure it's as safe as you can make it.

## What if I can't stay hydrated?

If staying hydrated isn't easy for you, employ some of these tips to help you hit your 102-ounce fluid goal:

- Create a fluid checklist for yourself and mark off your progress throughout the day.

- Carry a water bottle with you at all times. You'll be more inclined to drink up if you have water sitting in front of you.

- Set a timer to remind yourself to drink on average about 8 to 12 ounces every one to two hours.

- Add cucumber or fresh orange slices (or pineapple, berries, lemon slices, or lime slices) to keep your water interesting.

- Drink a tall glass of liquid at every meal.

- Fill up on liquid-containing foods, like soup, gelatin, fruits, and veggies.

- Drink water or sports drinks before, during, and after you exercise.

- Drink more fluid on hot days or if you're traveling by plane.

- Add more fluid to your daily diet if you've been sick with a fever, diarrhea, or vomiting.

Don't wait for thirst to tell you to drink. Once you feel thirsty, you're likely already at least slightly dehydrated.

# Living a Vegetarian Lifestyle while Pregnant

If you're a vegetarian, you can continue to live your lifestyle and have a healthy baby. I wouldn't recommend becoming a vegetarian right before or during your pregnancy, but if you've been one for some time, you've likely mastered the skills you need to plan properly nutritious meals.

The term *vegetarian* means different things to different people. For example, if you're a *lacto-ovo* vegetarian (meaning you eat dairy and eggs), you likely won't have any problem meeting your nutrient requirements as long as you're eating the iron-rich foods I list in the bulleted list later in this section. If you're *vegan* (meaning you don't eat any dairy or eggs), you'll likely have to take dietary supplements to ensure you're getting the proper nutrients.

Regardless of what being vegetarian means to you, make sure you're getting enough calories and gaining the proper amount of weight as your pregnancy progresses. As a vegetarian, focus on eating beans, soy, nuts, and seeds to get plenty of protein, and if you avoid dairy, choose calcium-fortified milk replacements like soy-based milk, yogurt, and cheese.

Vegetarian diets generally tend to be lower in a few key nutrients that are essential during pregnancy than traditional meat-containing diets. The following list breaks down these essential nutrients and explains how you can get more of them in your diet (to figure out the exact amount you need of each nutrient, see the earlier section "Getting the Nutrients You Need"):

- ✔ **Iron:** Choose fortified grains, dark leafy greens, dried fruit, tofu, prunes, beans, and blackstrap molasses. Or consider taking an iron supplement.

- ✔ **Vitamin B12:** Because only animal products like dairy and eggs contain this vitamin, vegans need to get their vitamin B12 from supplements or fortified foods.

- ✔ **Protein:** Incorporate a protein-rich food, like dairy, eggs, beans, nuts, seeds, or soy foods, into every meal.

- ✔ **DHA:** If you avoid fish, getting enough of this omega-3 can be a challenge. Look for algal-oil-fortified foods or choose eggs that have been laid by hens that eat special feed high in DHA. You can also look for an algae-based supplement (see the earlier section "Omega-3 fatty acids" for details).

- ✔ **Calcium:** If you eat your three servings of dairy per day, you'll likely meet your calcium needs. If you don't, look for fortified foods or supplements.

- ✔ **Zinc:** You find zinc in wheat germ, beans, nuts, seeds, milk, and fortified foods.

- ✔ **Vitamin D:** You find a small amount in fortified milk, seafood, and some mushrooms, but you probably still need to consider taking a vitamin D supplement to make sure you're getting enough of this important nutrient.

For more detailed information on good pregnancy nutrition for vegetarians, check out the latest edition of *Living Vegetarian For Dummies* by Suzanne Havala Hobbs (John Wiley & Sons, Inc.).

# Chapter 4

# Knowing What to Avoid during Pregnancy

**In This Chapter**

▶ Discovering which foods to avoid and which ones to use caution with while pregnant

▶ Preventing foodborne illnesses and reducing your exposure to food-related toxins

▶ Eliminating alcohol and cutting back on caffeine

*I* typically like to focus on what you should eat, but for safety's sake, when I talk about pregnancy nutrition, I have to shift the focus to what you shouldn't eat. This chapter gives you a rundown of exactly what foods (and substances) to avoid throughout your pregnancy to keep you and your baby safe. It also helps you reduce your chances of developing foodborne infections (you're at an increased risk for them now that you have a bun in the oven) and explains why cutting out alcohol and cutting back on caffeine are such important steps to take as soon as you see that positive pregnancy test.

## Foods That Aren't Safe during Pregnancy

If you look no further in this chapter than this section, you'll have a solid understanding of the foods and beverages that are of the most concern during pregnancy. Table 4-1 spotlights the foods and beverages that are dangerous when consumed while pregnant. Table 4-2 lists the foods that you don't have to completely avoid but that you do need to be cautious about when eating.

If seeing all the foods and drinks you can't enjoy during pregnancy gets you down, pay special attention to the last column in Tables 4-1 and 4-2. It highlights safe alternatives to the dangerous foods.

| Table 4-1 | Foods and Beverages to Avoid during Pregnancy | |
|---|---|---|
| *Don't Eat/Drink This* | *Why to Avoid* | *Alternative Strategy* |
| Agave nectar | Can cause uterine contractions | Use the safer sweeteners listed in Chapter 9. |
| Alcohol | Passes to the fetus; increases your risk of miscarriage or stillbirth; can result in fetal alcohol syndrome and brain damage if consumed in excessive amounts | Enjoy virgin cocktails. |
| Commercially prepared meat salads (ham, chicken, tuna salad) | Can be contaminated with *Listeria* bacteria | Make meat salads at home, using proper food safety techniques (see Chapter 10). |
| High-mercury fish (shark, swordfish, king mackerel, tilefish, golden/ white snapper) | Can have high levels of mercury | Choose low-mercury fish instead (see Chapter 9). |
| Raw eggs (like those found in cookie dough) | Can be contaminated with *Salmonella* bacteria | Cook all eggs until they're no longer runny and bake cookies without licking the spoon. |
| Raw honey | Can be contaminated with bacteria that causes botulism (a serious paralytic illness) | Look for the term *pasteurized* on the label and avoid raw honey at farmers' markets. Never feed honey to a child younger than 1 year old. |
| Raw shellfish (oysters, clams) | Can be contaminated with *Vibrio* bacteria | Cook all shellfish until it reaches 145 degrees or higher. |
| Raw sprouts (alfalfa, mung bean, clover) | Can be contaminated with *E. coli* or *Salmonella* bacteria | Ask for sandwiches without sprouts. |
| Raw or under-cooked fish (sushi made with raw fish) | Can be contaminated with various bacteria or parasites | Cook all fish until it reaches 145 degrees or higher. |
| Raw or under-cooked meat (pork, poultry, beef) | Can be contaminated with *E. coli* bacteria | Cook all meat until it reaches an internal temperature of 145–165 degrees or higher (see Chapter 10 for specifics). |

| Don't Eat/Drink This | Why to Avoid | Alternative Strategy |
|---|---|---|
| Soft cheeses from unpasteurized milk (Brie, feta, Camembert, blue cheese, queso blanco, queso fresco) | Can be contaminated with *E. coli* or *Listeria* bacteria | Check the ingredient lists of cheeses to make sure they say *pasteurized milk.* If they do, they're safe to eat. Hard cheeses, like cheddar and mozzarella, are safe. Avoid eating raw cheeses purchased at farmers' markets unless you're sure they're made with pasteurized milk. |
| Unpasteurized (or fresh-squeezed) cider or juice (like orange, cranberry, and other drinkable juices) | Can be contaminated with *E. coli* bacteria | Drink only packaged juice with the term *pasteurized* on the label or bring fresh juice to a rolling boil for one minute before drinking. |
| Unpasteurized (raw) milk | Can be contaminated with various bacteria | Buy commercial milk rather than fresh raw milk from a farm and look for the term *pasteurized* on the label. |

Adapted from `www.foodsafety.gov/keep/groupofpeople/pregnant/` `chklist_pregnancy.html`

### Table 4-2  Foods and Beverages to Be Cautious of during Pregnancy

| Use Caution with This | Why to Use Caution | Alternative Strategy |
|---|---|---|
| Albacore (or white) tuna | Can have moderately high levels of mercury | Limit intake to 6 ounces per week; choose light tuna instead. |
| Caffeine | Crosses the placenta and can increase the baby's heart rate; is linked to slowing fetal growth | Limit caffeine to 200 mg maximum or choose decaf beverages instead. |
| Deli meats (turkey, ham, roast beef), cold cuts (bologna), hot dogs | Can be contaminated with *Listeria* bacteria | Always cook these meats until they're steaming hot or 165 degrees or higher (even if the package says *precooked*). |

*(continued)*

## Table 4-2 (continued)

| Use Caution with This | Why to Use Caution | Alternative Strategy |
|---|---|---|
| Homemade ice cream, custard, eggnog, mousse, meringue, and Caesar dressing | Can contain raw eggs, which can be contaminated with *Salmonella* bacteria | Avoid eating it if you don't know whether raw eggs were used or use pasteurized eggs if you're making it yourself. |
| Liver (beef and chicken) | Contains high levels of vitamin A, which can be toxic, especially in the first trimester | Limit intake and enjoy other meats in place of liver. |
| Meat spreads or pâté | Can be contaminated with *Listeria* bacteria | Use canned versions. |
| Saccharin | Passes to the fetus and may remain in the fetal tissue; may increase cancer risk in offspring | Use the safer sweeteners listed in Chapter 9 or use small amounts of real sugar. |
| Smoked seafood | Can be contaminated with various bacteria or parasites | Cook all smoked seafood until it reaches a temperature of 165 degrees or higher. |
| Stuffing and gravy | Can be contaminated with various bacteria | Cook stuffing until it reaches a temperature of 165 degrees or higher; reheat gravy to a boil. |
| Undercooked eggs | Can be contaminated with *Salmonella* bacteria | Cook eggs until both the yellow and white parts are firm. |

*Adapted from* www.foodsafety.gov/keep/groupofpeople/pregnant/chklist_pregnancy.html

# A Warning on Herbals

When I say you need to avoid certain herbals during pregnancy, I'm not talking about the basil and thyme you may use in cooking. Those types of herbs are safe in the amounts used in normal food preparation. I'm more concerned about herbal preparations in supplement form that some people take in concentrated forms at higher doses.

Even though herbal supplements may appear to be "natural," they don't undergo the same safety testing that food products and over-the-counter and prescription medications go through. For that reason, you should avoid herbal products in food and supplements during pregnancy — a feat that's easier said than done these days because herbals are found not only in supplements but also in many foods. Read labels carefully and watch out for these common herbal products in particular:

✔ Aloe

✔ Agave

✔ Black cohosh

✔ Ephedra

✔ Ginseng

✔ Ginkgo biloba

✔ Goldenseal

✔ Saw palmetto

✔ Willow bark

✔ Yohimbe

# Focusing on Foodborne Illnesses Caused by Bugs

Throughout your pregnancy, you and your growing little one are at high risk for getting sick thanks to immune system issues. Your immune system is weaker because your body is so busy growing another person, and your baby's immune system is still developing and not even close to operating at full strength. Consequently, fending off the pesky, disease-causing bugs found on door handles, in the air, and in your food is much more difficult when you're pregnant.

*Foodborne illnesses,* which occur when you eat something that contains a type of bacteria, parasite, or virus that makes you sick, can cause miscarriage or premature delivery in serious cases. In really severe cases, exposure to these harmful organisms can cause death. The best-case scenario for you is a little bit of dehydration and fatigue, but your baby can suffer a variety of problems.

In the following sections, I fill you in on five pesky "bugs" — living organisms that are too small to see but can bring you to your knees — that pregnant women are particularly susceptible to. I also tell you how to protect yourself from contracting a foodborne illness from these little buggers.

# *Campylobacter*

*Campylobacter jejuni* bacteria are one of the major causes of diarrheal foodborne illness in the United States. These bacteria grow in raw or under-cooked poultry, other meats, and seafood as well as in unpasteurized milk and untreated water. In fact, some studies have found *Campylobacter* in up to 100 percent of the poultry tested in retail stores.

Symptoms occur two to five days after infection and include diarrhea, fever, muscle aches, vomiting, and nausea. In pregnant women, infection of *Campylobacter* can be transmitted to the placenta and can cause miscarriage, stillbirth, or preterm delivery.

The good news is that most modern water-treatment systems easily destroy *Campylobacter,* so the water you drink from your tap is completely safe. To prevent *Campylobacter* infection from spreading in your home, cook meats to proper temperatures and don't cross-contaminate cutting boards and knives (see Chapter 10 for the skinny on food safety).

# *E. coli*

*E. coli* bacteria have many strains, and all animals, including humans, have *E. coli* in their intestines. One specific strain — *E. coli O157:H7* — contains toxins that damage the lining of the intestines, causing hemorrhagic colitis, an acute disease. *E. coli* contamination typically happens when people don't properly wash their hands after using the restroom, when raw meats aren't properly handled, or when fruits and vegetables aren't properly washed. Manure (animal feces) is often used as a natural fertilizer, especially for organic produce, so it's no surprise that *E. coli* outbreaks often happen because of contaminated produce.

*E. coli* contamination typically affects the digestive tract the most; symptoms include diarrhea and bloody diarrhea. The biggest risk of *E. coli* infection during pregnancy is dehydration, which can cause miscarriage or premature labor in severe cases. *E. coli* bacteria are also the most common cause of urinary tract infections in pregnant women.

To prevent *E. coli* contamination, follow these simple steps:

- ✔ **Cook all meats well to their proper temperatures (see Chapter 10 for a list of these temperatures).**
- ✔ **Drink only pasteurized juices and milk.**
- ✔ **Wash all fruits and vegetables well, whether they're organic or conventionally grown.**
- ✔ **Wash all cutting boards and knives between uses with different foods.**

# Listeria

*Listeria* is a type of bacteria that can grow even below the "safety zone" of temperatures (less than 40 degrees), where most other bacteria can't. It can grow in unpasteurized milk and cheese, refrigerated ready-to-eat meats (like cold cuts and deli meat), poultry, and seafood. Fruits and vegetables that haven't been properly washed can also be contaminated, especially if manure was used as a fertilizer.

*Listeria* causes an infection known as *listeriosis.* Symptoms occur a few days to several weeks after infection and can include fever, chills, muscle aches, diarrhea, headache, stiff neck, and confusion. Pregnant women are 20 times more likely to get listeriosis than other healthy adults. In fact, about one-third of listeriosis cases in the United States involve pregnant women. Listeriosis is especially dangerous in the first trimester because it can cause miscarriage, but it also poses a risk to the baby after birth. It can cause mental retardation, paralysis, seizures, and developmental problems in the brain, heart, and kidneys.

Here are some steps you can take to reduce your risk of contracting listeriosis:

- ✓ **Heat deli meats, cold cuts, hot dogs, and smoked seafood to steaming hot if you choose to eat them.** Even when these meats are fresh and cold out of the refrigerator, they can have high levels of listeria, so don't eat 'em unless you heat 'em.

- ✓ **Check the labels on soft cheeses like Brie, Camembert, feta, blue cheese, Gorgonzola, and queso blanco or fresco to make sure the ingredient list includes *pasteurized* milk.** If it doesn't, don't buy the cheese! The only exception is ricotta cheese. You won't see *pasteurized* on the label because pasteurized milk isn't used to make the cheese. However, the heat treatment used during curd formation meets (and actually exceeds) the heat and time requirements for pasteurization.

- ✓ **Avoid refrigerated pâtés or meat spreads.** Only eat them if they're canned and shelf stable (meaning they're safe to shelve without refrigeration).

- ✓ **Wash fruits and vegetables prior to eating them.** Simply rub your produce well while holding it under running water.

If you enjoy making your own soft cheese (like queso fresco), be sure to use pasteurized milk.

# Salmonella

*Salmonella* bacteria is carried by animals that you find in raw meats. It also exists in soil, so it can contaminate fresh fruits and vegetables. *Salmonellosis* is one of the most common foodborne illnesses in the world. In pregnant women, it can pass to the fetus and cause miscarriage or developmental delays in the baby. Symptoms for Mom include fever, nausea, vomiting, diarrhea, and stomach cramps, but a woman can be infected without experiencing any symptoms.

Raw sprouts, like alfalfa and broccoli sprouts, are one of the most common produce items to carry *Salmonella*. Because sprouts are so difficult to wash properly, you should completely avoid them while pregnant. Eggs are another major source of *Salmonella* contamination. Only eat pasteurized eggs, and cook your eggs thoroughly until both the whites and yolks are firm. If you're eating a dish that contains raw eggs, make sure it's cooked well.

Other ways to prevent *Salmonella* poisoning include washing all fruits and vegetables thoroughly and cooking meats to their proper temperatures. (I list the minimum safe temperatures for cooking meats in Chapter 10.)

## Toxoplasma

*Toxoplasma gondii* is a parasite found in undercooked or raw meats that causes an illness called *toxoplasmosis*. It lives in the soil, so unwashed fruits and vegetables can also be contaminated. This parasite is the main reason water can make you sick in some countries; fortunately, the water supply in the United States is treated and safe.

Pregnant women are at a 20 to 50 percent higher risk of developing the toxoplasmosis infection. Symptoms include swollen glands, muscle pain, a stiff neck, and fever, but not all pregnant women experience symptoms. Even if you don't experience signs of toxoplasmosis infection, your baby could be infected. Infection in babies can cause mental retardation, blindness, and hearing loss.

Heating meats to their proper temperatures before eating them is key to preventing toxoplasmosis because heat destroys the infection-causing parasite (see Chapter 10 for a table of proper meat temperatures). Make sure you separate raw meat in the grocery cart and your refrigerator, and use a separate cutting board and clean knife when preparing meat at home. Also wash all fruits and vegetables before eating them.

Cat feces can also carry *toxoplasma* (especially if your cat is a mouse hunter outside), so if you can, ask someone else to change out the cat litter or use disposable gloves and give your hands a thorough wash if you're doing it yourself. Also be sure to wash your hands after handling your cat, especially before preparing meals, and keep your cat off all food preparation and eating surfaces in your home. Keep your cat's risk low by feeding him dry or canned food, not raw meat scraps.

Because *toxoplasma* exists in the soil, use gardening gloves while digging in the soil outside and wash your hands thoroughly before touching your mouth or your food.

## Myth busters: Foods that supposedly cause miscarriage

During your pregnancy, you're likely to hear all sorts of myths. For example, you may hear that certain foods will induce labor (not true) and that certain foods can cause miscarriage. While certain foods can indeed harm you and your baby (I cover those foods in this chapter), many of the scary tales you hear are just that — tales! Allow me to set the record straight:

**Myth:** Papayas, mangoes, and pineapples can cause miscarriage or premature dilation.

**Truth:** You don't have to avoid these nutritious fruits while you're pregnant; they don't

actually cause miscarriage. Just make sure you eat them when they're ripe and only after you've cleaned them properly.

**Myth:** Sesame seeds cause miscarriage.

**Truth:** Some cultures consider certain foods to have a "heat" that supposedly harms the baby. No scientific basis supports this claim, so you don't have to avoid sesame seeds.

If you're concerned about any particular food, talk to your doctor about your concerns. He or she can tell you the latest research and calm your fears.

# Tackling Food-Related Toxins

The microorganisms that cause foodborne illnesses aren't the only things that can harm you and your baby. Toxins can also be found in foods, as well as in the containers that house them. In the next sections, I reveal three toxins that are of particular concern during pregnancy and explain how you can reduce your (and your baby's) exposure to them.

A recent study conducted by the Environmental Working Group (EWG) found more than 230 toxins in the cord blood (the blood in the umbilical cord after delivery), specifically those of racial and ethnic minority groups. Another study found that almost all pregnant women they looked at had detectable levels of eight types of chemicals in their blood and urine from pesticides and flame retardants to some industrial chemicals that have been banned since the 1970s but still exist in the environment. Despite the fact that people are exposed to more than 83,000 different chemicals in their everyday lives, not much research exists on the exact effects of those chemicals during pregnancy.

## Mercury

*Methylmercury,* commonly known as *mercury,* is a metal that exists naturally in the environment, but industrial pollution produces high levels that enter the air and water supply in large amounts. Humans typically come into contact with mercury by eating fish. Mercury builds up in your bloodstream and passes to your baby, and although it does eventually leave your body naturally, it can take more than a year to do so. For that reason, limiting your exposure to high-mercury fish is vital, ideally even before you become pregnant (I list the most popular high-mercury fish in Table 4-1).

Nearly all fish have some mercury because they feed on mercury-containing organisms. But some fish have decidedly lower mercury levels than others. I tell you all about these low-mercury fish in Chapter 9.

Symptoms can include itching, burning skin, sensitivity in hands, feet, and mouth, lack of coordination, impairment of peripheral vision, muscle weakness, and speech impairment. However, you may not notice any symptoms at all from mercury poisoning. But even if you don't have any symptoms, your baby will. Mercury can affect your baby's developing nervous system, and the effects can carry on through childhood. To play it safe and still satisfy your seafood craving, eat no more than 12 ounces of low-mercury fish each week throughout the course of your pregnancy.

## Pesticides

To protect food from insects, rodents, bacteria, mold, and weeds, farmers use substances called *pesticides* to limit or kill these unwanted pests. Very little evidence connects pesticides to significant risk to unborn babies. However, large amounts of pesticides can lead to low-birth-weight babies, premature labor, or miscarriage.

One surefire way to reduce your exposure to pesticide residue on the produce you're eating is to go organic when it comes to the fruits and vegetables that tend to have the most pesticide residue. Flip to Chapter 9 for a list of these Dirty Dozen foods. If you don't go organic with your fruits and vegetables, be sure to wash all dishes, cutting boards, and utensils that may have been exposed to any pesticide residue before using them again.

## Plastics

Many of the foods people consume, especially ready-to-eat meals and milk and other beverages, are packaged in plastic containers. Unfortunately, plastics contain several potentially harmful chemicals, with biphenol A (BPA) and phthalates leading the pack. Here's what you need to know about these chemicals and how they relate to your pregnancy:

  ✔ BPA makes plastic clear and stronger. You find BPA in food containers, water bottles, and the lining of many metal food cans. BPA has been linked to miscarriage and negative effects on the brain and prostate gland in fetuses and children.

- ✔ Phthalates are responsible for softening plastic and making it more flexible. You find them in many food containers used in packaging. Phthalates have been connected to birth defects, specifically in male genitals, and after-birth exposure to these harmful chemicals can still have negative effects on the reproductive systems of baby boys.

Heating plastics can leach some of the BPA and phthalates from the containers into the food you consume. So heat only those plastics that are made specifically for cooking or transfer your food to a ceramic or glass container before warming it up.

To reduce your (and your baby's) exposure to toxins found in plastics, follow these steps:

- ✔ Avoid any plastics that have the number 7 or the letters *PC* (which stand for polycarbonate) in a triangle on the container.

- ✔ Don't microwave food in plastic containers; use glass instead.

- ✔ Wash plastics by hand to prevent exposing them to high heat in the dishwasher.

## Tips for staying chemical-free

Everyone is exposed to some chemicals every day, but pregnancy may be a good time for you to limit that exposure as much as possible. Here's how to do just that:

- ✔ Avoid participating in renovating your home or painting the nursery. Opt for a girl's day out while your partner handles these duties. Choose a paint with low or no volatile organic compounds (VOCs) to minimize your exposure to solvents in the paint.

- ✔ Use cleaning supplies that have fewer toxins. Use vinegar, baking soda, and hydrogen peroxide rather than harsh chemicals such as bleach.

- ✔ Use glass and ceramic pots and pans and limit your use of nonstick varieties. Or choose an environmentally friendly brand, like Scanpan, that's free of harmful chemicals.

- ✔ Choose organic and free-range produce and meats.

- ✔ Choose skincare and toiletry products that don't contain triclosan, fragrances, or oxybenzone.

- ✔ Choose low-mercury fish.

- ✔ Use glass containers for food and beverages. Reuse steel water bottles rather than plastic bottles.

- ✔ Avoid air fresheners and fabric softeners and other overly fragranced products.

- ✔ Wash new clothes before wearing them to reduce factory pollutants.

# Going without Your Daily Alcohol or Caffeine Fix

For most women, two of the hardest things to give up during pregnancy are alcohol and caffeine. Passing on the raw-fish sushi seems to be much easier than turning down a glass of wine or cup of coffee. Although you don't have to completely eliminate caffeine from your diet, reducing your normal intake to the recommended pregnancy intake may indeed be a challenge. In the sections that follow, I help you understand why eliminating alcohol from your diet and cutting back on your caffeine intake are so important to a healthy pregnancy. I also provide you with some coping strategies that you can turn to as you form your new nonalcohol- and noncaffeine-related habits.

## Lose the booze

No level of alcohol has ever been proven to be safe during pregnancy. Even women who drank on average one drink per week had babies with a smaller head circumference (indicative of small brain size) and children who had behavioral problems as they grew up. Children who are born to women who drink during pregnancy are also more likely to have problems with alcohol abuse as they get older.

When I use the term *alcohol,* I mean all of it: beer, wine, vodka, rum, tequila, gin, and all other liquors. Even those sugary wine coolers contain a good deal of alcohol, so you need to scratch them off the list, too. Alcohol can also appear in foods like rum balls and some desserts or sauces. (Although some alcohol can be baked or cooked off, to be safe, you should avoid all forms while pregnant. If you're not sure whether a particular food contains alcohol, ask someone who knows or just avoid it.)

Drinking alcohol, even small amounts of it, during pregnancy can cause fetal alcohol syndrome (FAS) and fetal alcohol spectrum disorders (FASDs), including mental retardation. Alcohol passes directly through the placenta to your baby, where it breaks down very slowly. The effects of even just a few drinks can include the following:

- Miscarriage or stillbirth
- Premature birth
- Low-birth-weight babies
- Learning disabilities
- Difficulty with attention, memory, and problem solving
- Speech and language delays and poor performance at school

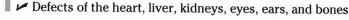

> ✔ Hyperactivity disorders
> ✔ Psychological disorders
> ✔ Defects of the heart, liver, kidneys, eyes, ears, and bones

If you had a drink before you knew you were pregnant, you can't do anything about it now, but as soon as you get the positive pregnancy test, avoid alcohol.

## Moderate your caffeine intake

Caffeine is a *stimulant,* which means it not only wakes you up but also increases your heart rate and blood pressure. (You know what I mean if you've ever felt your heart race or had jittery hands after one too many cups of coffee.) Caffeine is also a *diuretic,* which means it causes your body to urinate more often and can lead to dehydration.

Caffeine crosses the placenta and reaches your baby, decreasing blood flow to the placenta as it does so. Small amounts of caffeine don't seem to cause harm to the fetus, but excessive amounts have been shown to increase the risk of miscarriage, affect your baby's growth, and reduce fertility.

Exactly how much caffeine is too much during pregnancy is still up for debate. But all the research suggests that a moderate amount of caffeine — namely a maximum of 200 mg per day — is okay. That's equal to about 12 ounces of regular coffee. If you're hitting up your favorite coffee shop and the coffee tastes strong, it likely has more caffeine in it, so you may want to limit yourself to 8 ounces. To get an idea of exactly how much caffeine common foods and beverages contain, flip to Chapter 2.

## Coping strategies for life with less caffeine and no alcohol

If one of the hardest things about being pregnant is limiting your intake of caffeine and avoiding alcohol, remember that it's only temporary. You may have to wait more than a year when you include the 40 weeks of pregnancy (or more if you cut back while trying to conceive) and the weeks or months (or years) you spend nursing, but you will be able to drink what you want eventually. And after you go back to your life with caffeine and alcohol, you may find that you don't need it as badly as you did pre-pregnancy.

The most important thing to remember as you struggle with your alcohol-free, caffeine-reduced life is the reason why you're making the sacrifice. You're literally shaping a new life inside you, and the sacrifice of giving up alcohol or coffee for a little while is negligible compared to the huge return of a healthy baby. As someone who's committed to nourishing your baby in the best way possible, try to see your new lifestyle as an opportunity rather than a sacrifice, and you'll have no problem switching from wine to seltzer and regular to decaf.

You may also find these strategies helpful:

✔ If you have a hard time being around alcohol and not being able to indulge, ask your friends and family not to drink around you. Don't allow them to try to convince you that taking a few sips is okay. When it comes to alcohol, no amount is safe.

✔ Seek professional help if you're really struggling. A counselor may be able to help you talk through your struggles.

✔ Hang out with other pregnant women who are in the same boat. That way, you can all commiserate together. Go out for a walk and frozen yogurt instead of meeting for happy hour.

✔ If you're feeling tired and in need of the pick-me-up you normally get from a few cups of coffee, get some exercise, eat a healthy snack, and drink water for hydration. If you're really tired, take a nap! You probably need it.

✔ Find substitutes that satisfy your cravings. Try virgin cocktails or decaf coffee, tea, or soft drinks to fill the void.

✔ Switch to half-caff. If you make your own coffee at home, use one scoop of decaf coffee for every one scoop of regular coffee to cut the amount of caffeine in half. That way, you can have up to 24 ounces of coffee rather than just 12.

✔ Dump out or give away all the alcohol in your house if it's too tempting.

# Chapter 5

# Weighty Matters: Managing Pregnancy Pounds

*In This Chapter*
▶ Gaining the right amount of weight
▶ Avoiding excess fat storage
▶ Moving your body safely with exercise

**O**ne of the most difficult things to control during pregnancy is your weight — and the feelings you have about it. Many women feel "fat" even though most of the extra weight they carry consists of fluid and the developing baby. Many women also end up gaining too much weight, easily putting on 50 to 70 pounds during pregnancy by allowing themselves to eat whatever, whenever.

In this chapter, you discover just how much weight you should aim to gain and why gradual weight gain is best. You also find out how to avoid gaining more than your recommended weight range and how to engage in safe, effective exercise — one of the keys to a healthy pregnancy.

# Gaining Weight Gradually

The best way to gain weight during your pregnancy is to gain it gradually. Doing so ensures your baby is getting good nutrition throughout the entire 40 weeks.

Gradual weight gain isn't linear weight gain. In other words, you may gain 3 pounds in one week and none for the next few weeks. As long as you're trending a steady weight gain, don't worry if you find that you gain more in one week and less in others. (Some women even lose a pound or two occasionally throughout their pregnancy.)

The following sections fill you in on how much weight you should try to gain during your pregnancy and what to do if you have trouble hitting that number.

## How much to gain

The amount of weight you should gain during your pregnancy is based on your pre-pregnancy weight status, or body mass index (BMI). Because of emerging research on weight gain and pregnancy and because more women today start their pregnancies overweight or obese, the Institute of Medicine of the National Academies released new guidelines for optimal pregnancy weight gain in 2009. These guidelines appear in Table 5-1. (Turn to Chapter 2 to determine your pre-pregnancy BMI.)

| Table 5-1 | Optimal Weight Gain during Pregnancy | | |
|---|---|---|---|
| Pre-pregnancy Weight Classification | Pre-pregnancy BMI | Recommended Weight Gain Range (Total Pounds) | Rate of Weight Gain in 2nd and 3rd Trimesters (Average Pounds per Week) |
| Underweight | < 18.5 | 28–40 | 1–1.3 |
| Normal weight | 18.5–24.9 | 25–35 | 0.8–1 |
| Overweight | 25.0–29.9 | 15–25 | 0.5–0.7 |
| Obese | >/= 30.0 | 11–20 | 0.4–0.6 |

Adapted from the Institute of Medicine of the National Academies (www.iom.edu/ pregnancyweightgain)

If you're expecting only one baby, aim to gain 1 to 4 pounds during your first trimester. By your second trimester, try to gain weight at a rate of about 1 pound per week, a pace that will continue throughout most of your third trimester. (Flip to Chapter 18 for weight-gain recommendations if you're expecting twins or triplets.) If you find that you stop gaining weight in the final few weeks of pregnancy, don't panic; this situation is perfectly normal.

If you're gaining too much weight too quickly during the first and second trimesters, you may be on track for going way above the recommended weight range. Slow down your weight gain by paying close attention to your caloric intake and remember that exercising while you're pregnant is perfectly safe as long as your doctor hasn't given you any restrictions. (I provide some suggested exercises later in this chapter.)

If you suddenly gain 5 pounds or more in a week, check with your doctor. This weight gain may be a sign of sudden fluid gain, which could be associated with preeclampsia.

While weight gain is inevitable — and necessary — during pregnancy, it's also unpredictable. And although you do need to keep track of your weight and monitor your progress, weighing yourself every day may drive you crazy.

After all, your weight can fluctuate greatly from day to day thanks to fluid gain. So weigh yourself only every few days or once a week. Your doctor will also weigh you at every visit and will alert you if something's not right.

## What to do when you're not gaining enough

Losing weight isn't uncommon during the first trimester, especially if you experience a lot of morning sickness. But if you get well into your second trimester without gaining much, if any, weight, your doctor will likely inquire more about your nutrition and exercise habits. He or she may even refer you to a registered dietitian (RD) for customized guidance.

If you don't gain enough weight, your baby may not be getting the proper nutrients he needs to grow. The result can be a low-birth-weight infant or a premature delivery. Your baby may also be at risk of developmental delays if he doesn't get enough calories and nutrients in the womb.

Some women are afraid to gain weight during pregnancy for fear of not losing it afterward. If you're afraid of gaining weight to the point of restricting your calories to lower-than-recommended levels, seek out help from your doctor and a registered dietitian. Remember that if you're underweight before you even get pregnant, you likely need to gain a few more pounds than women who start their pregnancies at a normal weight.

# Preventing Excess Weight Gain

Although a handful of pregnant women have trouble gaining enough weight, most are at a higher risk of going overboard and putting on too many pounds. Typically, that extra weight comes in the form of 20 or 30 extra pounds of fat, resulting in a total weight gain of 50 or 70 pounds over the course of the pregnancy. This extra weight isn't just a nightmare to get off after the baby is born; it can also lead to some serious health complications. Don't worry, though. You can avoid the "pregnancy 50+" if you maintain the right outlook on fueling your body and keep a few helpful tips in mind (I go over these tips later in this section).

Women who see pregnancy as a meal ticket to frequent the all-you-can-eat buffet, eat plates of loaded chili cheese fries, or relax with an entire pint of ice cream in one sitting are the ones at risk of gaining too much weight. If you approach pregnancy as an opportunity to nourish your body with the best foods to grow and develop the new life inside you, you'll be at a lower risk of excess weight gain. Sure, you may have days when your ferocious appetite gets the best of you, but if you take every day in stride and follow your hunger and fullness cues (which I describe in Chapter 7), you'll get to your 40th week in good shape to give birth to your new baby.

## Potential complications from gaining too much

Whether you start your pregnancy overweight or obese or you gain too much along the way, the extra weight can cause several complications before, during, and after birth. Specifically, too much weight gain

- ✔ May make it more difficult for your doctor to hear your baby's heartbeat and measure your uterus to plot your baby's growth.

- ✔ May lead to backaches, leg pain, and varicose veins — side effects that can persist even after you deliver your baby.

- ✔ Automatically puts you at a higher risk for medical conditions such as gestational diabetes, hypertension, and preeclampsia. (I describe these conditions and the nutritional tactics for combating them in Chapter 18.)

- ✔ Increases your risk for delivering your little one via cesarean section (C-section) because your baby could be overnourished and grow too large to fit through the birth canal.

Of course, the negative side effects aren't limited to pregnancy. More and more studies are showing the long-term impact of a mother's diet choices and weight gain during pregnancy on the weight status (increased risk of overweight) and health conditions of her children. Also, women who gain too much during pregnancy have a harder time getting the weight off after pregnancy, increasing their risk of many chronic diseases, specifically diabetes, heart disease, and certain cancers.

If you started out your pregnancy overweight or obese, your doctor may not want you to gain *any* weight. Check with your doctor about his or her weight-gain recommendation and visit a registered dietitian for advice on how to meet that number the healthy way.

Some recent studies have shown better pregnancy outcomes when obese women maintained or even lost some weight while pregnant. That doesn't mean they were "dieting," per se, but they cleaned up their act from pre-pregnancy to include less junk and more nutrition, which resulted in fewer calories than their bodies were used to before. They filled up on nutritious foods and, thus, provided their babies with the nutrients they needed.

## How not to gain the "Pregnancy 50+"

In college, first-year students try to avoid gaining the "freshman 15." Now that you're expecting, your goal is to avoid gaining the "pregnancy 50" (or more). Although you may be tempted to give in to the theory that you're eating for two, doubling your calorie intake is a surefire way to keep the numbers on the scale climbing upward.

To avoid gaining more than your recommended weight range, follow these tips:

- ✔ Eat small meals to keep yourself from consuming too many calories at one time. Stop eating when you're satisfied, not full or stuffed.

- ✔ Fill up on fresh fruits and vegetables, whole grains, and lean proteins.

- ✔ Drink plenty of calorie-free beverages to stay hydrated.

- ✔ Limit "junk" calories (as in the sugary, high-fat, and fried kind) because they neither fill you up nor provide the nourishment you and your baby need.

- ✔ Stock your cabinets, purse, and desk drawers with nutritious foods so that you can satisfy your hunger the healthy way. Turn to Chapter 9 for a grocery list you can use to start your shopping.

- ✔ Bridge your hunger in between meals with frequent snacks that provide lasting energy. Choose snacks with plenty of fiber and protein; refer to Chapter 7 for ideas.

- ✔ Keep track of your calories using smartphone apps (like Calorie Counter Pro) and online nutrition tracking tools (like www.fitday.com) so that you can easily see when you've gone too high.

- ✔ Avoid turning to food for emotional support or stress relief. Call a friend to talk it out or go for a walk to blow off some steam instead.

- ✔ Join support groups for pregnant women who want to be healthy during their pregnancies. Meet to go for walks or do prenatal yoga, not to go out for ice cream.

- ✔ Stay active and aim to get at least 30 minutes of moderate exercise each day. (See the next section for details on what exercises are safe during pregnancy.)

# Adding Exercise to Your Routine: You've Got to Move It, Move It

One of the keys to gaining the right amount of weight (and being healthy) during pregnancy is exercise. Doing planned physical activity while pregnant helps keep your heart and lungs strong and, in turn, improves your endurance (which will come in handy during labor). Burning a few extra calories through exercise also helps prevent excess weight gain throughout your pregnancy.

The Physical Activity Guidelines for Americans (which are put out by the U.S. Department of Health and Human Services) recommend that pregnant women get at least 150 minutes of moderate-intensity aerobic exercise each week of pregnancy. If you exercise six days per week, that's like getting 25 minutes of exercise a day. Some examples of moderate-intensity exercise include brisk walking, water aerobics, or cycling slower than 10 miles per hour.

The Guidelines also suggest that if you were engaging in vigorous-intensity aerobic exercise pre-pregnancy, you can continue that activity as long as you don't develop any pregnancy complications and your doctor knows about your activity level. Vigorous-intensity exercise includes jogging, running, swimming laps, and cycling faster than 10 miles per hour.

The benefits of exercising during pregnancy include the following:

- Better mood and reduced risk of depression
- Better sleep
- Easier labor and delivery
- Easier post-pregnancy weight loss
- Healthier birth weight for your baby
- Less chance of constipation, bloating, and swelling
- Less excess weight gain during pregnancy
- Reduced anxiety
- Reduced risk of preeclampsia, high blood pressure, and gestational diabetes
- Stronger heart for your baby

## Knowing when moderate exercise isn't safe

Most women can exercise safely during pregnancy as long as they keep a few guidelines in mind (see the section "Safety guidelines to consider" for details). However, some women may be in a situation that makes moderate exercise unsafe. If you have one (or more) of the following conditions, your doctor will probably tell you not to exercise:

- Persistent bleeding
- Risk of premature labor
- Placenta previa (when the placenta is too close to the cervix)
- Low amniotic fluid
- Preeclampsia or high blood pressure (hypertension)
- Multiple pregnancy

If you have one of these conditions, talk to your doctor to see if any type of exercise is right for you.

If you weren't active before you got pregnant, you can still start exercising now, provided you have your doctor's consent. Don't start running marathons, but do consider going for walks, taking part in prenatal exercise classes, swimming, and/or performing some of the exercises I recommend later in this chapter. Start by doing 10 or 20 minutes of physical activity at a time and build up to 30 or more minutes at least three days per week. Work up to doing something active most days of the week. You can also split your time up throughout the day and do, say, one 10-minute burst of exercise in the morning, another one in the afternoon, and another one in the early evening and still get all the benefits of exercise.

The following sections tell you what safety issues you need to consider before you start exercising and offer some fun, safe exercises you can do to stay active during your pregnancy.

## Safety guidelines to consider

Before you take up any form of exercise, you need to consider some basic safety guidelines. Namely, you need to know how intense of a workout you can handle and how to keep your internal temperature from rising too high. I share guidelines for both in the next sections.

If at any time during exercise you experience dizziness, lightheadedness, chest pain, muscle pain, weakness, contractions, shortness of breath, calf pain or swelling, fluid leaking from the vagina, or headaches, stop exercising immediately and seek medical attention.

### Monitoring the intensity

Beginning just a few weeks into your pregnancy, you may find that you tire more easily or can't work at the intensity you used to. For example, I was a marathon runner before I got pregnant, and I continued to run throughout both pregnancies. However, my running times slowed significantly even when I was just a few weeks pregnant.

Because every woman is different, I suggest you follow your own perceived intensity levels and learn your limits for exercise. You can wear a heart rate monitor to help you figure out how intense your exercises should be. In the past, the American College of Obstetricians and Gynecologists (ACOG) recommended a heart rate of no more than 140 beats per minute while pregnant, but the ACOG has recently decided not to specify specific heart rate limits. Instead, you can use the "talk test" as a guide. No matter what exercise you're doing, you should be able to talk and carry on a conversation throughout the exercise. Of course, you'll be breathing heavier than you do when you're at rest, but you should still be able to talk without struggling. If you can't talk while exercising, you're working too hard and need to bring down the intensity.

### Protecting your core temperature

One of the most important things to remember when you're exercising during pregnancy is that you need to protect your internal core temperature. Increasing your core temperature can put your baby in danger by potentially increasing your baby's temperature, which theoretically can increase the risk of birth defects. Because you can't measure your temperature like you can monitor your heart rate, you need to take special precautions to keep yourself cool and avoid exercising in the heat.

To keep your internal temperature at safe levels during exercise, wear loose-fitting clothes and cool down immediately if you start to get overheated. Drink plenty of water before, during, and after every exercise session. Remember that you need more fluid while pregnant, anyway, and you need even more when you exercise, even if you don't sweat a lot.

## Suggested exercises for pregnancy

The best exercises to perform during pregnancy are the low-impact exercises that simultaneously strengthen your muscles and work your heart and lungs. These exercises fall into three categories: aerobic exercise, strength training, and yoga.

Do some basic stretches (such as stretching your quadriceps, hamstrings, calves, and chest) after you exercise when your muscles are warm. Also, make sure you eat a small snack before and another snack or meal after you exercise to refuel your body.

### Aerobic exercise

*Aerobic exercise* is anything you do to get your heart pumping. Some great baby-bump-friendly options are walking, jogging, and cross-country skiing. Whatever you do to safely get your heart pumping, aim for doing at least 30 minutes of aerobic exercise most (if not all) days of the week, but don't be afraid to go longer than 30 minutes if you have the energy and time. Just make sure you're wearing good supportive shoes if your exercise involves being on your feet (note that you may need to go up a size to accommodate swelling feet).

Swimming is one of the best exercises you can do while pregnant because you feel weightless in the water and can still get your heart pumping. Contact your local pool to see whether it offers any prenatal water exercise classes.

Working out on an elliptical machine (see Figure 5-1) is an excellent way to fit some low-impact aerobic exercise into your day. You can choose either the manual setting or one of the programs on the machine to follow. Either way, make sure you warm up by going at a slow pace for five minutes; then increase the intensity by increasing your speed or the resistance for 20 or more minutes. Finish up by cooling down for five minutes before getting off the machine.

Throughout the workout, remember that you should be able to carry on a conversation. If you can no longer talk during your workout, tone it down a bit.

For additional aerobic exercises that are safe to do while pregnant, check out *Fit Pregnancy For Dummies* by Catherine Cram, MS, and Tere Stouffer Drenth (John Wiley & Sons, Inc.).

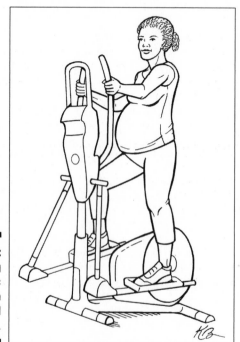

**Figure 5-1:**
Doing aerobic exercise on an elliptical machine.

### Strength training

*Strength training,* also called *resistance training,* is when you use weights, machines, resistance bands, or even your own body weight to build muscle. Recent studies have shown that low- to moderate-intensity weight lifting is safe for women in low-risk pregnancies. (If you have any doubts about your limitations, check with your physician before you start exercising.) Aim to do strength training two to three times per week. You can typically work out all major muscle groups (chest, back, arms, and legs) in about 20 minutes.

Figure 5-2 is an example of a strength training exercise that's simple and effective to perform if you have access to an exercise ball. To do this exercise, simply sit in a stable position on the ball with your back straight. Lift light (2- to 5-pound) dumbbells straight up over your head in a controlled motion and then return to the position shown in the figure. Repeat for 12 to 15 repetitions. You can do one or two sets. If you don't have an exercise ball, you can do the same exercise by standing with your feet shoulder width apart and a slight knee bend.

Avoid using heavy weights that force you to strain to lift them. To keep yourself from getting dizzy, remember to breathe in and out while lifting weights.

For a unique approach to strength training during pregnancy, pick up a copy of *Kettlebells For Dummies* by Sarah Lurie (John Wiley & Sons, Inc.).

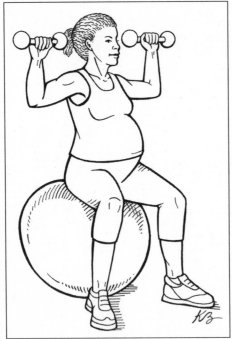

**Figure 5-2:** Lifting light weights while sitting on an exercise ball.

## Yoga

Yoga is a popular exercise to do during pregnancy, and many yoga studios offer prenatal classes. Not only does yoga help build muscle and increase flexibility, but it also teaches you how to control your breathing, which is a key skill to have when in labor. You can benefit from doing yoga daily or just once or twice a week.

Avoid Bikram yoga because it's typically done in a hot room that could be dangerous to you and your baby. Also avoid poses that twist at the waist and put pressure on the abdomen, require lying on your stomach or flat on your back, require you to stand on one leg (your center of gravity is off and you could fall), or cause you to be inverted.

TIP

If you're feeling tension in your back, try out the cat and cow yoga poses shown in Figure 5-3. To do the cat pose, get down on your hands and knees with your back straight. Make sure your hands are under your shoulders and your knees are under your hips. Inhale deeply and then arch your back toward the ceiling, exhaling as you arch and keeping your head down. Hold the pose for a few seconds, breathing deeply. When you're ready, relax down into cow pose by pulling your head up and flexing your back, exhaling as you stretch. When you're ready, go back to cat pose and repeat several times, going back and forth between the two positions. For additional prenatal yoga poses, check out *Yoga For Dummies,* 2nd Edition, by George Feuerstein and Larry Payne (John Wiley & Sons, Inc.).

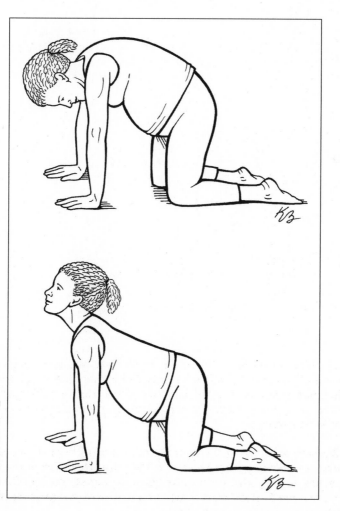

**Figure 5-3:**
Cat (top)
and cow
(bottom)
yoga poses.

## Exercises to avoid

Not all exercises are safe to engage in when you're sporting a baby bump (and even before you start showing). Anything that requires a lot of jumping and bouncing is a no-no because it can put undue stress on your baby, causing jarring and potential complications. If you love attending aerobics classes, just modify your movements so that you aren't jumping as high but are still getting some benefit from the class. Also avoid lying flat on your back during the second and third trimesters. If your doctor clears you to do abdominal exercises, do crunches with a small range of motion on an exercise ball (as opposed to full sit-ups).

Your center of gravity changes during pregnancy, so make sure to avoid any activities that may cause you to fall down, including outdoor cycling, horseback riding, rock climbing, downhill skiing, water-skiing, rollerblading, and ice skating. Also avoid contact sports, such as flag football, soccer, and basketball, that may get intense or wind up with you getting kicked or pushed.

# Chapter 6

# Overcoming Embarrassment: The Unpleasant Unmentionables of Pregnancy

## In This Chapter

▶ Coping with nausea and vomiting so you can still nourish your baby

▶ Preventing and treating all kinds of digestive issues

▶ Understanding why you feel so fatigued and what you can do about it

*P*regnancy is a time of joy and excitement, but it can also be a time of some unpleasant and quite possibly embarrassing side effects. You may wonder at times what exactly has taken over inside your body. For example, you can go from feeling so nauseous you can't even stand the smell of food one minute to feeling a burst of energy and a ferocious appetite the next. You may also pass gas, get stopped up, and be so tired you feel like a truck ran over you. But don't worry; this, too, shall pass.

In this chapter, I help you cope with the uncomfortable side effects of pregnancy. First, I reveal how to deal with the nausea and vomiting that's often called morning sickness. Then I help you figure out how to prevent and treat several conditions related to your digestive tract, including heartburn and constipation. Finally, I wrap up the embarrassing topics of this chapter by showing you how to fight off the fatigue that happens to many pregnant women.

## Morning Sickness Can Happen Morning, Noon, or Night

If you're feeling a bit nauseous, you're not alone! The majority of pregnant women experience nausea and vomiting at some point in their pregnancy, typically beginning in the first month of pregnancy and ending around 14 to

16 weeks (though some women do experience it longer). Nausea and vomiting may be due to low blood sugar and hormone fluctuations that occur in early pregnancy. Most women haven't spilled the beans that they're pregnant in these first few weeks or months, yet they walk around looking green at the smell of their co-worker's tuna fish sandwich. Feeling sick is bad enough, but trying to hide it from everyone around you is even worse!

Even though pregnancy-induced nausea is called *morning sickness,* it can actually happen at any time of the day. A completely empty stomach contributes to feelings of nausea, so many women do feel it more in the morning. But nausea can strike at any time, even after you're all ready for bed. To make matters worse, just the sight or smell of food can send a woman running to the bathroom to lose her lunch (or breakfast . . . or dinner). The good news is that nausea and occasional vomiting is not harmful to you or your baby.

*Note:* If you don't feel nausea at all, count yourself as one of the lucky 20 to 30 percent who don't experience it. It doesn't mean that something's wrong in your pregnancy. And just in case you're curious, the idea that you have more nausea if you're having a girl is just a myth, so don't try to guess the gender of your baby yet, either!

If you are experiencing nausea and making the occasional mad dash to the restroom, check out the following sections. They offer advice on coping with pregnancy-related nausea, help you realize how getting sick can affect your nutrient intake, and spell out when your nausea may require medical attention.

## Dealing with nausea

Feeling sick to your stomach is one of the worst feelings. Sometimes you actually wish you could throw up just to feel better, even if the relief is only temporary. If you're experiencing even mild nausea, try these tips (which are in order of effectiveness) to feel better fast:

- ✔ **Go bland early.** Eat something bland (like plain toast or soda crackers) within 15 minutes of getting up in the morning. You may even want to have them on your bedside table to munch on before you get out of bed.

- ✔ **Avoid having a completely empty stomach at any time of the day.** When your stomach is empty, the acids in your stomach signal nauseous feelings to your brain. Keep snacks handy so you don't find yourself hungry without something to munch on.

- ✔ **Eat small portions.** Of course, you don't want to get too full either. Limit portions at meals to only small amounts of food and follow those small meals with frequent snacks so you don't get hungry. Don't let your stomach get completely empty, but also avoid filling it too full.

✔ **Eat foods that are low in fat and sugar.** Avoid greasy, creamy, or high-sugar items. I love donuts, but when I was pregnant, I just couldn't eat them because they made me feel sick to my stomach for hours. Fat takes a long time to digest, and sugar can cause a spike and subsequent drop in energy levels.

✔ **Stay hydrated.** Nausea can be a side effect of dehydration during pregnancy. To avoid becoming dehydrated, suck on ice chips or sip cold water to count toward your recommended 102 ounces of fluid per day. Why cold water? Not only is it refreshing but it can also help decrease nauseous feelings and keep you hydrated after you vomit. (For additional tips on staying hydrated, flip to Chapter 3.)

✔ **Keep cool.** Getting too warm or overheated can make nausea even worse! Keep cool in comfortable, loose-fitting clothing that doesn't press on your stomach (stomach pressure can increase feelings of nausea).

✔ **Relax and rest up.** Get plenty of rest at night and nap throughout the day as needed and when possible. Sometimes sleep is the best escape from feeling nauseous because your body is worn down and needs the recovery.

✔ **Take your vitamins at night.** Prenatal vitamins have iron, which can aggravate nausea, but if you take yours at night, you may not experience any. Remember to have a small snack with the vitamin so you aren't taking it on an empty stomach.

✔ **Suck on lemon drops or sour candy.** Sour foods can stimulate digestion, starting with saliva in the mouth and moving into the stomach. I had a bag of sour gummies in my purse for the first few months and would pop one whenever I felt the watery buildup of saliva in my mouth that signaled an attack of nausea.

The preceding tips are some of the standard ways of relieving nausea, but some women swear by less mainstream tactics, such as

✔ **Using ginger:** People have used ginger to combat nausea for centuries. Scientists aren't completely certain how it works, but it has something to do with the unique compounds found in ginger and their effect on the stomach. Look for lowfat gingersnap cookies, ginger tea, or ginger gum.

✔ **Smelling lemon scents or eating lemon-flavored foods:** Lemon is a refreshing scent, and many women report feeling less nauseous when eating, drinking, or even smelling lemon. Some companies have special lollipops, lemon drops, and gum just for pregnant women. But plain old lemon drops can do the trick without the premium price tag.

✔ **Undergoing hypnosis or acupressure:** These techniques can be beneficial for really severe nausea in some women. Hypnosis works by training the unconscious mind to suppress the involuntary feelings of nausea. Acupressure has been used in traditional Chinese medicine to relieve nausea, and acupressure bands for the P6 pressure point on the wrist work for many pregnant women.

If your nausea is strong enough to interfere with your daily life, talk to your doctor about certain nausea-reducing medications that are safe to use during pregnancy.

If smells bother you, take action to head them off. Gently let the people around you know which smells tend to trigger your nausea. Sometimes you don't know what those smells are until they cause an incident — like your best friend's perfume that sends you running to the bathroom one day. If at all possible, avoid visiting places or people that are too fragrant for your fragile stomach.

Food smells are often the worst offenders for setting off nausea. Ask someone to help you with food preparation if just smelling food prevents you from eating. Use fans and open windows in the house to get strong smells out as soon as possible. Also, stick with cold foods because they don't have as much aroma as warm foods.

## Understanding how vomiting may prevent you from getting enough nutrients

Obviously, no one likes to feel or be sick to her stomach. When you're pregnant, you're even more concerned because you're now growing another life inside you. If you're throwing up daily or several times a day, how is that affecting your ability to provide nutrients to your baby?

Believe it or not, your baby doesn't suffer from your occasional or even daily vomiting. Your body has reserves of nutrients and energy that the baby can use to grow and develop if food is unavailable in the short term. If you experience vomiting on a regular basis, try to stay hydrated and well nourished when you're feeling good. Doing so can help build up your fluid and nutrient stores.

The main risk of vomiting is dehydration. Mild dehydration can lead to fatigue and headaches, and severe dehydration can cause an imbalance in electrolytes, including sodium and potassium, which can be serious. To prevent either scenario from happening, sip on sports drinks to replenish sodium, potassium, and fluids. If sports drinks don't appeal to you, simply drink water and eat salted crackers or pretzels and fresh, frozen, or dried fruit.

## Determining when medical intervention is necessary

For a few women, vomiting becomes so excessive that it can harm them or their babies. This condition is called *hyperemesis gravidarum*. Typically, hyperemesis gravidarum is characterized by severe nausea, vomiting, weight loss of more than 5 percent, and evidence of dehydration. See Table 6-1 to recognize the difference between morning sickness and serious illness.

| Table 6-1 | Distinguishing between Morning Sickness and Serious Illness |
|---|---|
| *Morning Sickness* | *Serious Illness* |
| Your nausea goes away after 14–16 weeks. | Your nausea doesn't go away. |
| Your nausea leads to occasional vomiting. | Your nausea leads to severe vomiting (several times per day). |
| Your vomiting doesn't cause dehydration. | Your vomiting causes severe dehydration. |
| Your vomiting still allows you to keep some food down. | Your vomiting doesn't allow you to keep food down. |
| Your nausea and vomiting are annoying. | Your nausea and vomiting disrupt your life. |
| You don't experience any significant weight loss. | You experience weight loss of more than 5% of your body weight. |
| Nausea and some vomiting are your only symptoms. | Dizziness, weakness, and fatigue accompany your vomiting. |

Treatment for severe nausea and vomiting can be as simple as taking antinausea medications prescribed by your doctor, getting enough fluids, and resting. If your symptoms become severe enough, you may have to be treated with intravenous fluids and electrolytes. Some serious cases require hospital stays and bed rest. When in doubt, call your doctor for advice on how to deal with your nausea and vomiting.

Even though some vomiting is normal during the first 14 weeks or so of pregnancy, other symptoms that sometimes accompany vomiting are not. Call your doctor or visit your local emergency room for immediate assistance if you

✔ Have a fever, diarrhea, and/or severe abdominal pain

✔ Experience prolonged vomiting and are also weak, dizzy, or faint

✔ Can't keep liquids down for more than 24 hours

# Your Digestive Tract Acquires a Mind of Its Own

If you haven't already discovered it for yourself, forgive me for bearing the bad news: Pregnant women are known to have problems with their digestive tracts. You can pretty much blame all your digestive tract woes on hormones — specifically progesterone and estrogen.

- ✔ *Progesterone* is one of the most important pregnancy hormones. Some of the side effects of increased levels of progesterone include water retention, sluggish digestion, and nausea. The result of these side effects is feeling bloated, gassy, and constipated.

- ✔ *Estrogen* is to blame for your expanding uterus, which, as the pregnancy goes on, also causes pressure on the digestive tract. This pressure can lead to heartburn and constipation.

Of course, knowing about these wonderful hormones won't make you physically feel better, but I like having someone or something to blame for feeling stopped up or as big as a hot-air balloon. At least then I know what to yell at when I'm in the midst of a particularly bad bout of constipation. (In fact, when in doubt, blame hormones for everything in pregnancy!) The following digestive tract issues may or may not affect you during pregnancy, but if they do, reading the next sections will arm you with what you need to know to deal with them.

## Avoiding heartburn with the help of some nutrition tricks

*Gastroesophageal reflux disease* (GERD) is the technical term for that burning sensation in your throat and chest, but you probably just call it plain old *heartburn*. Heartburn is quite common during pregnancy and can happen any time throughout your 40 weeks, although it often gets worse in the second and third trimesters.

Heartburn has two causes, and both are related to the sphincter muscle that connects the esophagus to your stomach. The progesterone your body produces relaxes that sphincter muscle, and your growing uterus presses on it. The result is that gastric acids, liquids, and food from the stomach travel back up your esophagus, leaving you uncomfortable. Heartburn typically worsens as your belly grows and puts more pressure on your stomach, causing the sphincter muscle to allow acid back into the esophagus (see in Figure 6-1).

You can lessen the symptoms of heartburn by trying the following tips:

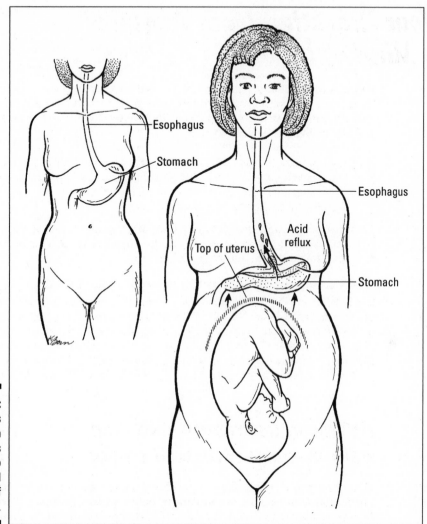

**Figure 6-1:**
Your baby's
position in
the uterus
can lead to
increased
feelings of
heartburn.

✔ **Stop eating two to three hours before lying down for bedtime or a nap.** The less you have in your stomach, the less likely you are to experience acid reflux.

✔ **Sleep propped up to avoid lying flat.** By elevating your upper body, gravity helps keep your stomach acids down. (If you're past your first trimester, you shouldn't lie flat, anyway, to avoid cutting off circulation to your baby and your legs. Lie on your left side for optimal circulation).

✔ **Practice good posture when sitting.** When you slouch, you put more pressure on your esophagus, which can lead to heartburn.

✔ **Avoid big meals.** Eat small portions so that you don't overfill the stomach and cause extra food to come back up the esophagus.

✔ **Sip liquids with meals instead of drinking large amounts.** Because you want to avoid having large amounts in your stomach at one time, drink small amounts at meals and stay hydrated by spreading your liquids out between meals.

✔ **Avoid greasy or fatty foods.** High-fat foods, specifically fried foods, tend to trigger heartburn because they don't stimulate digestion but do take longer to digest (because they just sit in your stomach).

✔ **Skip spicy and acidic foods.** Acidic foods, like tomatoes, citrus, and peppers, can be problematic for many women. Onions and garlic are also on some women's problem-foods list. For example, pizza gave me heartburn every time I ate it while pregnant.

✔ **Avoid caffeinated and carbonated beverages.** These drinks have been known to cause acid reflux. Sorry to say, but chocolate can also irritate the esophagus, so you may want to avoid it, too.

✔ **Take an antacid when you're uncomfortable.** Talk to your doctor about which one to choose or about a safe prescription medication if over-the-counter antacids don't work for you.

## Reducing gas with an antibloating diet

Burping and farting are two of the worst unmentionables of pregnancy. Who knew such an innocent-looking pregnant woman could produce so much gas? Again, you can blame this unpleasant side effect of pregnancy on the hormones.

The bacteria in your intestinal tract that help you digest carbohydrate-containing foods produce gas. (Fat and protein foods don't produce much, if any, gas.) Those fun pregnancy hormones (which I describe earlier in the section "Your Digestive Tract Acquires a Mind of Its Own"), combined with certain foods, can cause your body to produce more gas, so you may want to adjust your lifestyle to avoid producing even more. Limit your consumption of the following if you find that they cause more gas:

✔ Cruciferous vegetables, such as broccoli, cauliflower, cabbage, Brussels sprouts, and bok choy

✔ Legumes and beans, such as pinto, kidney, black, cannellini, and garbanzo beans, black-eyed peas, and lentils

✔ Onions and garlic

✔ Soy and soy-containing foods

✔ Sugar-free items that contain sugar alcohols (Avoid foods that have maltitol, xylitol, sorbitol, mannitol, and isomalt on the label. Erythritol is also a sugar alcohol, but it doesn't produce gas like other sugar alcohols tend to do.)

✔ Inulin (*Inulin* is a type of fiber added to many processed food products.)

✔ Whole grains, nuts, and seeds

As you can see, most of these common gas-producing foods are good for you, so you still need to be able to enjoy them. To do so while reducing gas production, eat small portions of these (and really all) foods and spread out portions throughout the day. Also, eat slowly so you don't swallow large amounts of food, and chew with your mouth closed.

One of my favorite gas-reducing tricks is to take Beano, an over-the-counter supplement that contains an enzyme that helps you digest certain parts of carbohydrate-containing foods that cause gas. The trick is to take Beano at the start of the meal, not after you finish. To prevent gas from forming, it needs to be present in the stomach while you're eating gas-inducing food. Beano is considered to be safe for pregnant women because it's isolated to the digestive tract.

## *Preventing pregnancy constipation*

The digestive tract becomes sluggish during pregnancy, causing the body to eliminate waste at a slower rate, which, in turn, can lead to constipation. If you're anxious about your pregnancy, don't exercise at all, or don't eat healthy, high-fiber foods, pregnancy constipation can become a lot worse. Iron supplements or the iron found in prenatal vitamins may also be to blame for some of your constipation.

About half of women experience constipation during pregnancy, but you can definitely do something about it! Follow these tips to keep things moving in your body:

✔ **Drink, drink, and drink more water.** Stool needs water to keep it moving through the digestive tract. (Refer to Chapter 3 for tips on how to stay hydrated during pregnancy.)

✔ **Eat lots of fiber.** Choose whole grains, beans, and plenty of fruits and vegetables. (Chapter 3 explains how to get more fiber into your diet.)

  If fiber hasn't been at the top of your must-eat list in the past, increase your fiber intake slowly and spread it out throughout the day to avoid a lot of gas and bloating. For example, have a small amount of high-fiber cereal for breakfast, a few additional servings of fruits or vegetables throughout the day, and some whole grains and beans for dinner.

✔ **Move your body to move your bowels.** Exercise, even a low-key activity like yoga, has been shown to stimulate your digestive tract. Stay active throughout all phases of pregnancy. (Flip to Chapter 5 for some exercises that are safe to do while you're pregnant.)

✓ **Spread out your iron supplement throughout the day.** Your prenatal pill has a high iron level, so cut it in half and take half in the morning and half in the evening. Your doctor may also be able to recommend an iron supplement that's easier on the stomach.

✓ **Consider taking over-the-counter fiber supplements or a stool softener.** Turn to over-the-counter items only as a last resort and talk to your doctor about which one is best for you before making a purchase.

✓ **Get "good" bacteria from probiotics.** Your digestive tract is full of bacteria, and some of the bacteria (commonly called *probiotics*) help support immune and digestive health. You can get probiotics by eating yogurt, drinking *kefir* (a type of fermented milk), or taking a probiotic supplement. Unlike stool softeners that you may take only as needed, probiotics are good to have on a daily basis.

Don't take a laxative to relieve constipation because doing so can cause uterine contractions and may also leave you dehydrated. Also, avoid taking mineral oils (which are natural laxatives) because they may inhibit absorption of some important nutrients during pregnancy.

## Dealing with hemorrhoids

*Hemorrhoids* are one of the most embarrassing unmentionables of pregnancy. They're essentially dilated, swollen veins in the rectum.

The best way to prevent hemorrhoids is to avoid becoming constipated. Read through the recommendations in the preceding section to discover how to avoid constipation. If you find yourself with hard stools that don't pass easily, don't strain yourself trying to get them out. Simply drink lots of fluid and boost the fiber in your diet to 28 grams per day. (For more tips on bumping up your fluid and fiber intake, check out Chapter 3.) Go for a walk to get things moving naturally, and avoid sitting for a long time, which puts additional pressure on the rectal area.

Nutritionally speaking, you can also prevent or deal with hemorrhoids by following the dietary guidelines for reducing swollen veins. Basically, these guidelines include the following:

✓ Limit the sodium in your diet to less than 2,300 mg per day.

✓ Avoid processed foods and high-salt condiments, like pickles, salad dressing, and soy sauce.

✓ Avoid adding salt to your food. (For more reasons to limit your sodium intake, see Chapter 18.)

Hemorrhoids can bleed and be quite painful. If you have hemorrhoids already, take a warm bath with baking soda in the water to help soothe pain, reduce itching, and assist in healing. Witch hazel also helps reduce the swelling.

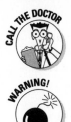

Visit your doctor if hemorrhoids become a concern. If you're losing a lot of blood or if it's too painful to have a bowel movement, you may need medical help.

However you choose to deal with hemorrhoids, don't avoid eating because you're afraid of having a painful bowel movement. Starving yourself during pregnancy is especially worrisome because you need to keep your body properly nourished.

## Steering clear of urinary tract infections

Pregnancy puts you at an increased risk for another pesky problem: urinary tract infections (UTIs). In case you don't remember anatomy and physiology from school, your *urinary tract* includes your kidneys, bladder, and the tubes that connect them.

During pregnancy, your kidneys work overtime to get rid of all your waste products and produce more urine. However, your bladder may not fully empty because your uterus is constantly pressing on it, leaving room for bacteria to multiply and grow until you have a full-blown UTI.

To reduce your chances of developing a UTI, follow these tips:

- ✔ Drink plenty of water to flush out the kidneys.
- ✔ Drink cranberry juice, especially if you're prone to kidney infections.
- ✔ Eat fruits, vegetables, and whole grains to get plenty of antioxidants to boost your immune system.
- ✔ Eat yogurt, drink kefir, and look for other products with added probiotics (or take a probiotic supplement) to increase "good" bacteria in the urinary tract.
- ✔ Avoid caffeinated beverages, which act as a diuretic.
- ✔ Wear cotton underwear.
- ✔ Avoid tight-fitting pants.
- ✔ Wipe front to back when using the bathroom to prevent bacteria from entering the urethra.
- ✔ Urinate when you first feel the need to do so instead of trying to hold it.
- ✔ Urinate before and after having intercourse.

UTIs are easy to treat with antibiotics that are safe during pregnancy, so don't despair if you have any of the symptoms in the following list. Instead, call your doctor.

- Blood or mucus in the urine

- Pain or burning when urinating

- Feelings of urgency to urinate

- Fever or chills

- Urine that looks cloudy or has an unusual odor

- Pain or tenderness in the bladder

An untreated UTI is more likely to develop into a kidney infection in pregnant women. So if you have back pain, nausea, vomiting, fever, and chills, don't wait to report these symptoms, all of which can signal a kidney infection.

# Fatigue Drains Your Energy Dry

If you're feeling unusually tired, you're not alone. Most women don't just feel a little bit tired when pregnant; they literally feel exhausted. It makes sense that in the third trimester you'd be tired from the extra weight you're carrying, but what could possibly make you feel so tired in the first trimester? The answer to that $50 million question? Hormones! Between the surge of hormones and the increase in your blood supply, your body is going through a lot of change. Your breasts and uterus are growing, and your baby is already getting a lot of your energy. The resulting fatigue is also your body's way of telling you to slow down and get plenty of rest.

The good news is that the second trimester is well-known for bursts of energy. Even though their bodies are still working overtime, many women find themselves cleaning and organizing in preparation of the baby's arrival. The third trimester brings some fatigue again, but this time it's mostly because of your larger size.

Don't listen to those well-intentioned people who say, "If you think you're tired now, just wait until the baby comes!" Your fatigue right now comes from the physical drain on your body, and you need to take it seriously so that you take care of yourself properly.

Follow these tips to beat fatigue:

- **Take a nap when you need it.** Even resting for 20 minutes without sleeping can make a world of difference.

- **Ask for help.** Don't be a superwoman and try to do everything yourself. Ask your partner, friends, and family for assistance. Don't be afraid to delegate!

- **Move your body regularly.** Exercise regularly (unless your doctor has told you not to). Women who exercise tend to have more energy and sleep better at night. See Chapter 5 for recommendations on safe ways to get moving.

> ✓ **Take your prenatal vitamin to ensure that you're getting enough iron.**
> Fatigue is a major symptom of iron deficiency because iron plays a role
> in transporting oxygen to the cells.

The most powerful ways to combat fatigue involve eating (specifically, paying
attention to how and what you eat) and sleeping (as in getting the amount
of sleep your body really needs). I delve into the details of these two fatigue-
fighting activities in the sections that follow.

## Eating to have energy

Most women think that fatigue and exhaustion are just part of the territory
called pregnancy. What you may not know is that what you eat and, even
more important, when you eat it can make a big difference in your energy
levels throughout the day. I've been studying and teaching people how to
have more energy for many years, and many of the people I work with have
incredible changes in their energy levels as a result of changing just a few
simple things in how they eat. Putting into practice even just one or two of
the tips in the next sections can help boost your energy levels.

### Eating small amounts

Eating small amounts rather than large meals has so many benefits in pregnancy. You can reduce your risk of getting heartburn, prevent excess weight
gain, improve sleep, and decrease feelings of nausea, just to name a few. But
the biggest benefit may be in the fact that you simply feel more energetic to
face your day.

By limiting portions, you fuel your body with just the right amount of food and
subsequent energy to get through your day. Eating large quantities can make
you feel sleepy and lethargic, preventing you from having enough energy for
you and your developing baby.

### Eating frequently throughout the day

When you eat smaller meals, you naturally have to eat more often, which really
just means you get to enjoy some yummy snacks. Snacks act like a bridge
between meals, preventing you from getting too hungry and making poor food
choices. When the snacks you choose are also nutritious, you provide you and
your baby with more nutrients to properly fuel your activities and your baby's
growth. To see a list of good snacks to choose, turn to Chapter 7.

### Eating foods that provide lasting energy

Certain foods give your body sustained energy throughout the day, but some
foods can cause a crash in energy. Avoid foods that are high in simple sugars
and refined carbohydrates, like cookies and other sweets, many crackers, and
regular soft drinks. Instead, choose foods that contain whole grains. Read labels

on breads, crackers, tortillas, rice, and cereals, and look for the words *whole grain*. Whole grains have more complex carbohydrates (starches) that take your body longer to digest than simple sugars, resulting in more lasting energy. (For more information about whole grains and fiber, head to Chapter 3.)

For lasting energy in a meal or snack, combine foods rich in complex carbohydrates with protein-rich foods. Aim to include protein, such as a piece of meat, poultry, fish, dairy, eggs, or a vegetarian alternative, at every meal. Protein keeps you feeling full for a longer period of time and prevents blood sugar from rising too quickly, leading to the inevitable crash of energy when it drops back down. Look for snacks that have either protein or fiber in them to prevent this type of energy crash at snack time.

## Getting the sleep you need

Most people don't get enough sleep on a regular basis. If you're one of them, you may need to take a serious look at getting the sleep you need during pregnancy. Adults need between seven and nine hours of sleep per night, but you may find that your body needs more sleep while you're pregnant. Plus, poor sleep can affect your labor when you're ready to deliver. Some studies suggest that women who get six hours of sleep or less have longer labors and increased risk of C-section deliveries.

Many pregnant women face a variety of problems, like those in the following list, that cause significant disruption to their sleep (and therefore help increase feelings of fatigue):

✓ **The need to urinate:** Many women get up several times each night to visit the bathroom, disrupting their ability to get continuous, restorative sleep.

✓ **Heartburn:** This condition, which I tell you how to prevent in the earlier section "Avoiding heartburn with the help of some nutrition tricks," can make some women very uncomfortable when they lie down to catch some zzz's.

✓ **Restless leg syndrome (RLS):** RLS is a condition that causes discomfort in the legs when you're lying down. You relieve the discomfort by moving your legs. To help minimize RLS, exercise regularly and be sure to stretch after exercise. Also, get checked for iron deficiency because it can sometimes contribute to RLS.

Follow these tips to get a more restful night's sleep:

✓ **Drink liquids during the day and limit your intake three to four hours before bedtime.** Limiting liquids later in the day may help cut down on the number of trips to the bathroom you need to make in the middle of the night.

✔ **Develop a good bedtime routine.** Take a warm bath, relax with a book, and dim the lights. Get the TV, computer, and phone out of your bedroom. Use the bedroom for sleep and sex only.

✔ **Go to bed at approximately the same time each night.** If at all possible, don't set an alarm so you can allow your body to naturally wake up when you feel you've gotten the sleep you need.

✔ **Sleep on your left side, especially after the first trimester.** Use a body pillow or just a small pillow in between your knees or under your belly to get more comfortable.

✔ **Sleep with your head elevated to keep stomach acids down and avoid eating two to three hours prior to bedtime.** Doing so helps minimize the possibility of heartburn.

Pregnant women, particularly those who are overweight at conception, may develop *sleep apnea,* a disorder in which breathing is repeatedly disrupted during sleep. Untreated sleep apnea is a serious medical condition and increases risk of gestational diabetes, preeclampsia, and having a low-birth-weight baby. If your partner notices that you snore much louder or seem to have long pauses between breaths while asleep, alert your doctor.

---

# Avoiding balloon-like feet and hands

Swelling happens because of the increase in fluid in your body. It can also lead to varicose veins and spider veins as your uterus puts pressure on the veins that send blood back up to your heart from your legs, feet, face, and hands. If you're prone to swelling, follow these tips:

✔ Prop up your feet whenever you can.

✔ Limit your salt/sodium intake.

✔ Drink plenty of water and avoid alcohol, of course.

✔ Avoid standing or sitting for too long. Take breaks if you have a job that requires you to sit or stand a lot.

✔ Sleep on your side and elevate your legs with pillows.

✔ Swim laps or join a water aerobics class to take the pressure off your legs. Or just enjoy being weightless while floating in the water.

✔ Wear medical-grade compression stockings. Get advice from your doctor on the right ones for you.

*Remember:* Call your doctor if swelling is severe or comes on suddenly. Dramatic or sudden swelling could be a sign of one of the more serious medical conditions I cover in Chapter 18.

# Part II
# Eating Right for Pregnancy

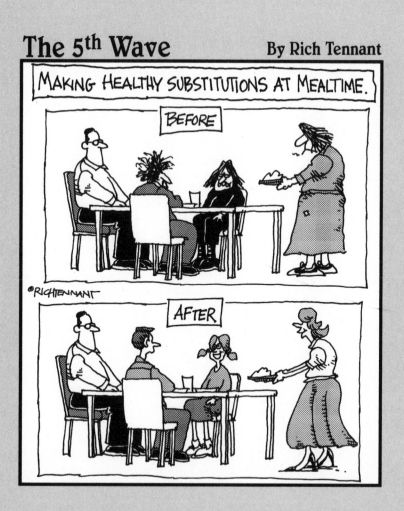

# In this part . . .

In this part, I take you through a typical day, mealwise, and show you how often to eat and what to munch on between meals. If you've heard about pregnancy cravings or are experiencing them yourself, you can use this part to help guide you through those cravings.

I show you how to deal with common restaurant temptations and help you make good decisions at the grocery store, including whether to go organic and which fish to buy. I also reveal how to stock your kitchen and prepare (and store) food safely. If you still have doubts as to what to eat and when, check out the sample meal plans I include at the end of this part.

# Chapter 7

# Completing the Puzzle: Discovering How to Eat while Pregnant

*In This Chapter*

▶ Eating small meals and frequent snacks to curb hunger and fuel your body

▶ Snacking the smart way with delicious go-to pregnancy snacks

▶ Knowing why you get cravings and what you can do to manage them

Knowing what to eat and what to avoid to help your baby grow is essential, but it's only one piece of the puzzle. Because pregnancy often comes with a host of experiences — including filling up quickly because your baby is fighting for room in your belly, feeling content one minute and hungry the next, and having a serious hankering for an ice cream sundae — you also need to know *how* to eat.

This chapter has you covered with the information you need to know. You discover a new approach to eating (here's a hint: small meals are your friend), and you find out why snacking between meals is critical. You also discover how to deal with cravings that may at times seem impossible to deny.

## *Adopting a New Dining Strategy: Eat Small Amounts Frequently*

If you adopt any new mantras over the course of your pregnancy, I strongly encourage you to adopt this one: Eat small amounts frequently. Here's why:

✔ **Your body is designed to have food on a regular basis.** Think about the actual size of the human stomach: It's only about as big as a softball or grapefruit. Although it will stretch to accommodate more food, too much stretching makes you feel bloated and uncomfortably full.

Eating small amounts is especially important when you're pregnant. You may find that as your belly grows, your stomach shrinks. Well, your stomach isn't really shrinking, but your baby is pressing down on your stomach, causing it to feel full quickly. You can minimize the discomfort you feel after eating by eating small meals. When you cut back on meal size, you get hungry more frequently, leading you to eat more often.

✓ **Your body needs food all day long while you're awake.** If your body doesn't get the energy it needs because you're not eating, it can't function at the best of its ability. As a result, it'll begin to break down stored fat and muscle tissue — not an ideal scenario when you're pregnant.

Giving your body the fuel it needs starts with eating breakfast. Your energy needs go up the minute you've silenced the snooze and your feet hit the floor. When your energy needs increase, your food intake should do the same (in other words, you need to supply food to the body when it demands it). To start your day off right, either eat breakfast right away and then have a midmorning snack or, if you're not hungry for breakfast right away, eat a snack (like a few handfuls of dry cereal or crackers, a cup of milk or yogurt, a banana, or one slice of toast) within an hour of getting up and then follow that an hour or two later with a more substantial breakfast.

If you're experiencing nausea, which is often caused by having too much stomach acid, eat a little bit of food (even though you don't feel like eating) to help keep that queasy feeling at bay. See Chapter 6 for more on combating nausea and other unpleasant side effects of pregnancy.

You can't only eat small amounts or only eat frequently. You have to do both. After all, if you just eat small portions but don't eat often, you'll be hungry all the time. If you just eat more frequently but don't cut back on portions, you may end up with too many calories and undesired excess weight gain.

The following sections help you figure out how to read your body's signals so that you can more easily know when to eat and when to stop eating and how to tame the ravenous hunger that can sometimes strike during pregnancy.

## Using the hunger gauge to interpret your body's signals

Many people have learned to effectively ignore or suppress the signals their stomachs so diligently send to their brains in favor of telling themselves stories like these:

✓ "I don't have time for breakfast; I just deal with the hunger."

✓ "This food tastes so good that I can't stop."

✓ "There's always room for dessert!"

✓ "I've had a hard day; I deserve it!"

✓ "I'm pregnant; I need the extra calories."

If you really want to master the eat-small-amounts-frequently technique, I suggest using a hunger gauge to become more in tune with the ways your body signals that it's running on empty. One sign you're probably already familiar with is that growl in your tummy — you know, the one you're sure everyone around you can hear although they're too polite to comment on it. If you don't provide your body with some food fuel within 15 minutes of that growl, you may start to experience other symptoms of hunger, including

- ✔ Feelings of being really irritable, unfocused, and/or lightheaded
- ✔ The inability to stop thinking about food
- ✔ Headaches
- ✔ Nausea
- ✔ Shakiness

As you reacquaint yourself with your body's hunger signals, think of them like the gas gauge on your car. To see what I mean, take a look at Figure 7-1, which shows what the feelings in your body would look like if you had a gas gauge installed in your body.

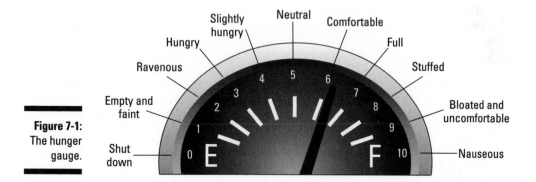

**Figure 7-1:**
The hunger gauge.

The first four levels of the hunger gauge deal with varying degrees of hunger. When you're at level three (hungry), eat a small meal. When you're at level four (slightly hungry) and a meal is still a long time off, have a snack to tide you over (see the later section "Being prepared with a go-to pregnancy snack list" for some yummy snack ideas). If you wait to eat until you're at level two (ravenous), you're much more likely to make bad food choices, eat too quickly, and not know when to stop. If you get all the way to level one (empty and faint), you may start to feel physically ill. If you get to level zero (shut down), your body is so hungry that you don't even feel hungry anymore; at that point, your body starts to shut down metabolism and may break down muscle for energy. A number five on the hunger gauge represents a neutral feeling, neither hungry nor full.

The other end of the hunger gauge deals with the levels of fullness. Ideally, you stop eating when you reach level six (comfortable) but definitely by the time you reach level seven (full). If you keep eating until you reach level eight (stuffed), your stomach stretches, telling your body there's an excess energy supply that it must store as fat. At level nine (bloated and uncomfortable), you feel tired and possibly guilty about how much you ate, and at level ten (nauseous), you're so full that you feel sick.

Figuring out the difference between being comfortable and being full or stuffed takes practice. By practice, I mean being aware of the sensations in your stomach and paying attention to how you feel, not just physically but also emotionally and mentally. When you're at level six on the hunger gauge and feeling pretty comfortable, you should feel about 80 percent full. At this point, the food you just ate should last you about two to three hours before you're hungry again. When you're at level seven on the hunger gauge, you should be feeling full (but not uncomfortable), and your food should last you about three to four hours. When you're comfortable or full, you're still alert, focused, and happy. When you go beyond fullness and into the feelings of stuffed and bloated, you're in what I call a "food coma," where you'd like to just take a nap or unbutton your pants. At this point, you can't concentrate on the things around you because you're feeling tired and guilty about eating too much.

To keep from feeling more uncomfortable than you may already be feeling, avoid going above level seven (full) on the hunger gauge.

## Keeping your hunger from becoming ravenous

Many pregnant women complain that they're hungrier than usual and that their hunger can sometimes become quite ravenous (often with very little warning). During both of my pregnancies, I'd find myself quite content and not hungry at all one minute and literally ravenous the next minute.

Becoming aware of what being hungry feels like so you know when to start eating is just as important as knowing when to stop eating. If you allow your-self to become ravenous, you'll attack that bread basket as soon as you sit down to a meal at a restaurant or immediately grab a bag of chips when you walk in the door at home. So eat when you first start to feel hungry. Don't wait to dig in until you're either sick or so hungry that you feel like you could eat everything in sight.

If you find that your hunger is utterly unpredictable, carry healthy food with you at all times and make snacking your secret weapon. I provide a list of go-to pregnancy snacks later in this chapter.

# *Knowing when to stop*

Pushing away a plate of tasty food takes discipline and enough self-awareness to know where you're at on the hunger gauge (a tool I describe in the preceding section). Developing both is well worth the effort, especially if you're one of the many pregnant women who experience heartburn — a pregnancy side effect that's often exacerbated by large portions of food.

I know that saying no to an extra piece of pizza or turning down dessert can be tough, but skipping out on this extra food has two big benefits: You may wind up feeling better, and you (and your developing baby) will wind up healthier when you don't gain excess weight during your pregnancy.

Follow these tips to become more mindful while eating so that you know when to stop:

- ✔ **Eliminate distractions while you eat.** Always sit down at a table to eat and don't do anything else (like working, reading, or watching TV) while you're eating. Eating delicious food is a pleasure in life, and it should get your full attention. Plus, if you're distracted, you won't pay attention to your body's hunger cues, and before you know it, you'll be overfull.

- ✔ **Eat from a smaller plate.** The average plate size in America has increased by 36 percent since the 1960s. Eating from larger plates usually means piling on larger portions, so eat from smaller plates to help you eat smaller portions. A smaller plate holds less food, but when you fill it up, your brain still sees a plate full of food.

- ✔ **Don't be part of the "Clean Plate Club."** Just because you still have food in front of you doesn't mean you have to finish it, especially when the portion was too big to begin with.

- ✔ **Eat slowly by putting your fork down between bites.** By consciously putting your fork down, you force yourself to slow down. Your stomach takes about 20 minutes to signal fullness to your brain, so eating slowly helps you know when to stop eating before you end up feeling stuffed.

- ✔ **Chew well and drink fluids with your meal.** Chewing your food well promotes good digestion. Similarly, drinking fluids (like water, milk, and juice) helps your body break down food while you're eating.

- ✔ **Be aware that some foods are more filling than others.** Protein, fiber, and water all fill you up faster than simple carbs, like sugars or refined starches. Fill half your plate with fruits and vegetables (which provide water and fiber) and the rest with complex carbohydrates (preferably whole grains) and lean protein. (To find out which foods are the best sources for the nutrients you need during pregnancy, see Chapter 3.)

- ✔ **When you're dining with others, engage in conversation so that you slow down the pace at which you eat.** However, don't allow that conversation to distract you too much from enjoying the tastes and textures of your food!

# Snacking Is Sensible

Snacks are a must-have during pregnancy. Think of them like little bridges that help carry you over from one meal to the next, leaving you with the energy you need to get through the day and keeping you in a good mood.

If the bridge image doesn't sell you on the idea of snacking, consider that snacking allows you to fill in small nutrient gaps throughout your day. If you're not getting all the nutrients you need during your regularly scheduled meals, you can eat nutrient-rich snacks that provide you with some of the nutrients you need more of when you're expecting. (If that doesn't sound too exciting, don't fret. You don't have to eat only "healthy" food as snacks. Chocolate, ice cream, and chips can have their place at the snack table, too!)

In the sections that follow, I clue you in to the wonderful world of healthy snacking. Prepare to discover what kinds of foods are worth snacking on and when snacking fits best in your day.

One important note about snacks: Snacks aren't intended to fill you up. Eating a banana mid morning won't fill you up, but if the banana bridges you from breakfast to lunch so you don't arrive at lunch feeling ravenous, the banana did its job.

## Presenting guidelines for smart snacking

The main rule of thumb for snacking is to eat something that has nutritional value. Focus on foods that have high fiber or protein. (I introduce you to high-fiber and high-protein foods in Chapter 3.) These nutrients take longer to digest, which means you won't crash shortly after consuming them and your energy will last longer. Read food labels if you're not sure whether something has fiber or protein in it. For fresh foods, you can find the nutrient data you need at nutritiondata.self.com.

To provide lasting energy, avoid foods that are high in sugar or refined flour, including rice cakes, pretzels, donuts, sugary drinks, cookies, and candy. All of these foods can cause a spike and drop in your blood sugar, leading to a major energy crash. Also stay away from high-fat foods that may be greasy or full of cream because they may be difficult to digest, leading to heartburn or a queasy stomach.

Aim for eating between 100 and 150 calories per snack. Anything more than this could be considered a small meal. Remember that a snack is intended to bridge you from meal to meal; in other words, it should curb your hunger enough so that you can make it to the next meal, not fill you up. If the snack contains fiber or protein, 100 to 150 calories should be enough to last you for one to two hours. If you're really hungry or need that snack to last longer, go for a 200-calorie snack. (See Chapter 3 for more on your calorie needs during pregnancy.)

# Being prepared with a go-to pregnancy snack list

The biggest issue most people have with snacking is a lack of preparation. They forget to pack snacks and then don't have them ready when hunger strikes. So get into the habit of keeping your purse, briefcase, car, desk drawer — basically, everywhere you go — stocked with nonperishable snacks.

Eventually, you'll develop your own go-to list of snacks, but for now, consider the foods on this list as a jumping-off point:

- **Beans:** Edamame is probably the bean that's most commonly eaten as a snack, but other beans make good snacks, too. I've been known to eat chickpeas (or garbanzo beans) right out of the can as a snack, but you can also eat them toasted like in the Crunchy Garbanzo Beans in Chapter 13. Or save some leftover bean salad (like the Three-Bean Artichoke Salad in Chapter 17) from lunch for a snack the next day!

- **Canned/jarred fruit:** Look for individual containers of fruit packed in its own juice for convenience. Avoid fruit that has been packed in light syrup so you don't consume extra sugar.

- **Cheese:** Go for string cheese or mini individually wrapped cheeses like mini Babybel or Laughing Cow. Always check labels to make sure the cheese is pasteurized.

- **Chocolate:** If you're craving chocolate, have some for a snack. Chocolate has fiber, so it's not a completely empty-calorie food, but, of course, try to limit your portion to about an ounce. For an even more satisfying chocolate snack that won't leave you crashing, have chocolate-covered nuts (think Peanut or Almond M&Ms and go for the snack-sized bag with about 10 pieces in it).

- **Cottage cheese:** Look for the 1% or 2% milk or fat-free varieties. Also consider buying the individual cups for convenience.

- **Dried fruit:** Dried fruit — think raisins, cherries, blueberries, cranberries, pineapple, apples, bananas, and so on — is denser than fresh fruit, so a little goes a long way (a quarter cup is a tad over 100 calories for most dried fruit). Mix your favorite dried fruit with nuts for a tasty trail mix.

- **Dry cereal:** I often snack on dry cereals, like Cheerios, Frosted Mini-Wheats, Kashi cereals, Cracklin' Oat Bran, and Quaker Oatmeal Squares. Look for cereals with at least 3 grams of fiber per serving. Put a serving of cereal into a snack-sized resealable bag and throw it in your purse for a midmorning snack.

- **Fresh fruit:** Fruit has fiber, especially if you eat the peel (when appropriate, of course). So pick up staples such as bananas, apples, oranges, pears, berries, grapes, melon, peaches, and plums, but don't be afraid to experiment with different fruits like kiwi or Medjool dates.

✔ **Greek yogurt:** Get twice as much protein as regular yogurt when you eat Greek yogurt. Stick to the fat-free or lowfat kind.

✔ **Half of a sandwich:** Eating something more substantial that's still low in calories can help keep you feeling satisfied longer. Heat some turkey to steaming hot in the microwave and put it on a slice of whole-grain bread. Add the veggies of your choice, fold it over, and enjoy.

✔ **Nut butters:** Peanut butter, almond butter, and soy nut butter are all delicious snack ideas. Spread them on celery, apple slices, whole-grain crackers, or brown rice cakes, or simply eat them with a spoon (just be sure to limit yourself to one tablespoon!).

✔ **Nut or cereal mixes:** Make your own snack mixes with your favorite nuts and cereal. Check out the Apple Cinnamon Trail Mix and the Quinoa Nut Mix in Chapter 13 for ideas to get you started.

✔ **Nutrition bars:** Choose a bar that has fiber or protein or both. KIND, SOYJOY, LÄRABAR, PowerBar Pria, Clif Bar Luna or Mojo, and ZonePerfect are just a few of the brands you have to choose from.

✔ **Nutrition shakes:** Shakes are delicious and often come in the perfect size for a snack. EAS AdvantEDGE, Slim-Fast, Carnation Breakfast, and Mix1 are just some of the brands you can choose.

✔ **Nuts:** Almonds, pistachios, pecans, walnuts, peanuts, and cashews are full of fiber and protein, and the fat they contain is heart-healthy fat. But beware of portions when you're eating nuts because a little bit can add up fast. For 150 calories, you can get 22 almonds, 45 pistachios, 15 pecan halves, 11 walnut halves, 25 peanuts, or 16 cashews.

✔ **Oatmeal:** Just add hot water or milk and you've got yourself a tasty snack. Or look for Seneca Oatmeal and Fruit cups, which don't require adding milk or water and take just 45 seconds in the microwave.

✔ **Popcorn:** You can get a lot of volume (3 or more cups) of this whole grain in a serving for relatively few calories. Pop it on the stove in a small amount of canola oil or use the snack-sized microwavable bags for convenience.

✔ **Raw veggies and hummus:** Slice or chop up some red pepper, celery, broccoli, cauliflower, or mushrooms, or go for the more convenient baby carrots or sugar snap peas. Eat them by themselves or dip them into a few tablespoons of premade hummus.

✔ **Salad:** Who says salad is only for meals? Have a small salad loaded with lots of veggies for a satisfying midafternoon snack.

✔ **Smoothies:** Throw some frozen berries, milk, and a banana into the blender for a quick and satisfying smoothie. Check out the Chocolate Banana Blast Smoothie or Pomegranate Power Smoothie in Chapter 12.

> ✔ **Whole-grain crackers and chips:** Kashi crackers, Triscuits, Wheat Thins, SunChips, Tostitos, and many tortilla chips are made with whole grains. Look for the phrase *whole grain* on the ingredient list and check the label for 2 or more grams of fiber. Add nutrition by dipping your crackers and chips into bean dips and fresh salsas, like the Minty Watermelon Salsa in Chapter 13.

## Determining how many snacks you need

To determine the number of snacks you need in a day, take a look at your current eating patterns. The typical recommendation you may hear of eating three small meals and three snacks per day may or may not apply to you. For example, you may need more than three snacks, depending on how big or small your meals are and how many calories you need. If you don't mind snacking frequently or you don't have a problem pushing the plate away to eat smaller meals, then you may need four or five snacks each day. If you don't want to be bothered with very many snacks, just plan on having two or three to bridge your hunger between meals.

Generally, you want to eat something within an hour of waking. Follow that up by eating a meal or snack every two to four hours throughout the day, as indicated by the following sample eating schedule. (For sample meal plans that include specific food recommendations for each meal and snack according to the trimester you're in, flip to Chapter 11.)

✔ 7:00 a.m. — Out of bed

✔ 8:00 a.m. — Breakfast

✔ 10:45 a.m. — Snack

✔ 12:30 p.m. — Lunch

✔ 3:00 p.m. — Snack

✔ 5:00 p.m. — Snack

✔ 6:30 p.m. — Dinner

✔ 9:30 p.m. — Snack

✔ 10:30 p.m. — Bedtime

The fuel you get from meals (400 to 600 calories) typically lasts your body about two to four hours, whereas the fuel you get from snacks (100 to 150 calories) may last only one to two hours.

# Get Me Some Ice Cream . . . NOW!: Understanding and Managing Cravings

Sending your partner out at midnight for an ice cream run? Dying for a summer sausage and cheese sandwich on rye with grape jelly? Welcome to the land of pregnancy cravings. Cravings in pregnancy are normal. In fact, most women experience them at some point in their pregnancy. The extent of the cravings is what you may need to worry about. If the junk food you're craving is filling you up and you're not hungry for healthy foods, you have a problem. And too much junk food in addition to healthy food can lead to excess weight gain and pregnancy complications. The next sections offer some insight into why cravings occur and how you can manage them so that you don't gain a ton of extra weight throughout the course of your pregnancy.

## Why am I craving this food, anyway?

Lots of theories exist for why pregnant women tend to crave certain foods during pregnancy. Emotions — happy, sad, stressed, anxious — can cause many people to turn to food to calm down or reward. One emotion many pregnant women feel is a sense of entitlement or reward. You figure that because you're working hard carrying your baby, you need (and deserve) the extra calories, so why not give in to every craving you experience? Because, if you do, you may end up with more pounds than you bargained for in your pregnancy. After all, your body stores every unneeded calorie you take in as extra fat, and that extra fat is much harder to get rid of when you're trying to get back down to your pre-pregnancy weight.

Sometimes people (pregnant women included) crave foods because of the power of suggestion; they see, smell, or even just hear about a particular food and then have a real hankering for it. As a dietitian, I talk about food all day long, so I've definitely experienced this type of craving. For example, if a client talks about chocolate chip cookies hot out of the oven, two days later I may find myself craving warm chocolate chip cookies. Have you been to the movies, mall, or airport lately and, all of a sudden, found yourself craving popcorn, cinnamon buns, or pizza? If so, you, too, have fallen victim to the power of suggestion.

One craving cause scientists have proven to be true is hunger. When you're hungry, you crave food. The hungrier you get, the worse the cravings can be. For example, if you feel low on energy, your brain's natural reaction is to crave something sweet because sugar provides instant energy. Similarly, fat provides lasting energy, so if your body senses that energy levels have been running low for a while, it signals you to eat something with fat. Thus, chocolate and ice cream are the perfect craving foods because they offer sugar for energy right away and fat for energy long-term.

# When cravings are bad

Not all cravings are good cravings. For instance, a condition called *pica* is when someone craves and eats nonfood items. It's actually more common in children, but it does occasionally strike pregnant women. If you suffer from pica, you may have intense cravings for (and subsequently eat) nonfood substances like paper, chalk, dirt, sand, laundry starch, cornstarch, coffee grounds, clay, mothballs, plaster, soap, charcoal, ashes, stones, paint, soap, and animal feces.

Eating these substances is dangerous and can harm you and your baby because these nonfoods can interfere with nutrient absorption and some of them are toxic. If your cravings have turned to nonfood substances, contact your doctor immediately for help. Some people believe that zinc and iron deficiencies cause the cravings, so get your blood tested. Also, look for alternatives to calm the cravings. Chew sugarless gum and suck on strong mints. Keep yourself properly fueled with real food so that you don't feel hungry. You may need to seek professional help from a therapist to take a behavioral approach to stopping the behavior.

## How can I get through my cravings without gaining 70 pounds?

You may have discovered that many food cravings don't go away until you eat the specific foods you crave. Say you're craving olives wrapped in cream cheese and pepperoni. Eating a carrot stick instead probably isn't going to cut it. Sometimes you just need to fulfill that craving, as weird or normal as it may be.

If you give in to every craving, you may end up putting on more pounds than you planned during your pregnancy. If you're determined to survive your cravings without experiencing excess weight gain, follow these tips:

- ✔ **Figure out how to distinguish between physical hunger and psychological hunger.** Ask yourself whether you're truly hungry or just bored, sad, happy, or stressed. If you're truly hungry, eat a snack or meal. If you're not, stall and distract yourself (see the next bullet).

- ✔ **Stall and distract yourself.** Instead of giving in right away to a particular craving (if you're not physically hungry), buy yourself some time by engaging in another activity (call a friend or go for a walk, for example) to see if the craving goes away. A lot of times it does, but if you come back still wanting the particular food, then have it for your next meal or snack to satisfy the craving.

- ✔ **Figure out what you really want.** For example, if you're craving a strawberry milkshake, ask yourself what you're really craving. Are you craving the strawberries or the creamy, cold, sweet taste of the milkshake? Could you satisfy the craving with some fresh berries and whipped cream? What about a half cup of strawberry sorbet or lowfat ice cream?

Would a strawberry-banana smoothie do the trick? Any of these options would be much lower in calories or have more nutritional value than the strawberry milkshake.

✔ **Substitute if possible.** Always choose the healthiest version of the foods you're craving, For example, if you're craving potato chips, you may be able to substitute lowfat popcorn for the full-fat chips. But don't substitute if no good substitute exists. For example, if you're craving pickles, eating a plain cucumber won't be very satisfying! Just eat the pickles and be done with the craving.

✔ **Eat a variety of foods throughout the day.** If you eat nothing but protein, you'll probably crave carbs. If you eat only carbs, you may find yourself craving a steak. Eat some carbs, protein, and fat at every meal and get a variety of grains, meats or meat alternatives, fruits, and veggies every day. Doing so helps you (and your baby) stay healthy! (See Chapter 3 for the lowdown on proper pregnancy nutrition.)

✔ **Be aware of your portions.** With foods like cake, ice cream, chocolate, cookies, chips, and other high-calorie foods, pay attention to the portions you eat. Serve yourself one serving on a plate and put the rest of the package away instead of plopping down on the couch with the entire container. Eat slowly and enjoy every bite.

✔ **Avoid trigger situations.** If your favorite donut shop is on the way home from work, take an alternate route to avoid craving donuts simply because you drove by the shop. Get rid of the candy jar at work. Ask your partner and those close to you to avoid tempting you unnecessarily.

✔ **Rest up and pamper yourself.** When you're tired, you may crave food for energy. If you find yourself unusually tired or you're not getting the proper sleep at night, do everything you can to give yourself a break. Get a massage or pedicure, take a nap, or simply put your feet up with a good book or magazine. That way, you won't find yourself craving high-sugar, high-fat foods that'll just lead to energy crashes and excess weight gain later.

# Chapter 8

# Making Safe and Healthy Choices When Dining Out

**In This Chapter**

▶ Figuring out how to find the healthiest items on the menu and then how to order them

▶ Overcoming the potential pitfalls of restaurant eating

▶ Keeping you and your baby safe when dining out

**P**regnancy lasts a long time, so even if you're diligent about preparing meals at home, chances are you're going to dine out at least a few times. The good news is that pregnant women aren't limited in their choice of restaurant. You can find something to eat at any type of restaurant — American, Italian, Mexican, Korean, fast-food, sit-down, or coffee house. What you choose from the menu, however, can make a difference in providing you and your baby with safe and healthy food. Don't start panicking, yet. This chapter is here to help you make good food choices while dining out. In it, you discover how to navigate any restaurant menu, no matter how complex it seems; prevent common restaurant temptations from getting the best of you; and keep food safety in mind, whether you're enjoying your restaurant meal outside the home, on your couch, or in a doggie bag.

## First Things First: Navigating the Menu

The first step in ordering right at any restaurant is knowing how to read the menu. After all, restaurant menus can be rather deceptive thanks to their tantalizing, mouth-watering descriptions. The restaurant's main goal is to get you to love its food so that you keep coming back — preferably with every known friend or relative in tow. But what tends to make most restaurant dishes so yummy is an excess of fat, salt, and sugar. The following sections reveal how to translate those delicious-sounding menu descriptions so that you can decide which dishes are best for you and your baby.

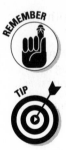

If you can't tell how a dish is prepared from its description in the menu, be sure to ask! If you're at a sit-down restaurant and the server doesn't know, ask to talk to the chef so you can find out whether that dish is a good choice for you (and your baby).

If you want to guarantee you won't be fooled by a restaurant menu, take advantage of modern technology and browse menus and nutritional information online. Most major chain (and even some family-owned) restaurants offer menus and nutritional information on their websites. Or you can pick up a copy of *Restaurant Calorie Counter For Dummies,* 2nd Edition, by Rosanne Rust and Meri Raffetto (John Wiley & Sons, Inc.). Browse through and make your dinner decision before you even set foot in the restaurant!

## Spotting high-sodium foods

Sodium is linked to high blood pressure and can increase swelling during pregnancy (see Chapter 18 for more on both of these conditions). But because sodium provides flavor, you can bet that pretty much all restaurant food has a good deal of sodium in it. The following foods are especially high, so try to limit your intake of them when you're dining out:

- Anything pickled (think pickles and olives)
- Sauces like soy, teriyaki, cocktail, marinara, gravy, and salad dressing
- Broths, including soups and au jus
- Processed meats (think deli meats and bacon)
- Anything smoked

## Picking out high-fat foods

High-fat foods are high in calories, which could cause excess weight gain during pregnancy (see Chapter 5 for tips on avoiding excess weight gain). You don't need to eat everything fat-free while carrying your little one, but you should limit how many high-fat foods you eat and how often you eat them. So when you're at a restaurant, try to avoid ordering meals with the following menu terms; although they may sound yummy, they basically mean "high in fat":

- **Pan-fried, deep-fried, sautéed:** These terms are just another way to say something is cooked in a good deal of oil.
- **Crispy, breaded, battered, tempura, golden:** These terms warn you that whatever foods they're describing are fried.
- **Alfredo, cream sauce, aioli, béarnaise, hollandaise, mayonnaise:** These terms mean the dish is creamed or creamy. (Note that even dishes with "light" cream sauce can contain more fat than you should eat in one sitting.)

✔ **Smothered:** This term typically means that the dish is served with a creamy sauce, oily vegetables, or a whole lot of cheese.

✔ **Fondue:** This term means that you dip individual pieces of food in cheese, oil, or chocolate — all of which are loaded in fat. Dipping in broth won't add the fat, but it'll add a good deal of sodium to your meal.

✔ **Cheesy, au gratin, scalloped:** These terms indicate that the recipe is full of either cheese or cream.

## Zeroing in on good-for-you descriptions

To protect your health and weight when eating out, choose menu items that involve healthier cooking techniques. The end result will be less extra fat and calories and, in some cases, less sodium, too. Foods bearing any of the following descriptions are typically good bets during pregnancy:

✔ Baked

✔ Broiled

✔ Grilled

✔ Lean

✔ Poached

✔ Roasted

✔ Steamed

# Placing Your Order

As you mentally prepare your order, bear in mind that a well-rounded meal consists of complex carbs, protein, and some fruit and/or vegetables. So if, for example, you're thinking about ordering a salad, which naturally has lots of vegetables, consider whether it includes any protein. Also consider whether it comes with a roll or some starchy vegetables as toppings to provide you with complex carbs.

Most restaurants don't automatically give you a lot of fruits and vegetables (salads are the exception), so you may need to order a side of veggies or a fruit cup to get your quota for the meal. Ask to sub the ever-present fries for vegetables. If your server tells you veggies cost a little more, just smile and say, "They're worth it."

Skip items like raw fish, undercooked meat, runny or undercooked eggs, and sprouts, and keep in mind that undercooked eggs may be an ingredient in custards, certain sauces (such as hollandaise and béarnaise), and cookie dough.

Also pass on freshly made Caesar dressing because you don't know whether it contains pasteurized eggs. When in doubt, ask your server how certain foods are prepared or what kinds of ingredients are used in the dishes you're considering so that you can make healthy decisions for you and your baby. (See Chapter 4 for the lowdown on which foods you need to avoid during pregnancy.)

Also avoid ordering freshly squeezed juices. Although they taste delicious, they haven't been pasteurized and could contain harmful bacteria. If you're unsure, ask the server whether the juice you're thinking about is freshly squeezed or comes out of a container.

If you want to ensure your meal is exactly the way you want it, just ask. Don't be bashful. The wait staff at most restaurants is used to having customers make special requests when ordering. If you want sauces on the side or less oil in your veggies, just ask. If you're not sure whether your special request is feasible, consider whether another dish on the menu contains the ingredient you're requesting. For example, if a restaurant has a salad with black beans in it, you know they have black beans in the kitchen in case you want to special order something that contains them.

# Standing Strong in the Face of Common Restaurant Temptations

Going out to eat should be a pleasurable experience, and everyone deserves to indulge occasionally. However, if you choose the greasy, creamy, high-fat dishes every time you go out, you may end up gaining a lot more weight than you bargained for. The next sections help you steel your reserve for when you encounter common restaurant temptations — from the bread basket to dessert — so you don't wind up gaining 100 extra pounds during your pregnancy.

## Dealing with appetizers

Although appetizers seem like a good idea when you arrive at a restaurant starving, they really just add extra calories to your meal. And because most restaurants offer portions that are already too big, adding more food with appetizers simply doesn't make sense. Add to that the fact that many appetizers top off at 1,500 or more calories (that endless bread or chip basket alone can add 300 calories to your meal!) and the case for just saying no to appetizers gets even stronger.

Resist the temptation to overindulge in appetizers by asking the server not to bring that bread or chip basket over in the first place. If your dining companions object, try to limit yourself to one piece of bread or just a few chips.

## Facing down the biggest temptation of all: The endless buffet

Food tastes good when you eat out, so it's no wonder that controlling how much you eat is sometimes the hardest part. If you choose a buffet-style restaurant, you have to have discipline of steel if you want to walk away without unbuttoning the top button of your pants. Don't let those elastic bands on your maternity pants be your excuse for not knowing when to stop!

Buffets are dangerous for two reasons: They offer an unlimited supply of food, and they have a large variety. Studies have proven that when people are exposed to a large variety of food, they tend to eat more because they want to try a little of everything. For instance, if you weren't planning on having dessert and the restaurant where you're eating had only one option, you'd probably be able to pass it up (unless it was one

of your favorites). But if you're faced with a table full of dessert options at a buffet, chances are good that something on that table will tempt you.

If you find yourself at a buffet restaurant, survey the entire buffet before you pick up a plate so you know all your options. Then take small portions of a few of the dishes and sit down to enjoy them. Skip "filler" foods that you can get anywhere, like bread and rolls. Use the buffet to try new things and enjoy foods you don't normally eat. Before going up for a second plate, wait five to ten minutes for the food to settle and then determine how hungry you still are for another helping. The key to walking (rather than rolling) out of a buffet is to eat slowly and limit your portions, convincing yourself that you don't have to get your money's worth.

If you absolutely must have an appetizer, make it your meal. As long as you steer clear of the fried options, you can find some delicious and nutritious offerings that are plenty big enough to count as your meal. Another alternative is to have soup or salad as your premeal snack. Both can be excellent ways to get your quota of vegetables. Choose broth- or bean-based soups (rather than the cream-based varieties) because they start to fill you up without adding too many calories. If you go the salad route, get your salad dressing on the side and choose a low-calorie option if possible.

## Handling oversized portions

Although some restaurants serve reasonable amounts of food, many tempt their customers with oversized portions. Just how oversized are those portions? Studies have found that the jumbo-sized portions offered by some restaurants are consistently 250 percent larger than the regular portion. The effect on customers is that when the portions offered are bigger, people tend to eat more. Consider the bagel. A restaurant bagel in the 1980s was 3 inches in diameter and provided about 140 calories. Today's restaurant bagels are 6 inches in diameter and weigh in at about 350 calories each!

Just because you're entitled to consume more calories during much of your pregnancy (you are growing another human being, after all) doesn't mean you should clean your plate every time you dine out. If you do, you may well consume excess calories from fat and sugar that neither you nor your baby need. Rely on your fullness cues to tell you when to stop eating (follow the hunger gauge in Chapter 7). Aim to get 2 ounces of grain, 3 to 4 ounces of lean protein, and 1 cup (or more) of combined fruits and vegetables at each meal (visit www. choosemyplate.gov for an in-depth look at recommended portion sizes).

Figure 8-1 illustrates the discrepancy between the common portion size served at a Mexican restaurant and the amount of food you should actually eat. Plate A shows a typical meal with quite a few tortilla chips, a large burrito, a big scoop of rice and beans, and a small amount of lettuce and tomatoes. Plate B depicts a more ideal scenario with a smaller burrito and more vegetables (lettuce, tomatoes, guacamole, and beans). Because you get enough grains from the burrito, you don't need the chips and rice.

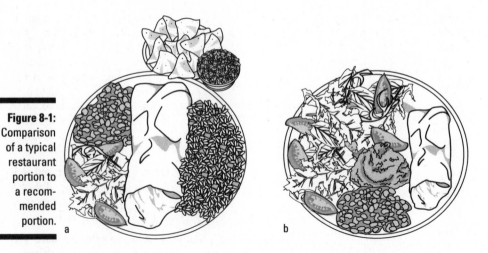

**Figure 8-1:**
Comparison
of a typical
restaurant
portion to
a recom-
mended
portion.

a                                              b

To help you eat healthier, more appropriate portions in restaurants, give these tips a try:

✔ Ask your server for a box right when you get your meal. Put half of your meal into the box so you're not tempted to keep picking at it after you're full.

✔ Forget the "clean your plate club" and focus on how much food you can save for another meal while still feeling satisfied after the first meal.

✔ Order the smallest size possible. Order your meal from the kid's menu if your server will let you and the menu offers something other than chicken nuggets and fries.

- Split meals with a friend or your partner.

- Eat slowly so your brain can register the food you're eating and so you can push your plate away before you're overfull. (I help you distinguish your body's hunger cues in Chapter 7.)

- Order an appetizer as your main course, as long as it's a smaller portion and a nutritious choice.

- Choose tapas-style restaurants that serve smaller portions. Go with a few friends so you can order several things and share. Don't get carried away with ordering more than one plate per person, though!

- Ask your server if you can order the lunch portion at dinnertime.

# Travel tips

When you travel, you likely eat out a lot. But even though I enjoy eating out as much as the next person, after a few days I'm always ready to get back home to my normal routine of eating and exercising. In an attempt to stay healthy on the road, follow these tips:

- **Plan ahead.** If you're flying, find out whether you'll get a meal on the plane. If you're driving, check out what kinds of restaurants are available along your journey.

- **Bring water with you.** Take a reusable water bottle with you so you always have water to stay hydrated.

- **Move frequently.** Whether you're traveling by plane, train, or automobile, take frequent breaks to stretch your legs and move around to help with blood circulation. If you drink lots of water, you'll probably need to go to the bathroom a lot, which will force you to get up and move around.

- **Pack food.** I always, always, always have food with me. When I was 22 weeks pregnant, I was stuck on the tarmac in a plane for 11 hours and the flight attendants couldn't serve us food or water. Fortunately, I had my water bottle and snack bars with me; otherwise, I would've been one unhappy and extremely hungry pregnant lady! You never know when you'll be delayed or when food won't be as available as you'd planned. Be prepared with nutrition bars, nuts, and fresh fruit (for more go-to pregnancy snacks, see Chapter 7).

- **Eat when you're hungry and don't wait until a designated time on the clock.** If you're traveling across time zones, don't try to fit your meals into the new schedule.

- **If you're traveling abroad, be sure you know the safety precautions of drinking the water and eating the unusual food in that culture.** Don't worry about offending anyone; the health of you and your baby is more important! If the water isn't safe, don't forget to use bottled water to brush your teeth and rinse your toothbrush. Pack several toothbrushes with you just in case you forget!

## *Being smart about beverages*

Take a minute to think about your beverage choice before the server comes around to take your drink order. As you peruse the drink menu, keep in mind that hydration is of utmost importance during pregnancy because of your increased fluid needs (to support your added blood volume). Also, be aware that most beverages have calories that you need to take into account.

Water is always the best beverage choice. It offers plenty of fluid with zero calories. If you get tired of plain water, try adding a simple slice of lemon or cucumber to help it go down a bit easier.

Seltzer, or sparkling, water is also a good option as long as it doesn't contain any added sugar. After all, even with a bit of carbonation, it's still water.

Following are some other beverages you're welcome to enjoy during pregnancy as long as you do so in moderation:

- ✔ **Soft drinks:** A 12-ounce can of regular soda has about 150 calories, but good luck finding one that size in a restaurant. These days, many restaurants serve soda in 20-ounce glasses, which contain about 250 calories each. If you choose to drink the whole thing, cut back on your portion of grains at that meal (less potatoes or bread) and definitely skip dessert to try to keep your calories under control. Also beware of how much caffeine is in your soft drink of choice (see Chapter 2 for details).

  Calorically speaking, diet soda is a much better option because it has zero calories, but you need to consume diet soda in moderation during your pregnancy (think no more than a few a week) because of the artificial sweeteners it contains. Turn to Chapter 9 for the lowdown on sweeteners.

- ✔ **Unsweetened tea or lemon water:** Healthy-sounding drinks like lemonade and sweet tea are no better for you than regular soft drinks in terms of calories. The problem with these sugary beverages is that they're just that — sugar! They don't contain any nutrients, so they just add empty calories to your overall daily intake. Bottom line: Choose unsweetened tea or lemon water instead.

- ✔ **Coffee:** Neither regular nor decaf coffee has any calories when you pour it from the coffee maker to your cup, but after the barista at your favorite coffee shop works her magic, you could walk away with a 500-calorie drink! If you have to have your flavored coffee drink, choose nonfat milk and one pump of syrup (or sugar-free syrup) and leave off the whipped cream. Just remember to limit your caffeine intake to 200 mg per day; you may want to order a mix of regular and decaf or just go decaf all the way (flip to Chapter 2 for caffeine amounts in coffee and espresso).

✔ **Milkshakes and smoothies:** These drinks do have some nutritional value thanks to the milk or fruit they contain, but you need to be aware of how big the portions are. Stick to the smallest size offered, preferably about 12 ounces (or less).

Smoothies can be an excellent choice for a snack or even a small meal when you're pregnant. Just be sure to seek out smoothie shops that use real fresh or frozen fruit and not just sugary syrup.

Of course, alcohol is completely off-limits during pregnancy (see Chapter 4 for the reasons why). Order a seltzer water with a twist of lime or a virgin mixed drink if you want to feel like part of the crowd.

## Saving room for dessert

You can be completely satisfied and done with a meal, not even thinking of eating any more food, and then someone mentions or brings out dessert and somehow you make room for it.

As a sweet lover myself, I'd be a hypocrite if I told you not to eat any sugar or dessert during your pregnancy. So instead of eliminating dessert entirely, I encourage you to eat it on occasion; just do your best to keep the portion in check.

Aside from simply ordering mini desserts (one of the best introductions in the dessert world in recent years!), try these tricks to help you have dessert without overindulging:

✔ **Budget for dessert.** If you know you're going to get dessert, eat less at the meal to save calories (and room in your stomach) for dessert. In other words, skip the bread basket and box a big portion of your meal.

✔ **Savor every bite.** Eat every bite of dessert as slowly as possible. If no one else is looking, close your eyes and really pay attention to the flavors and textures of that decadent treat so you can fully enjoy it and, therefore, be satisfied with a smaller amount and avoid overindulging.

✔ **Split up the dessert.** Often you need just a few bites of yummy dessert to satisfy your sweet tooth. Order one dessert for the table and enjoy a few forkfuls.

✔ **Choose lowfat or fruit dessert options — sometimes.** For example, you may find that fresh fruit with a dollop of whipped cream satisfies your sweet craving. Then again, you may find that occasionally a lowfat or reduced-sugar dessert just doesn't cut it. (Personally, I know I'd rather have one piece of high-quality chocolate than half a box of lowfat cookies.)

When a dessert is particularly decadent, you can get away with eating it in a small amount. If you try to eat something that misses the mark, you'll keep searching until your sweet tooth is satisfied. So why not satisfy it the first time?

# Keeping Food Safety in Mind at Your Favorite Restaurant

Unlike when you're in your own kitchen, when you're at a restaurant, the servers and cooks are the ones responsible for following proper cleanliness and food storage guidelines. Consequently, you have to trust that they're doing their job.

You can certainly choose not to visit a dining establishment whose public areas look dirty (because if these areas are dirty, chances are the kitchen is even worse). You can also check up on your favorite restaurants by looking up the health reports conducted by the local health department. Simply visit the department's website and search for the health reports applicable to your particular area.

The following sections outline some additional ways you can gain more control over food safety matters after choosing where you want to eat.

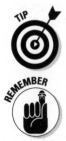

The best time of the day to eat at any restaurant is when it's busy. Food is freshest when it's made right then and there. During slow periods, food has a tendency to sit for too long.

Wherever you decide to eat, be sure to wash your hands before touching your food or drink. This is especially true if you're going to touch any food that will go into your mouth — bread, crackers, pickles, chips, and more. Even a straw that you unwrap and drop into your drink touches your hands before you use it, and you certainly don't want any dirt from your hands swimming around in your drink! At the very least, use an alcohol-based sanitizer to disinfect your hands prior to digging in.

## Send back food that isn't right

When you're at your restaurant of choice, make sure you emphasize to your server how important it is for you to get safe food. Be clear about how well-done you want your eggs or steak. If your meal arrives lukewarm or undercooked, don't be bashful; send it back and don't accept it until it's cooked right. If your dish arrives with something you know you're not supposed to eat (like sprouts or soft cheese) even though you asked that it be omitted, send the whole dish back and have them remake it. (I fill you in on these and other unsafe foods in Chapter 4.) Don't worry what others think about your high-maintenance attitude; remember that you're just doing what's best for you and your baby. Besides, who's going to argue with a pregnant woman?

Trust your instincts. If something doesn't taste quite right and you think it may have gone bad, send it back and order something completely different. Sometimes food has turned bad but no one besides a pregnant woman with heightened senses can detect it. Tell your server that you're pretty sure the food is spoiled so the chefs can take care of it before making other customers sick.

## Reheat takeout and delivery food before you eat it

When you order takeout, try to get to the restaurant a little earlier than when it's supposed to be ready. The worst thing from a food safety perspective is prepared food that sits at room temperature for too long, waiting for you to pick it up. By the time you finally get it home and dig in, it may have been in the temperature danger zone (between 40 and 140 degrees) for an hour or more. Although, technically speaking, food should be safe as long as it's not in the danger zone for two hours or more, you may still want to reheat it before eating. (You can never be too safe, right?)

You run into the same problem with delivery. The delivery driver may have had three or four stops before yours, and your food may have been sitting at room temperature for most of the trip. When you open up your food containers, check to see how hot the food is. The good news is that you can always microwave it to make it steaming hot (and safe to eat) again.

## Keep your leftovers safe

You're enjoying a date night that includes dinner and a movie. You don't finish your dinner and get it boxed up. Those leftovers will be okay for the two-hour movie as long as you refrigerate them when you get home, right? Nope!

The food safety countdown clock starts when the food leaves the kitchen, not when you leave the restaurant with the leftovers.

Beginning as soon as the food is prepared, the maximum amount of time it should be at room temperature is two hours. If it's been sitting out for longer than two hours, throw it out!

If room temperature means more than 70 degrees because it's a hot day, your two-hour window shrinks to one hour. This hour includes the car ride home and any stops you make along the way.

When reheating leftovers (that you've stored safely, of course), bring them to steaming hot (about 165 degrees) by doing one of the following:

- ✔ **Zapping them in the microwave:** First, transfer your leftovers to a microwave-safe container. (I assure you, the takeout container your leftovers came in is *not* safe to zap in the microwave.) Then use a microwave-safe lid to keep moisture in.

- ✔ **Warming them in the oven:** Set the oven to at least 325 degrees to allow the food to reheat safely. Just make sure you transfer the leftovers to an oven-safe container before you heat them.

# Chapter 9

# This or That: Making Grocery Shopping Decisions

........................................................................

## In This Chapter

▶ Evaluating the pros and cons of eating organic food

▶ Reviewing the various sweeteners and their safety in pregnancy

▶ Identifying which fish to avoid and which fish is best for you and your baby

▶ Choosing safe, healthy convenience foods when you're in a hurry

▶ Creating a grocery list of nutritious and safe foods

........................................................................

The world of nutrition can be quite confusing. As you enter the grocery store, you may find yourself asking questions like these: Do I need to eat organic? Are artificial sweeteners safe to use? What about those frozen meals I love to eat for lunch? These questions alone can make grocery shopping a tedious task. But when you're pregnant, the confusion multiplies thanks to a plethora of unsolicited advice from well-intentioned mothers, in-laws, and even complete strangers. They're all trying to tell you what to eat and what not to eat.

The goal of this chapter is to clear up this confusion so you can feel confident that you're stocking your grocery cart with foods that are safe and nutritious for you and your baby. I also share some ideas to make your next trip to the store go a little more smoothly.

## Choosing to Go Organic

Organic foods have popped up in most supermarkets and produce stands. But even though they're readily available to you, you may be tempted to pass them by and continue toward the conventionally grown foods when you see the price of many of the organic options.

Now that you're pregnant, though, should you pay the premium for organic foods? Generally speaking, health professionals don't agree on whether choosing organic while pregnant is necessary. So the choice is ultimately up to you. To help you make your decision, the following sections present some basic information about organic foods, show you how to read an organic food label, and reveal the pros and cons of going organic.

## Organic food basics

*Organic* means something slightly different depending on whether you're talking about produce or animal foods:

- ✔ **Organic produce:** Organic produce farmers must grow their fruits, vegetables, herbs, and grains without using any conventional pesticides or fertilizers that contain synthetic ingredients or sewage sludge. They also can't use bioengineering or ionizing radiation to produce their plants. However, organic farmers can treat their plants with pesticides and fertilizers that are found naturally in the environment and that appear on a list approved by the United States Department of Agriculture (USDA).

- ✔ **Organic animal foods:** Organic meat, poultry, dairy, and eggs have to come from animals that weren't given any growth hormones or antibiotics. To be considered a certified organic farm, an organic farmer has to have a certified inspector from the USDA National Organic Program (NOP) come and inspect the farm to ensure that the standards are being met. In addition, an inspector must certify handlers and processors of organic animal foods.

For both produce and animal products, organic regulations restrict the use of food additives, fortifying agents, and processing aids to a certain approved list of allowed substances. For example, organic farmers and processors can't use artificial sweeteners, certain preservatives, artificial colors, artificial flavors, or monosodium glutamate (MSG).

Organic standards don't address food safety. Just because organic produce doesn't contain pesticides or conventional fertilizer doesn't mean you don't have to wash it. In fact, many organic farms use manure to fertilize, which can increase the risk of *E. coli* contamination. Remember to wash *all* fruits and vegetables before you eat them, whether they're organic or not. Even if something says it's prewashed (like salad greens), I recommend giving it a quick rinse just to be safe.

## What the different types of "organic" labels mean

For a food to have the word *organic* on its label, it needs to meet certain standards. First, all the organic ingredients in the food must come from certified organic farms and processing plants. The specific amount of organic ingredients the food contains (not including water and salt) dictates which organic label claim it can use. Here's a cheat sheet to what the various label claims mean:

✓ **100 percent organic:** The food contains only organic ingredients.

✓ **Organic:** At least 95 percent of the food's ingredients are organic.

✓ **Made with organic ingredients:** At least 70 percent of the food's ingredients are organic.

If you're looking for 95 to 100 percent organic ingredients in your food, look for the USDA Organic symbol (see Figure 9-1); this symbol indicates that the food has passed the USDA's organic certification standards. If you don't see the organic symbol or a claim on the front of the package, check out the food's ingredient list because it's likely that fewer than 95 percent of the ingredients are organic. The manufacturer likely calls out all the organic ingredients by name. For example, if you're looking at a can of soup, the ingredient list may simply list each organic food, like so: organic tomatoes, organic corn, and so on.

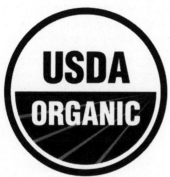

**Figure 9-1:**
The USDA
Organic
symbol.

## Why some pregnant women consider going organic

One major factor that gets many pregnant women considering whether they should go organic is pesticide residue. Pesticides can harm health, especially during fetal development. The USDA has thresholds for pesticide residue on both organic and conventionally grown produce, and no produce can exceed those thresholds and still be sold to consumers.

However, not all foods have the same amount of pesticide residue. The Environmental Working Group (EWG), a nonprofit group dedicated to protecting public health and the environment, regularly evaluates the pesticide residues in commonly consumed produce. Its most current lists are the "Dirty Dozen" (12 fruits and veggies you should always buy organic) and the "Clean 15" (15 fruits and veggies that are safe to buy conventionally grown). The EWG based its clean and dirty designations on the amount of pesticides remaining on the foods after you wash, rinse, and peel them. I've recreated these lists for you in Table 9-1. Note that the foods in the left column go from the ones with the most pesticide residue to the ones with the least; the order is the opposite in the right column.

| Table 9-1 | EWG's Shopper's Guide to Pesticide Residue |
| --- | --- |
| *Dirty Dozen* | *Clean 15* |
| Celery | Onions |
| Peaches | Avocado |
| Strawberries | Sweet corn |
| Apples | Pineapple |
| Blueberries | Mangos |
| Nectarines | Sweet peas |
| Bell peppers | Asparagus |
| Spinach | Kiwi |
| Cherries | Cabbage |
| Kale and collard greens | Eggplant |
| Potatoes | Cantaloupe |
| Grapes (imported) | Watermelon |
| | Grapefruit |
| | Sweet potatoes |
| | Honeydew melon |

*Source:* www.foodnews.org

The EWG estimates that people who eat five servings of fruits and vegetables from the Dirty Dozen list each day ingest an average of ten pesticides. Those who eat from the Clean 15 list ingest two or fewer pesticides daily.

As for the foods that come from animals, pesticide residue is low whether you're talking organic or conventional. In particular, a recent study found no significant difference between the amount of pesticide residue in organic milk and that in regular milk.

Although organic food does have less pesticide residue than conventionally grown food, the extent of the health risk of pesticides to you and your baby in the quantity normally consumed is still unclear. Of course, if there's ever a time to be aware and try to reduce your exposure to pesticides, it's when you're pregnant (and breast-feeding). If you want to do everything you can to reduce your child's exposure to pesticides, go ahead and buy organic produce.

Still wondering whether it makes sense for you to go organic? The good news is that you don't have to make an all-or-nothing choice. You can review the pros and cons I present in the next sections and pick and choose the factors that weigh most heavily on your decision. Ultimately, you may choose to buy certain organic produce items but not organic dairy products. Or you may decide to eat only organic meats but opt for conventionally grown apples and grapes. Make the choice that feels right for you and your baby.

### The pros

Organic foods have some major advantages when it comes to the following:

- **They're better for the environment.** Just because something's organic doesn't necessarily mean it's environmentally friendly, but the production of organic food is based in environmental stewardship and conservation. Studies show organic farming to be better than conventional farming for maintaining or improving soil quality, reducing greenhouse gas emissions, conserving water and energy, reducing water contamination, enhancing biodiversity, and recycling waste.

- **The animals used to make organic meats haven't been treated with antibiotics.** Organic meats may help reduce the development of human antibiotic resistance. It's thought that the widespread use of antibiotics is causing bacteria and other microorganisms to develop new strains that resist those antibiotics, leading to infections that are more difficult to treat and that can be deadly.

- **Animals raised on organic farms are treated better.** Organic farms raise their animals with more concern for the animals' welfare. For example, free-range animals are free to roam, and they tend to have fewer infections compared to caged animals. Grass-fed animals are leaner and healthier overall than their grain-fed counterparts.

  Interestingly enough, some studies have shown that organically raised, grass-fed beef has a higher omega-3 content than the beef from grain-fed cows. (See Chapter 3 for details on omega-3 fatty acids and their role in keeping you and your baby healthy.)

### The con

The drawback of organic food is the cost. Due to the smaller scale of production on many organic farms, prices for organic foods are higher than the prices for conventionally grown foods.

The difference in price varies greatly from food to food. Organic meats can cost twice as much as conventional meats, but some produce or organic packaged food isn't as different in price. If you're buying organic produce in season or at a farmers' market, you can often find it at comparable prices.

# Being Selective with Sweeteners

If you've ever looked at the ingredient list for a box of cookies, can of soda, or even a loaf of bread or jar of peanut butter, you're probably well aware that sugar isn't the only sweetener out there. Many foods and beverages contain *nonnutritive sweeteners,* which sweeten food without contributing significant calories. (Nonnutritive sweeteners are also commonly referred to as *artificial sweeteners,* although not all of them are artificial.) Other foods are made with *nutritive sweeteners,* which do contribute calories.

It's important to note that in order to be in the food supply in the United States, a food ingredient or food additive must go through an approval process with the U.S. Food and Drug Administration (FDA). The agency is responsible for reviewing safety studies to ensure that every food ingredient and food additive is safe to eat. The safety data reviewed must include safety for everyone — children, adults, elderly, and pregnant and lactating women. The FDA uses panels of scientists to rigorously review all data available on that particular food ingredient in an objective and independent fashion.

That being said, you may still have some concerns about whether a particular sweetener is safe to consume during pregnancy. I'm not here to tell you "use this type of sweetener" or "steer clear of all nonnutritive sweeteners." My goal is simply to give you the information you need to make your own decision as to whether to include the following sweeteners in your diet.

Even if you never pick up a blue or pink packet of sweetener, you may be consuming nonnutritive sweeteners without realizing it, depending on the foods and beverages you're eating and drinking. If you prefer to avoid everything artificial (including artificial colors and flavors) throughout your pregnancy, you need to diligently read ingredient lists on food labels.

## Acesulfame K

*Acesulfame K* (brand name Sunett and commonly called Ace-K) is a nonnutritive sweetener that's used quite frequently in food products, often in combination with other nonnutritive sweeteners. You can find acesulfame K listed among the ingredients of more than 4,000 foods, including soft drinks, ice cream, chewing gum, baked goods, breakfast cereals, and canned fruits. Although you may also find packets of acesulfame K, it's not as popular as the other nonnutritive sweeteners in packet form.

The FDA has found acesulfame K to be safe for use in pregnancy in moderation. What's moderation? The acceptable daily intake (ADI) is set at an equivalent of 2 gallons of an acesulfame-K containing beverage every day.

# Agave nectar

*Agave nectar* is a natural, nutritive sweetener that comes from the tequila plant. You find agave as a sweetener option in natural food stores and in some coffee and tea houses.

Just because something is natural doesn't mean it's safe. In terms of pregnancy safety, agave is surrounded by controversy. For instance, some people link it to cramping or increased risk of miscarriage. Agave contains a large number of saponins, which are naturally occurring substances that can cause uterine contractions. For this reason, I recommend avoiding agave while pregnant. After all, it's better to be safe than sorry.

# Aspartame

*Aspartame* (brand names Equal and Nutrasweet) is one of the most widely known nonnutritive sweeteners. You find it in the blue tabletop sweetener packets, as well as in a wide variety of soft drinks, chewing gum, yogurt, and many reduced-sugar items. The FDA has approved the use of aspartame for pregnant women, but many experts still recommend using caution with how much you consume. In fact, the ADI for aspartame is set at 97 packets or 20 cans of diet soda each day. As long as you're not downing can after can of diet soda, you'll be fine adding a couple of blue packets to your foods or beverages and eating a few aspartame-containing foods per day.

Aspartame breaks down to phenylalanine, so if you have phenylketonuria (PKU), steer clear of this sweetener.

# High-fructose corn syrup

*High-fructose corn syrup* (HFCS) is an inexpensive nutritive sweetener that many manufacturers use to sweeten their foods. In recent years, HFCS has drawn a lot of blame for the ever-increasing number of diabetes and obesity cases in the United States. However, scientific studies don't support this theory. HFCS isn't the poison that many people lead you to believe it is; however, it does contain calories without nutritional value.

HFCS is simply syrup made from cornstarch mixed with fructose, another type of sugar found naturally in fruit. HFCS is actually very similar in composition to table sugar. You can find HFCS in a wide variety of products, including soft drinks, yogurts, candy, cookies, crackers, and condiments. Studies have determined that HFCS is safe to consume when you're pregnant, but remember that it does have calories. (To be exact, it has 16 calories per teaspoon — the same as table sugar.)

# Honey

*Honey* is a nutritive sweetener that's naturally created by bees. It contains trace amounts of minerals, as well as dormant *Clostridium botulinum* bacteria, which can cause a severe paralytic illness known as botulism. The honey you find on store shelves has been pasteurized to eliminate the toxins created by the bacteria, but you may find raw honey at farmers' markets.

Avoid eating raw, unpasteurized honey while pregnant. And don't feed children under age 1 any type of honey because they don't have mature enough immune systems to break down and destroy the bacteria.

If you want to eat pasteurized honey while pregnant, remember that it does contain calories (21 per teaspoon), so be careful how much you use as you sweeten your tea in order to control extra calories.

# Saccharin

The pink sweetener packets you see on many restaurant tables contain another well-known nonnutritive sweetener called *saccharin* (brand name Sweet'N Low). Saccharin isn't used in as many food products as other nonnutritive sweeteners, which is nice because the safety of saccharin during pregnancy is questionable. To date, no studies absolutely prove that saccharin is harmful in pregnant humans, but some animal studies have shown increased cancer risk in offspring when mothers consume the sweetener during gestation.

For many years, saccharin was on the National Institute of Health's list of possible cancer-causing agents because of some older studies. However, more recent studies haven't confirmed the cancer findings, so the Institute removed saccharin from the list in the 1990s. Even so, because saccharin crosses the placenta and may remain in fetal tissue, many health professionals recommend that you don't use it during pregnancy.

# Sucralose

*Sucralose* is one of the newer nonnutritive sweeteners out there, and it goes by the brand name Splenda. You find it in the yellow tabletop sweetener packets as well as in soft drinks, yogurts, ice creams, and other reduced-sugar items. The FDA has approved the use of sucralose in pregnancy, but as with aspartame, you should use moderation with the amount you consume. The ADI for sucralose is equivalent to about 28 packets of sucralose each day, so definitely stick with less than that amount.

Even though sucralose claims to be "made from sugar," it has been chemically altered to not be absorbed by the body, so it belongs in the classification of artificial sweeteners.

## Stevia

*Stevia* (brand names Truvia and PureVia) is the new kid on the block when it comes to nonnutritive sweeteners. You find it in the green tabletop packets as well as in many foods, including yogurts, soft drinks, juices, and ice cream. Stevia is a natural sweetener that comes from the stevia plant. This plant contains several sweet components, one of which is called rebiana. On food labels, you may see rebiana (rather than stevia) in the ingredient list. The ADI for rebiana is 29 packets or 64 ounces of rebiana-sweetened beverage every day.

# Hitting the Seafood Counter

Fish should definitely be on your weekly shopping list. After all, eating fish and seafood is especially good for your health during pregnancy (and while nursing). Fish contains protein and iron, two nutrients you need while pregnant (see Chapter 3 for why these nutrients are so important). Plus, eating fish has been linked to reduced risk of cardiovascular disease and reduced risk of dying from any cause in adults. The benefits you get from eating fish come mainly from the omega-3 fatty acids that are so prevalent in many fish and seafood. These same omega-3s, especially DHA and EPA, are part of the building blocks of the brain, which is why pregnant women and young children should get plenty of DHA and EPA. (Find out more about omega-3 fatty acids in Chapter 3.)

All these benefits sound great, but what about the bad things you've heard about fish, like mercury, polychlorinated biphenyls (PCBs), and dioxin (see the next section for more on these contaminants)? Although these contaminants are important to be aware of, many experts believe that the benefits of eating fish outweigh the potential risks. Just to be safe, though, the Environmental Protection Agency (EPA) and the FDA have come up with a recommendation that pregnant women eat no more than 12 ounces of seafood per week.

You can minimize any potential seafood-related risks even more by choosing the right kinds of fish to include in your max of 12 weekly ounces. I outline the fish to watch out for, as well as the safest fish to eat, in the following sections.

## Knowing which fish to be cautious of

The main concern with fish is mercury. Mercury occurs naturally in the environment and is present in trace amounts in almost all fish, but most of the mercury comes from industrial pollution that gets into the water. Bacteria in polluted water change the mercury into a form called *methylmercury,* which can be toxic. Fish consume the methylmercury by eating the organisms that live in and absorb the water.

Methylmercury passes from your blood to your baby and can have a negative effect on his developing nervous system. Fish that are highest in methylmercury are the larger, predatory fish because they spend their days eating smaller fish, who've eaten even smaller fish, who've eaten teeny-tiny fish, who've eaten the organisms that absorbed methylmercury. Avoid the following high-mercury fish while pregnant and nursing and don't feed them to small children:

- ✔ King mackerel
- ✔ Shark
- ✔ Swordfish
- ✔ Tilefish (also known as golden bass)

Although fish that contain moderate amounts of mercury are safe for most people to consume, I recommend that you avoid the following moderate-mercury fish while pregnant and nursing:

- ✔ Ahi tuna
- ✔ Chilean sea bass
- ✔ Grouper
- ✔ Mahi mahi
- ✔ Marlin
- ✔ Orange roughy
- ✔ Spanish mackerel

Aim to eat the lower-mercury fish that I list in the next section rather than their moderate- or high-mercury counterparts.

If you're worried about eating fish because of *PCBs* and *dioxins* (chemical contaminants found in the environment), keep in mind that the levels found in fish are similar to those found in beef, chicken, and pork. In fact, only 9 percent of the PCBs and dioxins in the U.S. food supply come from fish and seafood; the other 90 percent come from other foods. If you eat fish caught in local waters, check the local fish advisories to see whether they've issued any warnings about contaminated waters.

## Discovering which fish are best

The EPA and FDA recommend that pregnant or nursing women choose fish and seafood that are low in mercury to get the recommended limit of 12 ounces per week. Choose from these low-mercury options:

- ✔ Catfish

- ✔ Cod

- ✔ Light tuna (*not* albacore, or "white," tuna, which is only safe to consume in 6-ounce amounts per week as part of your overall fish allowance)

- ✔ Pollock

- ✔ Salmon (*not* smoked salmon or fresh salmon jerky, which may contain harmful bacteria)

- ✔ Shrimp, crab, clams, and scallops

- ✔ Tilapia

Not sure what 12 ounces of fish look like? A 3-ounce portion is the standard recommended portion size. For 12 ounces, you could have four servings of one of the following 3-ounce portions: six large shrimp, six large scallops, a tuna salad sandwich, or a 3-ounce fillet that fits in the palm of your hand.

# Going the Convenient Route with Convenience Foods

Convenience foods, such as packaged foods, frozen meals, and grab-and-go foods, can be great to have on hand when you're short on time or when you're feeling pregnancy fatigue set in. They sometimes cost you more financially, but if you follow the tips I present in the next sections, they don't have to cost you or your growing baby in the nutrition and food safety arenas.

## Selecting nutritious frozen meals

With the plethora of frozen meals available, you can eat a different frozen meal every day for months and never eat the same meal twice! Many of these frozen meals contain a convenient mix of protein, complex carbs, and vegetables all in one container, but some of them also contain a handful of not-so-good-for-you ingredients, like loads of saturated fat, sodium, or calories. When you're trying to make decisions in the freezer aisle, follow the guidelines I present in Table 9-2 to help you sift through all the choices.

### Table 9-2 Guidelines for Choosing the Most Nutritious Frozen Foods

| Nutrient | Amount to Look for |
|---|---|
| Calories | Up to 500 calories |
| Fat | 5–15 grams |
| Saturated fat | Less than 3 grams |
| Sodium | Less than 800 milligrams |
| Fiber | 3 or more grams |
| Protein | 10–20 grams |
| Vitamins and minerals | 10 percent or more of Daily Value (DV) for many vitamins and minerals listed |

You may want to look for the more nutritious frozen food brands that focus not only on the number of calories but also on the quality of the food and the nutritional value of the meal as a whole. Some of my favorites are Healthy Choice, Amy's (vegetarian line), Kashi, Lean Cuisine, and Smart Ones.

If the meal isn't filling enough, pair it with a piece of fruit or some cut-up veggies. Sometimes frozen meals, particularly the vegetarian varieties, don't have enough protein. Drink a glass of milk or have a yogurt with these meals to boost the protein content of your overall meal.

Whenever I start recommending frozen meals to clients, the question of sodium always comes up. Yes, frozen meals do contain sodium, but so do most other foods. Not buying it? Think about what you'd be eating in place of your frozen meal. Perhaps a grilled chicken sandwich with a side salad? That chicken and the salad dressing on the salad likely have much more sodium in just those two food items than the entire frozen meal.

## Making sure grab-and-go items are safe to eat

In today's world, most supermarkets offer grab-and-go food options for the hungry shopper. The main concern with eating these foods during pregnancy is food safety. Think about that rotisserie chicken that's packaged up and in the warmer at the supermarket. Sure it looks great, but what temperature is it? To be safe, check the temperature of the chicken before eating it. If it's not at the proper temperature (over 165 degrees for whole poultry), heat it in the oven or microwave until it reaches the safe temperature. Foods that sit for hours in the danger zone (between 40 and 140 degrees) harbor bacteria that can make you sick (flip to Chapter 4 for more on harmful bacteria). But as long as you reheat the chicken to the proper temp, it'll be safe to eat.

# Cutting costs at the grocery store

Now that you have a baby on the way, you're likely looking for ways to save money any way you can. Your weekly grocery trip is no exception! Here are some tips for cutting costs at the grocery store. Although they may require a little more planning on your part, the money they help you save will be well worth it.

✔ **Buy in bulk.** If you know you consume a lot of one particular item, consider buying it in bulk. The price per unit is lower, and the savings are huge. Afraid you can't eat all the food before it expires? You can always freeze the excess for a later date. (Chapter 10 tells you how long you can store food in the freezer before you need to toss it.)

✔ **Study up and then stock up.** Almost every grocery store publishes a weekly or monthly circular or ad that lists all the special sale items. Scan your local ads to see whether any items you regularly buy are on sale and then purchase as many as you can. Stock up on nonperishable buy-one-get-one-free (BOGO) sale items.

✔ **Rethink the name brands.** When buying a specific item, check to see whether your grocery store offers that item in its own brand. You can often find the same products (that are just as nutritious) for much less if you're willing to think outside the brand name.

✔ **Some assembly required.** While precut, pre-packaged foods are convenient, they're not always as cost-effective as the individual ingredients. As an added bonus, buying the individual ingredients and creating your own meals allow you to avoid all the preservatives that are in most already-prepared meals.

✔ **Do some clipping.** Coupons are a great way to save on groceries. You find these money-saving helpers in your newspaper, on coupon websites, and even on individual company and brand websites.

✔ **Skip the soda.** Not only is water the least expensive drink (it's free from the tap!), but it's also essential to you and your baby's health. Substituting water for soda in your routine keeps you hydrated, saves you from consuming too many empty calories, and leaves you with some extra cash in your pocket.

If you're eyeing a sandwich in the grocery store's deli case, be aware of deli meats that may not be at the proper temperature. While pregnant, you should heat deli meat to steaming hot before eating it. In other words, don't consume cold-cut sandwiches directly out of your grocery's deli case, especially one that's not kept at 40 degrees or colder. To be safe, choose hot foods rather than cold sandwiches during your pregnancy.

As for prepared salads, such as egg salad and tuna salad, these foods are also dangerous when they aren't kept at the proper temperature. Only eat meat and egg salads that you prepare at home, using proper food safety techniques (see Chapter 10 for details).

# Simplifying Your Next Trip to the Store

Grocery shopping is one of those things that people tend to either love or hate. (Case in point: My husband would rather scrub toilets than make a grocery run.) Regardless of where you fall on the love-hate scale of grocery shopping, following these tips can help you make the most of your trip:

- ✔ **Always, always, always shop with a list.** Keep an ongoing grocery list at home and add to it as you run out of things so you don't forget to buy them the next time you shop. Check out the section "Preparing your pregnancy grocery list" for details on what to put on your list. (As an added bonus, shopping with a list helps you avoid making high-calorie impulse buys.)

- ✔ **Create a meal plan.** If you know what you'll be eating for the week, you can easily make your list and stick to it. If you don't plan ahead, you'll probably be one or two ingredients short when you go to make a recipe in the middle of the week. Chapter 11 offers guidance on creating pregnancy-friendly meal plans.

- ✔ **Don't go grocery shopping hungry.** Shopping for food when you're hungry is like waving a dog treat in front of a pit bull. You'll attack the bag of chips before you leave the parking lot to go home!

- ✔ **Read food labels, including use-by and sell-by dates.** Labels contain all kinds of useful info, including the Nutrition Facts panel, ingredient list, and food-safety dates.

- ✔ **Keep raw meats separate from everything else.** Use extra plastic bags to contain the juices so they don't contaminate the rest of your food with potentially harmful bacteria.

- ✔ **Put groceries (especially perishables) in the backseat rather than in the trunk in the summertime.** Putting your groceries in the air-conditioned car keeps them cool until you get home.

- ✔ **Go straight home.** Make the supermarket the last errand on your list. Refrigerate (or freeze) cold foods immediately when you return home to keep things safe.

If you already have at least one child at home, try to grocery shop without your little one(s) if at all possible. Kids can make the grocery experience more stressful than it already is. When my son was almost 2, he grabbed a bottle of olive oil out of the cart and dropped it on the floor. It broke into a million pieces and oil flowed down the aisle. I was pregnant with my second child at the time, so I'd like to blame what happened next on pregnancy hormones. I literally started crying in the aisle of the grocery store because I was mortified and all I could think about was how hard it is to clean up oil. The manager kept reassuring me that it was okay, but I was too upset to finish my shopping and I didn't go back to that location until about a year after the event.

In the following sections, I explain what to look for on food labels so you can quickly decide what (and what not) to buy as you shop, and I offer you a sample grocery list to help make your next trip to the store as painless as possible.

## Deciphering food labels

You'd think the labels on food would help clear up the confusion of what to buy, but often food labels are packed with so much information that you don't know where to start, much less what to look for. The information in the next sections can help you make sense of those often-confusing food labels so you can use them to make your next shopping trip easy as pie.

### The Nutrition Facts panel

The Nutrition Facts panel, like the one shown in Figure 9-2, tells you what's in the food's package, nutritionally speaking. The panel is divided into the following three main parts:

- **Servings:** The first thing the Nutrition Facts panel highlights is what constitutes a serving of the food item and, if the container has more than one serving, how many servings you can expect to find. The panel typically shows the standard serving size for that particular type of food in volume (cups or tablespoons, for example), weight (grams or ounces, for example), or both.

- **Nutrient amounts:** Next, the Nutrition Facts panel tells you the number of calories per serving, which is important to know for weight control. Then it walks you through the per-serving amounts of fat, cholesterol, sodium, carbohydrates, fiber, sugars, and protein found in the food according to the Percent Daily Value (which is based on a 2,000-calorie diet).

- **Vitamin and mineral amounts:** Finally, the Nutrition Facts panel breaks down the per-serving amounts of the vitamins and minerals the food contains, again in terms of Percent Daily Value. Every food's panel must include these four vitamins and minerals: vitamin A, vitamin C, calcium, and iron. But many food producers choose to list more.

During your pregnancy, pay special attention to serving sizes so you know how much you're eating. For example, you need to double the numbers if you eat a double portion. Focus on getting complex carbohydrates (especially fiber), protein, unsaturated fats, and plenty of vitamins and minerals. For the scoop on the amounts of these nutrients you should be consuming per day to get your baby what she needs to grow, see Chapter 3.

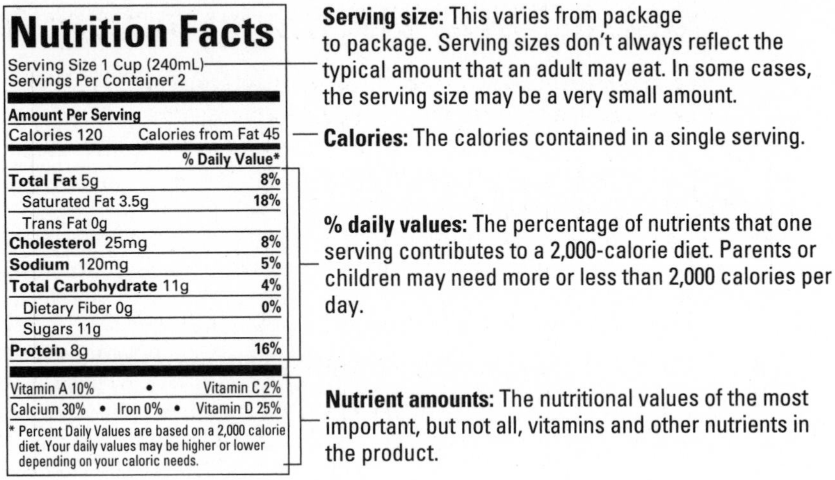

**Nutrition Facts**

Serving Size 1 Cup (240mL)
Servings Per Container 2

**Amount Per Serving**

Calories 120       Calories from Fat 45

| | % Daily Value* |
|---|---|
| **Total Fat** 5g | **8%** |
| Saturated Fat 3.5g | **18%** |
| Trans Fat 0g | |
| **Cholesterol** 25mg | **8%** |
| **Sodium** 120mg | **5%** |
| **Total Carbohydrate** 11g | **4%** |
| Dietary Fiber 0g | **0%** |
| Sugars 11g | |
| **Protein** 8g | **16%** |

| | | | |
|---|---|---|---|
| Vitamin A 10% | • | Vitamin C 2% | |
| Calcium 30% | • Iron 0% • | Vitamin D 25% | |

\* Percent Daily Values are based on a 2,000 calorie diet. Your daily values may be higher or lower depending on your caloric needs.

**Figure 9-2:**
A sample
Nutrition
Facts panel.

**Serving size:** This varies from package to package. Serving sizes don't always reflect the typical amount that an adult may eat. In some cases, the serving size may be a very small amount.

**Calories:** The calories contained in a single serving.

**% daily values:** The percentage of nutrients that one serving contributes to a 2,000-calorie diet. Parents or children may need more or less than 2,000 calories per day.

**Nutrient amounts:** The nutritional values of the most important, but not all, vitamins and other nutrients in the product.

## The ingredient list

Next on the food label is the ingredient list. If you have allergies or are trying to avoid certain ingredients, you must read this list. Food labels list ingredients from highest to lowest based on how much (in terms of weight) of the ingredient is present in the food. If the product contains any of the eight common food allergens (see Chapter 19 for what these are), they're listed in the main ingredient list and then again in **boldface** next to a statement like "this product contains . . . ."

## Dates

While pregnant, you need to pay special attention to dates on foods for your (and your baby's) safety. Here's what the different dates mean:

✔ **Sell-by:** Tells the store when to pull the product off shelves. The food is still safe to eat after this date as long as it's stored properly, but be sure to eat it within a few days.

✔ **Best-if-used-by:** Tells you the date by which the manufacturer recommends you consume the food for best quality. This date isn't for safety, and it's usually used in foods like chips or cereal. It's typically safe to eat food after the best-if-used-by date, but use your judgment and look for signs of spoilage.

✔ **Use-by:** Tells you the last date recommended for use of the product for peak quality. Use this date as a guide for when to throw out food during pregnancy.

# Preparing your pregnancy grocery list

Are you ready to start stocking your shelves with pregnancy-friendly foods? Use the following grocery list as a guide when you're preparing your shopping list or even when you're strolling down the aisles.

## Fruits and vegetables

❑ Staples like salad greens, carrots, potatoes, tomatoes, bananas, apples, oranges, and grapes

❑ Your favorite in-season fruits and vegetables

❑ 100% Concord grape, pomegranate, or orange juice

❑ Frozen broccoli, snap peas, carrots, corn, edamame, berries, or any of your other favorites

❑ Legumes (beans), stewed tomatoes, or other canned veggies of your choice

## Dairy products

❑ Lowfat milk (or milk alternative like soy)

❑ Lowfat Greek yogurt and cottage cheese

❑ Part-skim or reduced-fat cheeses (blocks and shredded)

❑ Individual cheeses for snacking, like string cheese or mini Babybel Laughing Cow cheese

## Grains

❑ Whole-grain cereal with more than 3 grams of fiber per serving

❑ Whole-grain bread, English muffins, bagels, pitas, or tortillas

❑ Quick-cooking oatmeal or instant oatmeal packets

❑ Whole-grain pasta and brown rice

❑ Other whole grains like quinoa and barley

❑ Whole-grain crackers

❑ Air-popped popcorn kernels or lowfat microwavable popcorn

### Proteins

❑ Peanut butter, almond butter, sunflower seed butter, or soy nut butter

❑ Almonds, pistachios, walnuts, pecans, and peanuts

❑ Canned light tuna, salmon, or chicken

❑ Frozen chicken breasts, 90% lean hamburger patties, or shrimp

❑ Fresh meat or seafood of your choice (for meals within the next day or two)

❑ Eggs that are enhanced with DHA

❑ Tofu and other meat alternatives (fresh or frozen)

### Mixed foods

❑ Frozen meals

❑ Reduced-sodium canned soups

### Staples

❑ Olive oil and canola oil

❑ Balsamic vinegar

❑ Ground flaxseed and wheat germ

❑ Herbs and spices

If you're into doing everything digitally, you can create your grocery list online. Check out the website of your favorite grocery store to see whether it has an online list you can customize. (Going to your local grocery store's website first is ideal because you can incorporate the deals of the week.) Alternatively, you can use www.ziplist.com (either the website or the smartphone app) or some other online grocery-list planner.

# Chapter 10

# Presenting Baby-Bump-Friendly Kitchen Basics

•••••••••••••••••••••••••••••••••••••••••••••••••••••

### In This Chapter

▶ Cleaning out and restocking your refrigerator, freezer, and pantry

▶ Making food safety a priority

▶ Discovering the tricks healthy cooks rely on

▶ Cooking comfortably in any trimester

•••••••••••••••••••••••••••••••••••••••••••••••••••••

*J*ust because you're pregnant doesn't mean your kitchen has to change drastically. But it does mean you have to get rid of expired foods and pay more attention to how to work (and eat) safely in the kitchen. After all, food safety is never more important than when you're expecting.

To get the most out of every meal, you also need to know how to turn your favorite high-fat, low-nutrient recipes into healthy, nutrient-rich recipes that are appropriate throughout your pregnancy (and beyond!). And because cooking tends to require you to be on your feet, at least for a little while, you probably want to know how to make that experience more comfortable for you as the weeks go on. I cover all these topics in this chapter.

## Stocking the Kitchen

One key to healthy eating during pregnancy is having the right types of foods on hand. Consequently, stocking your kitchen is a priority (and the sooner you do it, the better). You may find that you don't need to do much to stock your kitchen when you become pregnant. Or you may find that pregnancy is a good time to clean out your entire kitchen and start from scratch. Regardless, the next sections provide you with pointers on getting rid of old foods and stocking up on new, nutritious ones.

If you want to tackle stocking your kitchen during your first trimester but you're feeling too tired or grossed out by the idea of food, ask your partner to handle this project for you. It's a great, albeit indirect, way for him or her to do something baby-related early on.

## Out with the old

Most people don't even think about cleaning out their pantry, refrigerator, or freezer — let alone actually do it. But performing this bit of spring cleaning is especially important during pregnancy. Food safety is of course the main concern, but food quality can also suffer when food sits around for too long.

To make sure your kitchen is full of safe foods, spend an afternoon going through your refrigerator, freezer, and pantry, throwing out old items. The following sections offer guidelines for what to keep and what to toss.

When in doubt, throw it out! The safety of you and your baby is too important to gamble with when it comes to food that may not be safe to eat. If a food smells or looks weird, toss it. Even if a food is moldy only on the surface, it can be contaminated throughout, so don't take any chances.

### The refrigerator

You may be surprised at how little time food is supposed to spend in your refrigerator before you either consume it or toss it. Table 10-1 gives you an idea of how long you can keep certain foods in the fridge before you have to get rid of them.

| Table 10-1 | How Long to Store Food in Your Fridge |
| --- | --- |
| *Food* | *How Long It Can Stay in the Fridge* |
| Beef or pork (chops, steaks, roasts), raw | 3–5 days |
| Butter | 1–3 months |
| Cheeses (hard), opened | 3–4 weeks |
| Cream cheese | 2 weeks |
| Deli meat, opened | 3–5 days |
| Egg, macaroni, tuna, or chicken salad | 3–5 days |
| Eggs, hard boiled | 1 week |
| Eggs, raw in shell | 5 weeks |
| Ground beef, pork, or poultry, raw | 1–2 days |
| Ketchup, opened | 6 months |
| Margarine | 6 months |
| Mayonnaise, opened | 2 months |

| Food | How Long It Can Stay in the Fridge |
|---|---|
| Beef, pork, seafood/fish, or poultry, cooked | 3–4 days |
| Milk, opened | 1 week |
| Poultry and seafood/fish, raw | 1–2 days |
| Salad dressing, opened | 3 months |
| Salsa, opened | 1 month |

### The freezer

As you can see from Table 10-2, nothing should stay in your freezer for more than one year. The longer you keep a food in the freezer, the more you compromise its quality and safety. To help you keep track of exactly how long your food has been in the freezer, label each package with the date you put it into the freezer.

| Table 10-2 | How Long to Store Food in Your Freezer |
|---|---|
| Food | How Long It Can Stay in the Freezer |
| Bread products | 2 months |
| Cheese (hard) | 6 months |
| Fish, fatty (like salmon), raw | 2–3 months |
| Fish/seafood, lean (like cod), raw | 6 months |
| Ground beef, pork or poultry, raw | 3–4 months |
| Ham, cooked | 1–2 months |
| Beef or pork, cooked | 2–3 months |
| Poultry or seafood/fish, cooked | 4 months |
| Poultry, pieces (breast), raw | 9 months |
| Poultry, whole and raw | 12 months |
| Beef or pork (chops, steaks, roasts), raw | 12 months |
| Vegetables or fruit | 10–12 months |

*Freezer burn* (dry spots on your food) doesn't necessarily mean a particular food is unsafe, but it does mean the food probably won't taste good. To prevent freezer burn, wrap food tightly to keep air from getting into it.

### The pantry

Although your refrigerator and freezer contain the most perishable foods, you also need to clean out your pantry because foods such as spices and flour don't last forever. Keep the following guidelines in mind as you survey your pantry:

✔ Low-acid canned foods (such as corn, beans, and peas) can last two to five years.

✔ High-acid canned foods (like tomato products, fruit, and sauerkraut) last only 12 to 18 months.

✔ Dented or bulging cans get thrown away immediately! They could have a small leak, allowing air inside and causing spoilage.

✔ Unopened cereal, chips, and crackers are generally good until the date listed on their package. Keep opened boxes and bags of these foods sealed tightly with a clip in their original containers and eat them within a week for best quality.

✔ Spices can last up to one year when stored away from heat and sunlight.

✔ Baking powder and baking soda may lose their effectiveness after 12 to 18 months.

✔ Flour can last eight months when stored tightly closed (meaning don't leave it in the bag it comes in). If bugs appear, throw it out!

✔ Whole-wheat flour can last six to eight months when kept in the fridge or one year when kept in the freezer. Refrigerating or freezing this type of flour helps prevent the oils from going rancid. Just be sure to bring the flour to room temperature before using it in a recipe.

✔ Oils (olive, canola, and so on) can go rancid easily, so keep them away from sunlight and heat. Store them in a dark pantry rather than on the counter or stove and use them within three months of opening.

✔ Sugar has a long shelf life of two years as long as it's in an airtight container. Use brown sugar within four months to keep it from hardening.

## In with the nutritious

After you rid your refrigerator, freezer, and pantry of any questionable foods, you need to restock them with foods that are guaranteed to nourish you and your baby. Always have on hand a variety of choices from each of the various food groups: grains, fruits, vegetables, dairy, and meat or meat alternatives. Flip to Chapter 3 for guidance on which foods contain the vitamins, minerals, carbs, proteins, and essential fats that you need to keep your energy up and that your baby needs to grow and develop.

If you're wondering whether you should eat as many organically grown and produced foods as possible or whether you should steer clear of sweeteners such as aspartame, turn to Chapter 9. *Note:* That's also where I provide a handy grocery list of pregnancy must-haves that you can reference while shopping.

# Practicing Safety in the Kitchen

To cut down on the risk of acquiring a foodborne illness, you need to take all the steps necessary to protect your safety and the safety of your developing baby. I walk you through the specifics in the next sections, but basically you need to keep your hands and kitchen surfaces clean, avoid cross-contamination of foods, cook foods to the right temperature, and store food properly when you're done with it. (For details on foodborne illnesses and other food-related toxins, turn to Chapter 4.)

## Embracing cleanliness

There's no doubt about it: A clean kitchen is a healthy kitchen. What you may not realize is that having a clean kitchen starts with keeping your hands and kitchen surfaces clean while you work. *Always* wash your hands before preparing food or eating. Also wash them again whenever you handle raw meat or if you take a break from food preparation to use the restroom, tend to a pet, handle garbage, blow your nose — you get the idea.

I'm sure you know that the best way to wash your hands is to use soap and water and lather really well all the way up your wrists, covering all surfaces and folds in your hands and under your fingernails. But did you know you're supposed to rub your hands vigorously for 20 seconds to get them really clean? To make sure you scrub your hands as long as necessary, sing the song "Happy Birthday" twice in your head. From there, simply rinse well and, if possible, dry your hands on a disposable towel and use that towel to turn off the faucet.

Keeping your kitchen clean also means washing every surface that comes in contact with food, including the following:

- ✔ **Cutting boards:** Always wash your cutting board with hot, soapy water after preparing each food and before starting on the next food. If you have an old cutting board that's worn and difficult to get clean, toss it and buy a replacement.

- ✔ **Utensils:** These include knives, spatulas, and so on. Treat them the same way you do cutting boards.

- ✔ **Countertops:** Wipe your countertops down with a soapy cloth or a disinfectant wipe before you prepare food and throughout the food prep process. I recommend using paper towels because you can throw them out; cloth towels can harbor bacteria when you use them over and over again.

✔ **The refrigerator:** Clean your refrigerator often with hot soapy water. Be sure to wipe up spills immediately and always keep the produce drawers cleaned out (because produce is often stored unwrapped). Keep raw meats well-wrapped and wipe up any juice that leaks from them with a disposable disinfectant towel.

Always rinse fruits and vegetables (yes, even when they're organic) before you use them in a recipe or eat them raw. Even if something says *prewashed* on the label, I recommend giving it a quick rinse just to be safe. Use a small vegetable brush to wash foods like potatoes and carrots that have a rough outer skin. Even if you don't plan to eat the skin (like with a cantaloupe or watermelon), you need to rinse the fruit well because the outside germs will get into the fruit when you cut it open if you don't wash it first. (Speaking of cutting, be sure to cut away any bruised areas of fruit because bacteria can thrive there.)

Cross-contamination can happen easily when you're preparing raw meats and raw vegetables at the same time. Dedicate one cutting board to meats and another to produce. If you have only one cutting board, cut up the fruits and veggies first, wash the board and knife well, and then prepare the meat. And always use a clean plate to put cooked food on; in other words, don't reuse a plate that was previously occupied by raw meat.

## Cooking foods to the appropriate temperatures

Having the cleanest kitchen in the world doesn't do you much good if you don't cook foods, specifically meats, to a high-enough temperature to kill the pesky bacteria that can cause foodborne illnesses. Table 10-3 reveals the minimum safe temperatures for various types of meat; commit this list to memory or bookmark this page so you can easily refer to the proper temperatures when necessary.

---

### Soap and water alternatives

You can use a hand sanitizer when soap and water isn't available. Just make sure you choose one that contains at least 60 percent alcohol. Apply enough of it to wet your hands completely and then rub your hands together until they're dry, about 30 seconds.

*Note:* Antimicrobial wipes are also okay to use in a pinch, but they're not as effective as proper hand washing or as strong at killing bacteria as hand sanitizers.

| Table 10-3 | Minimum Meat Temperatures |
|---|---|
| *Meat* | *Minimum Temperature* |
| Precooked ham | 140 degrees |
| Fish | 145 degrees |
| Pork roasts and chops* | 145 degrees |
| Beef steak or roasts* | 145 degrees |
| Casseroles containing meat or eggs | 160 degrees |
| Ground beef, lamb, and pork | 160 degrees |
| Ground poultry | 165 degrees |
| Chicken breasts | 165 degrees |
| Whole poultry | 165 degrees |
| Leftovers containing meat or eggs | 165 degrees |

*The U.S. Department of Agriculture (USDA) recommends a three-minute "rest time" for these meats. In other words, allow the meat to sit (or rest) for three minutes before you carve or consume it.

The only true way to know whether your meat is at its proper temperature is to use a meat thermometer. As shown in Figure 10-1, insert the thermometer into the thickest part of the meat, being careful not to touch the bone if there is one, and leave it there until the temperature settles.

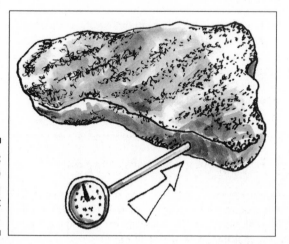

**Figure 10-1:**
How to insert a meat thermometer.

Using a meat thermometer on fish and seafood isn't always possible or practical because fish is flaky and sometimes doesn't hold the thermometer. Cook fish until it's milky white in color and flakes easily with a fork. Cook shrimp, lobster, and scallops until they're milky white in color and firm in texture. If you're cooking fresh clams, mussels, or oysters, you can trust that they're done when their shells open; if the shells don't open, throw them away.

When you're working with eggs, always cook them until the yolk and the white are firm. Don't use a recipe that calls for an egg to remain raw or only partially cooked. Also, look for eggs that have been pasteurized (they should have *pasteurized* on the label). You can find them raw in the shell as well as in liquid egg products in the refrigerator or freezer section of your local grocery store.

Having leftovers? Reheat them until they're steaming hot (about 165 degrees). If you're reheating meats, use a meat thermometer to check their temperature to make sure they're safe to eat (refer to Table 10-3). If you have leftover sauces, gravies, or marinades, bring them to a full, rolling boil before reusing them.

When you're defrosting food, whether it's leftovers or frozen chicken breast you're planning to use in tonight's dinner, you still need to pay attention to the food's temperature. Never defrost food on the counter at room temperature. Instead, use any of the following defrosting methods:

- **In the microwave:** Use the defrost setting and follow the instructions on your machine.

- **In cold water:** Change the water every 20 to 30 minutes to keep it cold. Defrosting meat in cold water takes about an hour per pound. Remember to make sure the meat is in a leak-proof package or bag. *Warning:* Never defrost in hot water because it encourages more bacteria growth.

- **In the refrigerator:** This method takes the longest amount of time, so plan ahead if you're going to use it. Remember that the larger the food item, the longer it takes to defrost. Thinner cuts of meat may defrost in one day, but some Thanksgiving turkeys take as many as three days to defrost (about 24 hours for every 5 pounds of bird)!

Always cook food as soon as possible after it defrosts. Freezing halts the growth of bacteria, but it doesn't kill it. Bacteria starts to grow again as soon as something is thawed. So after you thaw a particular food, treat it as if it's raw again and follow the guidelines listed in Table 10-1 for the maximum amount of time you can keep it in the refrigerator prior to cooking. If you've thawed your meat in the microwave, cook it right away because some areas may have started getting warm during defrosting.

## Storing your food properly

The final key to food safety is storing food at the proper temperature. That means keeping food chilled to prevent bacteria from growing and multiplying. Cold temperatures below the danger zone (that is, below 40 degrees) help keep food from spoiling because of high bacteria growth. So make sure you set your refrigerator at 40 degrees (or colder) and your freezer at 0 degrees.

You shouldn't let perishable foods sit out at room temperature for longer than two hours. If you're at a party and don't know how long a particular perishable food has been sitting out, avoid it or ask the host to get you some fresh food from the refrigerator. If you're the one doing the hosting, make sure never to replenish a dish of perishable food using the same container that has been sitting out. Instead, have two dishes prepared, swap out the entire old dish, and discard it. *Note:* If you're hosting an event outside in the heat, toss anything that has been sitting for more than one hour.

Always refrigerate food within two hours of preparing or eating it. In other words, don't listen to the advice you may have heard that says you need to give hot foods time to cool down on the counter before you put them in the refrigerator. This advice is actually a food safety nightmare! You don't want the food to reach the danger zone of between 40 and 140 degrees and stay there for a long time (the food will be in the zone briefly as it goes from hot to cold). Besides, your fridge will compensate and cool off the food as soon as it can. You just have to make sure you haven't packed the fridge so tightly that air can't circulate, because air circulation is what keeps the refrigerator cool in the first place.

To avoid putting large portions of hot foods in the fridge, simply transfer the food to several containers and get them in the fridge as soon as possible.

# Cooking the Healthy Way

By cooking the healthy way, you can ensure that the food you eat retains the most nutrients with a minimal amount of added fat, sugar, and salt. Cooking healthy requires you to look at two main aspects:

- ✓ **What you're cooking with:** The ingredients used
- ✓ **How you're cooking:** The method of cooking

When the called-for ingredients in a recipe don't strike you as the healthiest or when a recipe says to fry foods, be prepared either to make some ingredient substitutions or other modifications or to try a different cooking technique. I walk you through how to do both in the following sections.

## Modifying recipes to make them healthier

You may have a few favorite recipes that you know aren't the healthiest but that you love anyway. Well, guess what? Chances are you can easily make your favorites a bit healthier without sacrificing taste simply by swapping out (or reducing the amount of) the not-so-good-for-you ingredients. Take a look at some of your tried-and-true recipes and see whether you can swap an ingredient or two for something else to save some calories or to boost nutritional content.

If you're not sure where to start, take a look at Table 10-4 for some ingredient substitutions you can make to improve the overall nutritional quality of your recipes.

| Table 10-4 | Easy Ingredient Substitutions |
|---|---|
| *Original Ingredient* | *Substitute with* |
| Bacon | Turkey bacon, Canadian bacon, or imitation bacon bits |
| Breadcrumbs | Crushed bran cereal |
| Butter, margarine, oil, or shortening in baked goods | Half butter, margarine, oil, or shortening and half applesauce, prune puree, or mashed bananas |
| Butter or oil in pans to prevent sticking | Nonstick cooking spray |
| Cream | Fat-free half-and-half or evaporated skim milk |
| Cream soups | Reduced-fat, reduced-sodium soups, pureed silken tofu, or pureed vegetables (such as cauliflower, carrots, or potato flakes) |
| Ground beef | Lean (90% or greater) ground beef, ground turkey breast, or soy crumbles |
| High-fat dairy products (like sour cream, cream cheese, cheese, and milk) or full-fat mayonnaise | Light, reduced-fat, or fat-free dairy products or mayonnaise |
| Full-fat salad dressing | Flavored vinegars, lemon juice, or light, reduced-fat, or fat-free salad dressings |

| Original Ingredient | Substitute with |
|---|---|
| Seasoned salt | Salt-free herb mixes or fresh herbs |
| White bread, white rice, or white pasta | Whole-grain bread, rice, or pasta |
| White flour | Half white flour and half whole-wheat flour |

In addition to substituting ingredients, you can make other minor modifications to a recipe to beef up its rank on the nutrition scale. Here are just a few ideas to get you started:

- Use half of the amount of cheese a recipe calls for.

- Use half or three-fourths of the amount of sugar called for in a recipe and use more extract or spices to make up for the missing sugar. (Honestly, most recipes call for more sugar than you actually need.)

- Use half of the amount of salt called for if the recipe doesn't have yeast. (If the recipe has yeast, you can't reduce the amount of salt because it relies on the salt for leavening.)

- Add more herbs, spices, vinegar, or lemon juice to boost flavor, especially when you're cutting salt from recipes.

- Double the amount of vegetables. For example, if a recipe calls for a full pound of beef, use half that amount and double the vegetables. You can also add more vegetables to your sandwiches and go easy on high-fat condiments like oil and mayonnaise or high-salt condiments like pickles, olives, and ketchup.

- Add purees of fruits and vegetables whenever possible. To make a puree, simply toss your ripe fruit or vegetables (steamed until soft) of choice into a blender and blend until smooth. Pour the pureed mix into ice cube trays, cover with plastic wrap, and freeze. Use one or more cubes as you need them, but use them up within a month. My favorite purees are squash (for mac and cheese), broccoli (for soups), spinach (for pasta sauce), and raspberries (for homemade raspberry syrup).

## Trying healthier cooking techniques

In terms of cooking, the three main areas of focus are taste, safety, and nutritional quality. No one wants to eat food that doesn't taste good, but in pregnancy, you need to be especially concerned with the nutritional quality of the food you eat. To cook tasty, safe, and nutrient-rich dishes, you need to practice healthy cooking techniques like the following (notice that frying isn't one of them!):

✔ **Baking and roasting:** Baking uses dry, hot, circulating air (typically between 300 and 400 degrees) in an oven to cook things like bread, cookies, pies, casseroles, and potatoes. Roasting is the same as baking, but many people call it roasting when they cook things like garlic, vegetables, and meat. Roasting can also be done at a higher temperature, like 400 to 450 degrees.

Because baking relies on the circulating dry air, it can dry out some foods, so be sure to cover dishes when appropriate to keep the moisture in.

✔ **Braising:** This technique uses liquid and low heat to cook food for a long period of time. It's an excellent way to cook leaner meats to keep them moist. Slow cookers and Dutch ovens work well for braising. You just put the food in the slow cooker or Dutch oven with plenty of liquid (typically water or broth) and cook it on low for several hours.

✔ **Broiling:** Broiling uses high heat (typically 400 to 575 degrees) and works best for tender, thinly cut meats (like steak, pork, chicken, and fish) or certain vegetables (like peppers, onions, and zucchini). Place food on a high rack close to the broiling unit and keep the oven door cracked so the oven doesn't overheat and end up baking the food. Watch food carefully to avoid burning because it can happen quickly with the high heat.

✔ **Grilling:** Grilling is an excellent way to reduce the fat content in meat because some of the extra fat drips away during the grilling process. Grilling works well for whole steaks or chops, fish, hamburgers, and vegetarian burgers. You can also grill fruits and vegetables, but you may want to get a grill basket for those to prevent them from falling through the grates on the grill. Feel free to use charcoal or gas grills, and indoor electric grills work well, too.

✔ **Poaching:** Poaching food involves submersing the food either partially or completely in water or other liquid. Poaching cooks food quickly using very hot liquid; braising, on the other hand, uses smaller amounts of water and a long cooking time. Eggs are commonly poached, but you can also poach fish, poultry, or fruit.

✔ **Sautéing:** Sautéing uses a small amount of fat and relatively high heat to cook food. To sauté, spray a nonstick pan with cooking spray or a small amount of oil and allow it to warm up over medium to medium-high heat. Add foods that take a short time to cook, like bite-sized vegetables and shrimp or thin slices of beef, pork, or chicken. Stir frequently to avoid overcooking any one area of the food.

✔ **Steaming:** Steaming uses small amounts of boiling or simmering water or broth to cook food. This technique works best for vegetables. To steam food on the stove, put the food in a steamer basket and put the basket in a pot with a small layer of boiling water. To steam in the microwave, put the food in a microwaveable dish with a small amount of liquid at the bottom.

Steaming is preferred over boiling for cooking vegetables because it retains more nutrients. Boiling requires more water, and many nutrients can be lost in that water. Steaming, on the other hand, uses less water so the nutrients aren't lost.

# Making Cooking More Comfortable as Your Pregnancy Progresses

As your pregnancy progresses, you may have a hard time spending long periods of time on your feet (and that includes cooking in the kitchen!). In the first trimester, you may just be too tired. In the second and third trimesters, the extra weight may make you want to spend less time on your feet and more time with your feet propped up.

To make the cooking process more comfortable during your pregnancy, keep these tips in mind:

✔ Keep a stool or chair handy in the kitchen to take a break when you need it. Prolonged standing causes blood to pool in your legs, so don't feel bad about taking frequent breaks while you cook.

✔ Get a comfortable mat that you can stand on and wear comfortable shoes if you find yourself standing a lot while you cook.

✔ Use support hose if ankle swelling becomes a problem for you.

✔ Gather and premeasure your ingredients at the beginning of your cooking session so you don't have to run around the kitchen while the chicken (or whatever else you're cooking) burns on the stovetop.

✔ Make enough food to have leftovers or make two recipes on one day and store the second one for tomorrow's dinner. That way, you don't have to cook every day. If you're a morning person, cook a meal or two in the morning, store them, and heat them up later.

If you ever feel dizzy or faint, sit down immediately and call for help. Take a rest and don't push yourself so hard when you get back to cooking. Also, always keep the kitchen cool with good air circulation so you don't overheat, especially when you're preparing meals in the summer.

---

## Can I really kick-start labor with certain foods?

Overdue and wishing you could induce labor? Well, you can't turn to food to help you out. The idea that specific foods can help induce labor is a myth. You may have heard stories about how some women eat spicy foods, castor oil, or evening primrose oil to induce labor, but don't listen to them. No research backs up the idea that eating certain foods will guarantee labor. Letting it happen naturally is the best course of action.

# Chapter 11

# Meal Planning with Your Growing Belly in Mind

*In This Chapter*

▶ Planning ahead for best mealtime success

▶ Following sample meal plans during each stage of your pregnancy

*I*f you don't take some time each week to put together a pregnancy-friendly meal plan for yourself, you may wind up making poor nutritional choices and feeling guilty about not getting your baby the nutrients he needs. This chapter can help you out. It clues you in to the importance of meal planning so you can really understand why having a plan is valuable. It also offers sample meal plans to guide you in making a plan of what to eat each day, according to the trimester you're in. I'm confident that after you take a peek at these sample meal plans, you'll have a good idea of just how easy meal planning during pregnancy can be.

# *The Importance of Having a Plan*

Do you ever get home at the end of the day with no idea what you're going to make for dinner? Ever skip breakfast simply because you didn't plan for it? If you don't plan out the foods you're going to eat, you may find yourself relying too much on convenience foods or take-out — neither of which is typically as healthy as meals you cook yourself. Now I'm certainly not saying you have to cook every meal from scratch while you're pregnant. But with a little planning, you can make sure you get the nutrients you and your baby need through the food you eat instead of just grabbing whatever's edible and not nailed down when you feel the hunger callin'.

Planning your meals also helps you save time and avoid stress. If you have your meals planned and your snacks readily available, you don't have to waste time, holding open the door of the fridge, waiting for dinner to pop out at you. You also don't have to get stressed out, worrying about what's for dinner (or lunch or breakfast) as you move through your day. Instead, as soon as you start to feel hungry, you can get right to assembling (and eating) your next meal or snack. (Planning out your meals may also help you save some money because you won't be heading out to eat nearly as often.)

The following sections arm you with the basic info you need to plan out your meals and snacks, as well as some tips to help simplify the meal-planning process.

## Taking charge of your meals and snacks

Instead of haphazardly opening the fridge or pantry door and standing there until something screams, "Eat me!" take charge of your meals and snacks. Plan each meal using MyPlate, the food-guidance system developed by the United States Department of Agriculture (USDA), and make your grocery list based on your plan. (To see what the MyPlate tool looks like, refer to Chapter 3 or visit www.choosemyplate.gov.)

To use the MyPlate tool to plan your meals, follow these simple guidelines:

1. **Fill half of your plate with fruits and vegetables.**

2. **Fill one-quarter of your plate with grains (preferably whole grains) and one-quarter with lean protein.**

3. **Have a glass of lowfat or fat-free milk or yogurt with the meal.**

Always, always, always have a snack on hand for when the hunger urge strikes you. (After all, there's nothing worse than a really hungry pregnant woman with no food in sight.) Stash snacks in your purse or briefcase and always have extras at home or in the office. Choose a nutritious snack like fresh fruit, a handful of nuts, lowfat Greek yogurt, or a nutrition bar (see Chapter 7 for more ideas).

## Making meal planning easier with some tips and tricks

The key to successful (and stress-free!) meal planning is preparation. To get the most out of every meal, follow these simple tips:

- **Cook more than you need for a meal so you can have leftovers for lunch or dinner the next day.** By using leftovers, you reduce the number of meals you have to plan for the week. Plus, you save money by not having to make or purchase an additional meal. (After all, increasing the ingredients to make more of one recipe is usually cheaper than making a whole new recipe.)

- **Repurpose leftovers to make new dishes so that you don't get tired of having the same thing over and over again.** For example, you can use the chicken breasts you grill on Monday in a pasta dish on Wednesday.

> ✔ **Consider your schedule for the upcoming week as you plan your meals.** Will you get home early on Tuesday? Plan to make the dish that takes the longest to cook that night. Going to prenatal yoga on Thursday? Plan to heat up some leftovers when you get home. Just knowing you have a plan can motivate you to go straight home after class instead of hitting the drive-thru.

# Sample Pregnancy Meal Plans

Sometimes it helps to see a meal plan or two before you attempt to create your own. That's why I provide a couple days' worth of sample meal plans for each trimester of pregnancy in this section. The calories listed are an average for most women. If you need more than that, increase your portions slightly or add a few more snacks; if you need less, cut back a little bit. (See Chapter 3 for the scoop on how many extra calories you need during each trimester.)

Each sample meal plan includes breakfast, lunch, and dinner, as well as four snacks. Feel free to move the snacks around within your day or add or subtract snacks as needed, but aim to eat small amounts frequently. I recommend having a meal or a snack every two to four hours throughout the day; check out the sample eating schedule in Chapter 7 for details.

I encourage you to use the sample meal plans I include here as a guide to creating your own. Look at the examples and patterns and plug in foods that you enjoy (but remember to be aware of portion size and calories when you do).

*Note:* Each sample meal plan includes at least one of this book's recipes so you can see how to incorporate these tasty dishes into your daily routine. I include chapter references so you know where to go to find these recipes.

## 2,000-calorie sample meal plans for the first trimester

In your first trimester, you don't really need any extra calories. Most moderately active women (you're one of them if you walk between 1.5 and 3 miles per day in addition to your normal daily activity) need about 2,000 calories a day, so that's the number of calories you want to plan for when setting your meal plans in the first trimester. If you have a more active lifestyle (you walk more than 3 miles per day in addition to your normal daily activity), you may need more calories (100 to 300 or more, depending on how active you are).

## Day 1

### Breakfast

Spinach, Egg, and Cheese Sandwich (Chapter 12)

### Snack 1

Instant packet of oatmeal prepared with water

### Lunch

1 chicken salad pita with ½ of a 5-ounce can of white meat chicken, 2 tablespoons of light mayo, 1 whole-wheat pita (or 2 slices of whole-wheat bread), ¼ cup of raw spinach, and 1 slice of tomato

1 ounce of reduced fat potato chips

### Snack 2

45 pistachios

### Snack 3

1 piece of lowfat string cheese

1 kiwi fruit

### Dinner

Ratatouille with Cannellini Beans (Chapter 15)

1 cup of whole-wheat penne pasta, cooked

½ cup of marinara sauce

⅓ cup of shredded part-skim pasteurized mozzarella cheese

### Snack 4

1 cup of raspberries and ¼ cup of thawed frozen reduced-fat whipped topping

For dinner, you can melt the mozzarella on top of either the pasta or the ratatouille, or you can put a bit of cheese on both!

## Day 2

### Breakfast

1 cup of whole-grain flakes or O cereal

1 cup of sliced fresh strawberries

1 cup of fat-free milk

### Snack 1

1 stalk of celery, cut into three strips, with 1 tablespoon of almond butter

¼ cup of raisins

*Lunch*

2 slices of cheese pizza (⅛ of a medium pizza)

1 cup of cantaloupe

*Snack 2*

Minty Watermelon Salsa (Chapter 13) with 1 ounce of whole-grain tortilla chips

*Snack 3*

11 ounces of your favorite instant breakfast drink

*Dinner*

One 3-ounce lean hamburger patty on a whole-grain bun with romaine lettuce, 1 slice of tomato, and ketchup, pickle, mustard, or onion (if desired)

1½ cups of mixed salad greens with 2 tablespoons of low-calorie salad dressing

*Snack 4*

1 White Chocolate Berry Oatmeal Cookie (Chapter 16)

Use some leftover Minty Watermelon Salsa from your snack as a topping on your burger or salad at dinner.

# 2,300-calorie sample meal plans for the second trimester

The second trimester is a time of growth for the baby, so you need about 300 extra calories per day. I've added these extra calories by including some nutritious but slightly higher-calorie foods in the following meal plans.

## Day 1

*Breakfast*

1 whole-grain English muffin with 1 ounce of melted cheddar cheese and a sliced apple

6 ounces of 100-percent Concord grape juice

*Snack 1*

6 ounces of lowfat or nonfat Greek yogurt

*Lunch*

Asian Chicken Spinach Salad (Chapter 13)

### Snack 2

Mango smoothie with 6 ounces of lowfat milk or yogurt, ½ of a peeled mango, 1 banana, and ½ cup of ice (Mix all the ingredients in a blender.)

### Snack 3

½ cup of Crunchy Garbanzo Beans (Chapter 13)

### Dinner

5 ounces of baked salmon

1 cup of cooked brown rice

1 cup of cooked Brussels sprouts with 7 walnut halves and 1 teaspoon of olive oil

### Snack 4

3 cups of light microwave popcorn (or Truffle-Flavored Popcorn from Chapter 13)

## Day 2

### Breakfast

Cottage Cheese Pancakes (Chapter 12)

1 cup of raspberries and 1 teaspoon of sugar

### Snack 1

1 fruit and nut bar (such as a KIND Bar)

### Lunch

1 whole-wheat tortilla with 2 tablespoons of peanut or almond butter, ¼ cup of raisins or dried cranberries, 1 sliced banana, and 2 tablespoons of chocolate chips

### Snack 2

1 apple

### Snack 3

1 cup of mixed raw vegetables with ¼ cup of hummus

### Dinner

One 6-ounce Cocoa-Rubbed Grilled Steak (Chapter 14)

1 medium baked potato with 1 teaspoon of tub margarine and 1 tablespoon of light sour cream

1 cup (about 5 spears) of cooked asparagus

### Snack 4

1 Grilled Banana (Chapter 17)

# 2,450-calorie sample meal plans for the third trimester

Your third trimester is when you need the greatest number of calories. Aim to get about 2,450 calories each day to help you support your extra weight and to continue giving energy to your growing baby.

## Day 1

### Breakfast

Greek Omelet (Chapter 12)

2 slices of whole-wheat toast with 2 teaspoons of tub margarine

### Snack 1

1 pear

### Lunch

Sloppy Lentil Joe (Chapter 15) on a whole-grain hamburger bun

### Snack 2

1 ounce of (or 23) almonds

### Snack 3

1 banana

### Dinner

Parmesan-Herb-Crusted Pork Chop (Chapter 14)

1 medium cooked sweet potato with 1 teaspoon each of tub margarine and brown sugar and a sprinkle of cinnamon

1 cup of cooked collard greens

### Snack 4

1 ounce of Dark Chocolate Cherry Pistachio Bark (Chapter 16)

## Day 2

### Breakfast

Chocolate Banana Blast Smoothie (Chapter 12)

### Snack 1

½ of a whole-grain bagel with 1 tablespoon of light cream cheese

### Lunch

Egg salad sandwich with 2 peeled and sliced hard-boiled eggs, 2 tablespoons of light mayo, and 2 slices of whole-wheat bread

3 slices of raw tomato

### Snack 2

1 cup of cooked edamame

### Snack 3

Trail mix with ½ ounce of pecan halves, ⅓ cup of dried tart cherries (or cranberries), and ½ ounce of chocolate chips

### Dinner

Thai Scallops with Noodles (Chapter 14)

### Snack 4

1 cup of pudding

# Part III
# Cooking for Pregnancy

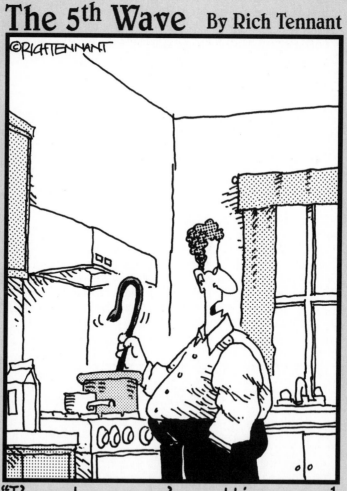

The 5th Wave    By Rich Tennant

©RICHTENNANT

"I'm not sure we're getting enough iron in our diet, so I'm stirring the soup with a crowbar."

# In this part . . .

Fortunately for you, eating while pregnant doesn't have to be boring. This part includes 100 recipes, all of which have been designed with you and your growing belly in mind.

Breakfast is an opportunity to get a jump start on fueling your body for the day, so I include several nutritious and delicious breakfast recipes at the beginning of this part. Because many women find that even though they need more calories during most of their pregnancy, they want to eat small amounts, I devote an entire chapter to recipes that can be either appetizers or small-plate main dishes from chicken wings to various salads. Whether you're a meat eater, pescatarian, or vegetarian, you're sure to find at least a few recipes that appeal to you in the chapters on main and side dishes.

Of course, I couldn't write a book on cooking for pregnancy without including some decadent desserts that are sure to please a sweets-craving pregnant woman's palate. Finally, because I know you may be tired or tight on time, I've also included ten recipes that are ready in ten minutes or less.

# Chapter 12

# Rise and Shine: Breakfast and Smoothie Recipes

## Recipes in This Chapter

- ☼ Oh, Baby! Banana Chocolate Chip Muffins
- ☼ Homemade Maple Berry Crunch Granola
- ☼ Apricot Oatmeal Bake
- ☼ Berries and Cream French Toast
- ☼ Cottage Cheese Pancakes
- ☼ Southwest Avocado Breakfast Burrito
- ☼ Spinach, Egg, and Cheese Sandwich
- ▶ Sausage Asparagus Frittata
- ☼ Greek Omelet
- ☼ Broccoli Hash-Brown Quiche
- ☼ Chocolate Banana Blast Smoothie
- ☼ Pomegranate Power Smoothie

🍸 ∅ ☼ ⌀ ≈ 🌿

## In This Chapter

▶ Getting energy from delicious grain recipes

▶ Filling up with incredible egg dishes

▶ Having breakfast on the go with smoothies

**C**hances are you've heard the phrase "Breakfast is the most important meal of the day" once or twice in your life. I'm not sure how to avoid sounding cliché when I reiterate these words, but you need to know that eating breakfast is especially important when you're sporting a baby bump.

Pregnant women who skip breakfast tend to

✔ Make up for the calories later in the day, typically at dinner or as snacks later in the evening

✔ Have more cravings for sweets and fat

✔ Make poor food choices because of excessive hunger later in the day

Not only is breakfast important to kick-start your metabolism, but many of the typical breakfast foods are also incredibly nutrient rich. They offer an excellent opportunity to check off quite a few of the nutrients you need for the day (I fill you in on these nutrients in Chapter 3). For instance, breakfast is a great time to get fiber and essential B vitamins from whole grains and plenty of antioxidants, vitamins, minerals, and more fiber from one of people's favorite breakfast items — fruit.

Every breakfast you eat needs to have a nice combination of carbohydrates and protein, as well as some healthy fat. Also, keep in mind that size matters. You don't have to — and really shouldn't — eat large quantities. If you don't have any appetite in the morning, simply start with a snack. Have a banana or a few handfuls of dry cereal within an hour of getting up. Then have either another snack or a more substantial meal an hour or two later.

In this chapter, you find a variety of recipes to fuel you and your baby throughout the morning, and each recipe has at least one benefit specific to you as a pregnant woman. So pick a dish and feel free to add other foods to your meal to create a well-rounded edible start to your morning.

# Glorious Grains

Carbohydrates are your body's preferred source of energy, so why not start your day with grains, a wonderful source of complex carbohydrates? Breakfast is an especially good time to eat carbs because they help replenish the energy your body used for fuel while you were sleeping.

Whenever possible, choose the whole-grain variety of grains you commonly eat, such as bread and cereal. When you're preparing grain-based breakfast foods from scratch, you can also experiment with using a mix of half all-purpose flour and half whole-wheat flour (or another whole-grain flour), as I do in the Oh, Baby! Banana Chocolate Chip Muffins recipe.

The recipes in this section are dedicated to providing you with grains. In addition to being good sources of carbs, these recipes also provide numerous other nutrients that are essential for you and your developing baby. Here's a sneak peak at those nutrients and the corresponding foods in the recipes:

- **Antioxidants:** Berries, whole grains, apricots, and flaxseed
- **Calcium:** Cottage cheese and milk
- **Fiber:** Whole grains, walnuts, almonds, pecans, seeds, bananas, berries, and dried fruit
- **Folate:** Apricots, berries, whole-wheat flour, and whole-grain bread
- **Iron:** Whole grains, sesame seeds, oatmeal, apricots, and almonds
- **Potassium:** Bananas, apricots, berries, and flaxseed
- **Protein:** Seeds, eggs, cottage cheese, walnuts, almonds, and pecans

# Oh, Baby! Banana Chocolate Chip Muffins

**Prep time:** 10 min • **Cook time:** 20–25 min • **Yield:** 12 servings

| Ingredients | Directions |
| --- | --- |
| Nonstick cooking spray | *1* Preheat the oven to 350 degrees. Line a 12-cup muffin pan with muffin liners or spray each muffin cup with nonstick cooking spray. |
| ¾ cup all-purpose flour | |
| ¾ cup whole-wheat flour | |
| ¼ cup ground flaxseed | *2* In a large bowl, sift together the all-purpose and whole-wheat flours, flaxseed, baking powder, baking soda, and salt. |
| 1½ teaspoons baking powder | |
| ¼ teaspoon baking soda | |
| ⅛ teaspoon salt | *3* In a medium bowl, beat the eggs with a fork and stir in the mashed bananas. Add the sugar and oil and stir the mixture with a spoon to blend well. |
| 2 eggs | |
| 1 cup mashed ripe bananas | |
| ¾ cup sugar | *4* Add the egg and banana mixture to the large bowl of dry ingredients. Stir the mixture with a spoon to combine well. Stir in the walnuts and chocolate chips. |
| 3 tablespoons canola oil | |
| ½ cup chopped walnuts | |
| ½ cup mini chocolate chips | *5* Fill the muffin pan cups ⅔ full. Bake for 20 to 25 minutes, or until the muffin tops are browned and a toothpick inserted into the middle comes out clean. Allow the muffins to cool and then serve one muffin per serving. |

*Per serving:* Calories 232 (From Fat 95); Fat 11g (Saturated 2g); Cholesterol 18mg; Sodium 106mg; Carbohydrate 33g (Dietary Fiber 3g); Protein 4g; Iron 1mg; Calcium 30mg; Folate 35mcg.

*Tip:* You can either purchase pre-ground flaxseed or grind your own using a spice grinder or a coffee grinder that's dedicated to grinding flaxseed. If you grind your own flaxseed and want to grind more than you need for this recipe, store the extra in an opaque container in the refrigerator. If you buy pre-ground flaxseed, store the extra in its original container in the refrigerator. Either way, your ground flaxseed should keep for about 90 days.

*Note:* If you have a nut allergy, leave out the walnuts. You'll still get a nutritious muffin, just without the nuts.

# Homemade Maple Berry Crunch Granola

**Prep time:** 15 min • **Cook time:** 45–50 min • **Yield:** 12 servings

| Ingredients | Directions |
|---|---|
| **3 cups rolled oats** | *1* Preheat the oven to 300 degrees. Line a large edged baking sheet with parchment paper. |
| ½ **teaspoon cinnamon** | |
| ½ **teaspoon salt** | *2* In a large bowl, combine the oats, cinnamon, and salt. |
| ⅓ **cup canola oil** | |
| ⅓ **cup maple syrup** | *3* In a small bowl, combine the oil, maple syrup, brown sugar, and almond extract. |
| ¼ **cup packed brown sugar** | |
| **1 teaspoon almond extract** | *4* Add the oil and syrup mixture to the oat mixture. Toss the ingredients with a spoon or your hands until the dry ingredients are well coated. Add the pumpkin seeds, flaxseed, sesame seeds, and almonds. Mix well. |
| ¼ **cup pumpkin seeds** | |
| ¼ **cup whole flaxseed** | |
| ¼ **cup sesame seeds** | |
| **1 cup whole almonds** | *5* Spread the granola on the prepared baking sheet, pressing the mixture down on the pan. Bake for 25 to 30 minutes, stirring occasionally. |
| ¼ **cup dried cherries** | |
| ¼ **cup dried cranberries** | *6* Remove the granola from the oven, sprinkle the dried fruit on top, and stir to mix. Bake the granola for another 20 minutes, or until the oats and nuts are toasted brown, stirring occasionally. |
| ¼ **cup dried blueberries** | |
| | *7* Allow the granola to cool in the pan. Break up the granola into chunks and serve (about ⅔ cup per serving). Store the leftovers in an air-tight container for three to four days. |

*Per serving: Calories 321 (From Fat 157); Fat 17g (Saturated 2g); Cholesterol 0mg; Sodium 107mg; Carbohydrate 36g (Dietary Fiber 6g); Protein 8g; Iron 2mg; Calcium 61mg; Folate 24mcg.*

*Tip:* This granola is delicious on its own with a glass of milk for breakfast or as a snack. But it also works well broken up on top of yogurt or in a bowl with milk. After you try this recipe, you'll never want granola out of a box again!

# Apricot Oatmeal Bake

**Prep time:** 15 min • **Cook time:** 40 min • **Yield:** 8 servings

| Ingredients | Directions |
|---|---|
| Nonstick cooking spray | *1* Preheat the oven to 375 degrees. Spray a 9-x-13-inch pan with nonstick cooking spray. |
| ½ cup applesauce | |
| ¼ cup maple syrup | *2* In a medium bowl, combine the applesauce, maple syrup, milk, brown sugar, and eggs. Use a mixer to mix well. |
| 2 cups lowfat or fat-free milk | |
| ¼ cup packed brown sugar | |
| 2 eggs | *3* Add the oats, baking powder, salt, and cinnamon. Beat the mixture on medium-low until well blended. |
| 3 cups rolled oats | |
| 1½ teaspoons baking powder | *4* Add the dried fruit and pecans and stir them into the mixture with a spoon. Transfer the oatmeal mixture to the baking pan. |
| ½ teaspoon salt | |
| 1 teaspoon cinnamon | |
| ¼ cup dried cranberries | *5* Bake for 40 minutes. Serve 1 cup of hot oatmeal per person and with additional milk (if desired). |
| ¼ cup chopped dried apricots | |
| ⅓ cup chopped pecans | |

*Per serving:* Calories 280 (From Fat 67); Fat 7g (Saturated 1g); Cholesterol 56mg; Sodium 269mg; Carbohydrate 46g (Dietary Fiber 5g); Protein 9g; Iron 2mg; Calcium 134mg; Folate 16mcg.

*Note:* Using applesauce rather than oil helps keep the calories down in this recipe.

*Tip:* Store the leftover oatmeal in a tightly covered container in the refrigerator. Heat a serving in the microwave each morning to enjoy hot baked oatmeal all week.

# Berries and Cream French Toast

**Prep time:** 10 min • **Cook time:** 6–8 min • **Yield:** 2 servings

| Ingredients | Directions |
|---|---|
| Nonstick cooking spray | *1* Heat a large skillet or griddle on medium heat and coat it with nonstick cooking spray. |
| 2 eggs | |
| ¼ cup fat-free milk | *2* In a small bowl, beat the eggs, milk, and vanilla with a fork. |
| ¼ teaspoon vanilla extract | |
| 4 slices whole-grain French bread | *3* Dip each slice of French bread into the egg mixture, soaking each side for 10 seconds. |
| ¼ cup cream cheese, softened | |
| 1 cup fresh berries (raspberries, strawberries, blueberries, or blackberries) | *4* Place the soaked bread slices on the skillet and heat them for 3 to 4 minutes, or until they're brown on the bottom. Flip the bread slices over and heat for 3 to 4 minutes, or until they're brown. |
| Powdered sugar (optional) | |
| Maple syrup (optional) | *5* Spread one side of each piece of bread with ¼ of the cream cheese and top with ¼ cup of berries. Dust the French toast with powdered sugar and serve two slices with syrup (if desired). |

*Per serving:* Calories 404 (From Fat 158); Fat 18g (Saturated 8g); Cholesterol 245mg; Sodium 420mg; Carbohydrate 36g (Dietary Fiber 7g); Protein 15g; Iron 3mg; Calcium 147mg; Folate 77mcg.

*Warning:* Cook your French toast until it's nicely browned so that the eggs in the batter are completely cooked through. No raw eggs during pregnancy!

*Vary It!* If berries aren't in season, improvise with thawed frozen berries or use your fruit of choice. And if you're not a fan of cream cheese, try using peanut butter instead for a PB&B (Berries) French toast.

# Cottage Cheese Pancakes

**Prep time:** 10 min  •  **Cook time:** About 15 min  •  **Yield:** 2 servings

| Ingredients | Directions |
|---|---|
| Nonstick cooking spray<br><br>1 cup lowfat cottage cheese<br><br>3 eggs, lightly beaten<br><br>2 tablespoons vegetable oil<br><br>⅓ cup whole-wheat flour | *1* Heat a large skillet or griddle over medium heat and coat it well with nonstick cooking spray.<br><br>*2* In a large bowl, combine the cottage cheese, eggs, and oil. Mix gently with a fork.<br><br>*3* Add the flour to the cottage cheese mixture and stir until all the flour is moist.<br><br>*4* Pour ⅓-cup servings of batter onto the skillet, cooking until bubbles appear on top of the pancakes. Use a spatula to gently flip each pancake and cook until it's browned on the other side.<br><br>*5* Serve four 2-inch pancakes per person with butter or soft spread, fresh fruit, jam, or syrup. |

*Per serving:* Calories 385 (From Fat 208); Fat 23g (Saturated 4g); Cholesterol 323mg; Sodium 554mg; Carbohydrate 18g (Dietary Fiber 2g); Protein 26g; Iron 2mg; Calcium 112mg; Folate 53mcg.

*Tip:* For a smoother consistency, put the cottage cheese in the food processor before you mix it with the eggs and oil.

*Note:* I've been making cottage cheese pancakes since I was a kid. Instead of using syrup I simply put a pat of butter on top and enjoy the savory flavor that the cottage cheese brings to the pancake.

*Tip:* To save time, simply add the cottage cheese to a premade pancake mix. Just be sure to use a bit less water!

# Incredibly Edible Eggs

Eggs are a wonderful choice for pregnant women, in large part because they offer a source of high-quality protein that doesn't cost you too many calories. Because of the amount of iron they typically contain — 0.9 milligrams (mg) — they're especially good if you're at risk of *anemia* (a condition in which you have low blood levels of iron). Eggs also provide choline, a little-known nutrient that's essential for your baby's developing brain. (In fact, eggs are one of the best sources of choline in a person's diet!) Finally, eggs have several B vitamins, including folate, which is vital for your baby's developing nerve tissue, brain, and spinal cord.

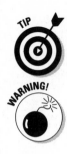

To get the most out of your eggs, be sure to eat the yolks. That's where a lot of the protein and essential nutrients are found.

Although eggs are a power food for pregnancy, they also require a word of warning. Because eggs can contain salmonella, make sure you cook all eggs well throughout your pregnancy. If you're used to runny yolks or softly scrambled eggs, make sure you cook those yolks (and whites) all the way through until they're hard. When dining out, order your eggs over hard or scrambled well (no more sunny-side-up or over-easy eggs).

This section features quite a few recipes that contain different ways to eat eggs. In addition, each recipe is packed with nutrients that are especially beneficial for you during your pregnancy. If you want to know which nutrients a particular dish offers based on its ingredient list, refer to the following list:

- **Antioxidants:** Spinach, artichokes, black beans, tomatoes, and peppers
- **Calcium:** Cheese, milk, and spinach
- **Fiber:** Whole grains, black beans, artichokes, and peppers
- **Folate:** Spinach, eggs, black beans, avocado, and asparagus
- **Iron:** Eggs, black beans, sausage, and whole grains
- **Potassium:** Potatoes, avocado, black beans, spinach, mushrooms, milk, and cheese
- **Protein:** Eggs, black beans, cheese, sausage, and milk

# Southwest Avocado Breakfast Burrito

**Prep time:** 10 min • **Cook time:** About 10 min • **Yield:** 2 servings

| Ingredients | Directions |
|---|---|
| Nonstick cooking spray | **1** Warm a nonstick skillet on medium heat and coat it with nonstick cooking spray. |
| 2 eggs | |
| 2 large whole-wheat tortillas | **2** In a small bowl, beat the eggs with a fork. |
| ½ cup canned black beans, drained and rinsed | **3** Add the eggs to the hot skillet and stir constantly to scramble them well. Cook until they're no longer wet, about 4 to 5 minutes. |
| ¼ cup shredded Mexican cheese blend | |
| ½ avocado, peeled and diced | **4** While the eggs are cooking, heat the tortillas in the microwave for 30 seconds. |
| ¼ cup salsa | |
| Cilantro, chopped (optional) | **5** Add the black beans and cheese to the eggs and cook until the cheese is melted, about 1 to 2 minutes. |
| | **6** Place half of the egg mixture on each tortilla. Top each tortilla with half of the avocado, salsa, and cilantro (if desired). Fold each tortilla and enjoy. |

*Per serving: Calories 449 (From Fat 174); Fat 19g (Saturated 7g); Cholesterol 225mg; Sodium 597mg; Carbohydrate 23g (Dietary Fiber 9g); Protein 23g; Iron 3mg; Calcium 165mg; Folate 123mcg.*

*Vary It!* Throw in mushrooms, peppers, tomatoes, or onions to add different flavors to your burritos. Sauté the vegetables in the same hot skillet before cooking the eggs for best results (and less cleanup!).

# Spinach, Egg, and Cheese Sandwich

**Prep time:** 5 min • **Cook time:** About 10 min • **Yield:** 1 serving

| Ingredients | Directions |
|---|---|
| Nonstick cooking spray | **1** Spray a small skillet with nonstick cooking spray and heat it over medium heat. |
| ½ cup fresh spinach, stems removed | |
| ½ cup chopped fresh mushrooms | **2** Add the spinach and mushrooms to the skillet and cook until soft, about 2 to 3 minutes. While the vegetables are cooking, mix the egg in a small bowl with a fork. |
| 1 egg | |
| 1 slice Swiss cheese | **3** Remove the vegetables from the skillet and set them aside. Add the egg to the hot skillet and cook it until it's no longer runny, about 4 minutes, flipping or stirring halfway through. Place the cheese on top of the egg and heat until melted, about 1 minute. |
| 1 whole-wheat bagel thin | |
| | **4** Toast the bagel thin in a toaster. |
| | **5** Add the egg and cheese to the bottom half of the bagel thin. Top that with the sautéed vegetables and the top half of the bagel thin. |

*Per serving:* Calories 305 (From Fat 128); Fat 14g (Saturated 7g); Cholesterol 239mg; Sodium 340mg; Carbohydrate 28g (Dietary Fiber 6g); Protein 22g; Iron 2mg; Calcium 354mg; Folate 75mcg.

*Vary It!* Use asparagus in place of spinach if you want a different flavor or if you want to take advantage of it while it's in season.

*Note:* A sandwich I eat quite often at a bagel place near my office inspired this recipe. It hits the spot for breakfast or lunch!

# Sausage Asparagus Frittata

**Prep time:** 15 min • **Cook time:** About 35 min • **Yield:** 6 servings

| Ingredients | Directions |
|---|---|
| Nonstick cooking spray<br><br>1 cup sliced reduced-fat smoked turkey sausage | *1* Preheat the oven to 400 degrees. Spray an ovenproof skillet with nonstick cooking spray and heat it on the stovetop over medium heat. |
| ¼ cup diced onion<br><br>½ cup thinly sliced red bell pepper | *2* Add the sausage, onion, bell pepper, and asparagus to the hot skillet. Cook until the sausage is browned, about 10 minutes. |
| ½ cup chopped asparagus<br><br>6 eggs | *3* In a medium bowl, whisk together the eggs, milk, sour cream, salt, and pepper. Mix in the mozzarella cheese with a fork. |
| ½ cup lowfat milk<br><br>¼ cup reduced-fat sour cream | *4* Pour the egg mixture over the sausage and vegetables in the skillet. |
| ⅛ teaspoon salt<br><br>⅛ teaspoon pepper | *5* Bake for 20 minutes, or until a knife inserted into the center comes out clean. |
| ½ cup shredded mozzarella cheese<br><br>½ cup grated Parmesan cheese | *6* Sprinkle the top of the frittata with the Parmesan cheese and return it to the oven for another 3 to 4 minutes. Cut it into 6 wedges and serve. |

*Per serving:* Calories 191 (From Fat 100); Fat 11g (Saturated 5g); Cholesterol 238mg; Sodium 486mg; Carbohydrate 7g (Dietary Fiber 1g); Protein 15g; Iron 1mg; Calcium 213mg; Folate 45mcg.

*Vary It!* Frittatas are quite simple and versatile. Play around with different meats, like turkey or Canadian bacon, and switch up the veggies with things like artichokes, sun-dried tomatoes, mushrooms, or whatever else your cravings call for.

*Note:* Frittatas are great any time of the day. Make a frittata for dinner and serve it with a side salad and whole-wheat roll for a well-balanced (and delicious!) meal.

# Greek Omelet

**Prep time:** 5 min • **Cook time:** About 6 min • **Yield:** 1 serving

| Ingredients | Directions |
|---|---|
| Nonstick cooking spray | *1* Spray a medium nonstick skillet with nonstick cooking spray and heat it over medium heat. |
| 2 eggs | |
| 1 egg white | *2* In a small bowl, scramble the eggs and egg white with a fork. Add the Italian herbs and salt and pepper to taste. |
| Pinch of Italian herbs | |
| Salt and pepper to taste | |
| ½ cup fresh spinach, stems removed | *3* Cook the spinach in the heated skillet until it's wilted, about 1 minute. Add the tomatoes, artichokes, and olives. Pour the egg mixture over the vegetable mixture. |
| ¼ cup chopped sun-dried tomatoes (not packed in oil) | |
| ¼ cup chopped artichokes | *4* Using a spatula, push the eggs away from the edges of the pan and tilt the pan to allow the eggs to run onto the empty portion of the pan. Let the omelet cook for about 3 minutes. |
| 2 tablespoons sliced kalamata olives | |
| 2 tablespoons pasteurized feta cheese, crumbled | *5* Carefully flip the omelet over and reduce the heat. Add the feta cheese to one half of the omelet and let it cook for another 1 to 2 minutes. Fold the omelet in half, enclosing the cheese. Slide the omelet from the skillet onto a plate and enjoy while hot. |

*Per serving:* Calories 317 (From Fat 170); Fat 19g (Saturated 7g); Cholesterol 442mg; Sodium 952mg; Carbohydrate 16g (Dietary Fiber 4g); Protein 23g; Iron 4mg; Calcium 189mg; Folate 152mcg.

*Tip:* Serve the omelet with whole-wheat toast and sliced tomatoes for a well-rounded meal.

*Note:* Greek omelets have been a favorite of mine since college when I worked at a Greek breakfast restaurant. I love the sharp salty taste of the feta combined with the flavors of the Mediterranean-inspired vegetables.

# Broccoli Hash-Brown Quiche

**Prep time:** 15 min • **Cook time:** About 1 hr 10 min • **Yield:** 4 servings

| *Ingredients* | *Directions* |
|---|---|
| Nonstick cooking spray<br><br>3 cups shredded hash-brown potatoes (fresh or frozen, thawed)<br><br>1 tablespoon olive oil<br><br>½ cup diced onion<br><br>¼ cup diced red bell pepper<br><br>1 cup chopped broccoli<br><br>½ cup diced zucchini<br><br>½ cup sliced mushrooms<br><br>4 eggs<br><br>½ cup lowfat milk<br><br>1 teaspoon Italian herb blend<br><br>¾ cup shredded cheddar cheese | *1* Preheat the oven to 425 degrees. Coat a pie plate with nonstick cooking spray.<br><br>*2* Press the hash-brown potatoes into the bottom and sides of the pie plate. Bake for 30 minutes, or until the potatoes are crisp. Remove the potatoes from the oven and set aside. Reduce the oven temperature to 375 degrees.<br><br>*3* While the potatoes are in the oven, heat the olive oil in a large nonstick skillet over medium heat. Sauté the onions until they're tender, about 3 to 4 minutes. Add the diced red pepper, broccoli, and zucchini and cook for another 4 minutes. Add the mushrooms and cook for 2 more minutes.<br><br>*4* In a medium bowl, whisk together the eggs, milk, and Italian herb blend. Stir in the cheese. Add the vegetable mixture to the eggs and stir everything with a spoon.<br><br>*5* Pour the egg and vegetable mixture into the potato crust. Bake for 30 to 45 minutes, checking the quiche for doneness after 30 minutes. (You can tell the quiche is ready when a knife inserted into the center of it comes out clean.) |

*Per serving:* Calories 326 (From Fat 209); Fat 23g (Saturated 10g); Cholesterol 236mg; Sodium 260mg; Carbohydrate 29g (Dietary Fiber 4g); Protein 17g; Iron 3mg; Calcium 262mg; Folate 87mcg.

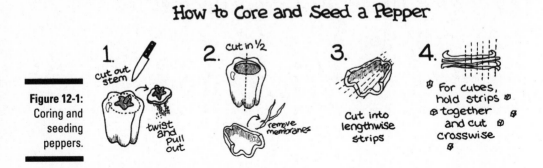

How to Core and Seed a Pepper

**Figure 12-1:** Coring and seeding peppers.

# On-the-Go Breakfasts — Smoothie Style

Morning is traditionally a very rushed time. Don't worry if you don't have a ton of time to cook! The most important thing is that you get something into your body, ideally within an hour of getting up. (If you wait longer than an hour to eat, your metabolism can take a nose dive and your risk of getting nauseous increases as those stomach acids take over an empty stomach.) A quick and easy way to get food into your body is by drinking your breakfast! Smoothies take just a few minutes to prepare, and you can pour them into a to-go cup to drink on your morning commute. This section contains some smoothie recipes that are sure to get you out the door fast with a healthy breakfast option in hand.

Smoothies can serve as your entire breakfast. As long as you include either milk, yogurt, or protein powder for protein and fruit for carbohydrates and fiber, you can actually get a well-rounded meal all in one glass!

To boost the nutritional value of your smoothie, consider some nutrient-dense add-ins. If you want extra protein, use a scoop of protein powder. Whey and soy-based powders are the most common, but you can also find unflavored, chocolate, and vanilla protein powders. (I typically use vanilla protein powder because it adds a bit of flavor without being overwhelming.) Other healthy additions include wheat germ, ground flaxseed, fresh spinach or other greens, and tofu. Have fun experimenting!

# Chocolate Banana Blast Smoothie

**Prep time:** 5 min • **Yield:** 1 serving

| *Ingredients* | *Directions* |
|---|---|
| **1 large banana, broken into chunks** | *1* Place all the ingredients in a blender and blend until smooth. |
| **½ cup frozen blueberries** | |
| **2 cups fresh spinach, torn into small pieces** | *2* Pour the chocolaty smoothie into a tall glass and enjoy! |
| **1 scoop unflavored protein powder** | |
| **1 tablespoon unsweetened cocoa powder** | |
| **1 tablespoon wheat germ** | |
| **½ cup lowfat or fat-free milk** | |
| **2 teaspoons honey** | |
| **½ cup ice** | |

*Per serving:* Calories 331 (From Fat 37); Fat 4g (Saturated 2g); Cholesterol 20mg; Sodium 128mg; Carbohydrate 67g (Dietary Fiber 10g); Protein 16g; Iron 4mg; Calcium 278mg; Folate 156mcg.

*Note:* Even though this recipe calls for 2 cups of spinach, you'll barely know it's there! This smoothie is packed in nutrients and is quite filling.

*Tip:* When your bananas start to turn brown, peel them and cut them into chunks. Put each banana into a resealable freezer bag and freeze it. That way, you'll always have a banana for smoothies ready to go! Keep in mind, though, that you may not need the ice in the recipe if you're using frozen bananas.

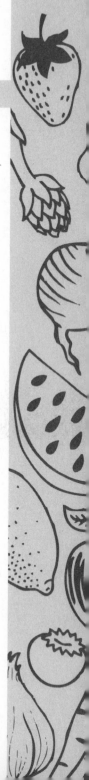

# Pomegranate Power Smoothie

**Prep time:** 5 min • **Yield:** 1 serving

| Ingredients | Directions |
|---|---|
| 6 ounces nonfat vanilla Greek yogurt | **1** Combine all the ingredients in a blender and blend until smooth. |
| 4 ounces 100% pomegranate juice | |
| 1 cup frozen mixed berries | **2** Pour the pomegranate smoothie into a tall glass and drink up! |
| ½ banana, broken into pieces | |
| 2 tablespoons ground flaxseed | |
| 1 teaspoon honey | |

*Per serving:* Calories 458 (From Fat 56); Fat 6g (Saturated 1g); Cholesterol 0mg; Sodium 90mg; Carbohydrate 85g (Dietary Fiber 11g); Protein 21g; Iron 3mg; Calcium 264mg; Folate 93mcg.

*Note:* Pomegranates are one of the highest antioxidant foods available. Drinking just 4 ounces of pomegranate juice daily is a good routine to get into whether you're pregnant or not!

*Source: Cindy Heroux, RD, and author of The Manual That Should Have Come with Your Body (Speaking of Wellness)*

---

## No time? Breakfasts in 5 minutes or less

If you find yourself in a rush to get out the door every morning, look for some fast and easy breakfast ideas so you can eat right for you and your baby even when you're in a hurry. Here are a few nutritious breakfast suggestions that require little to no preparation:

- Whole-grain frozen waffle topped with fresh mixed berries and a dollop of whipped cream and served with a glass of lowfat milk

- Whole-grain cereal of choice with lowfat milk and a sliced banana

- Whole-grain English muffin spread with almond butter and thinly sliced apples

- Greek yogurt with granola and fresh sliced peaches

- Two slices of whole-grain toast with 2 scrambled eggs and a glass of vegetable juice

- Hard-boiled egg with a bowl of oatmeal topped with blueberries

# Chapter 13

# Adding Fuel to Your Day: Snack, Appetizer, and Salad Recipes

**Recipes in This Chapter**

- Apple Cinnamon Trail Mix
- Quinoa Nut Mix
- Crunchy Garbanzo Beans
- Truffle-Flavored Popcorn
- Minty Watermelon Salsa
- Avocado Shrimp Martinis
- Fig and Olive Bruschetta
- Steamed Artichoke with Garlic-Herb Dipping Sauce
- Sun-Dried Tomato and Ricotta Stuffed Mushrooms
- Asian-Style Chicken Wings
- Sausage-Stuffed Baked Potato Skins
- Chicken Lettuce Wraps
- White Chicken and Pineapple Flatbread
- Mixed Greens with Chicken, Cantaloupe, & Red Grapes Salad
- Fruity Poppy Seed Salad
- White Bean and Portobello Salad
- Fresh Mozzarella, Tomato, and Pepper Salad
- Roasted Beet and Pistachio Salad
- Deconstructed Greek Salad
- Asian Chicken Spinach Salad
- Creamy Grape Salad
- Cranberry Gelatin Salad

## In This Chapter

▶ Whipping up healthy snacks to boost your energy between meals

▶ Savoring small meals with big nutrients

▶ Creating a colorful salad that's jampacked with the nutrients you and your baby need

I often hear pregnant women say that they can't eat very much at one time because they fill up faster than they used to. Whether that's due to hormones or the weight of the baby pressing on the stomach, many pregnant women simply gravitate toward eating smaller portions more frequently throughout the day as opposed to just a few large meals. Because you may find yourself among these women, this chapter provides you with 22 delicious ways to eat small bites — from trail mix to chicken wings to a variety of salads.

## Preparing Healthy Snacks

The days of thinking that all snacks are unhealthy or that you should avoid snacks are gone! Snacks provide you with an opportunity to add nutrients to your day. That's right. Snacks don't have to be empty-calorie foods. Don't get me wrong; I have nothing against digging into some chips or savoring some decadent chocolate. But even those seemingly unhealthy foods may create opportunities for boosting nutrients. For example, why not dip your whole-grain tortilla chips into the Minty Watermelon Salsa I describe later in this section? Expand your horizons by trying some new flavor combinations and thinking outside the box.

If you're looking for a quick snack that doesn't require any prep work, turn to Chapter 7 for some ideas.

The five recipes in this section provide a variety of crunchy snacks that are sure to satisfy, plus an assortment of essential nutrients to fuel your pregnancy. Here are just some of the nutrients you can expect to find in this section's recipes, along with the ingredients that contain them:

- **Antioxidants:** Whole grains, nuts (especially pecans), flaxseed, apples, watermelon, and peaches
- **Calcium:** Flaxseed and nuts
- **Fiber:** Whole grains, garbanzo beans, flaxseed, apples, and peaches
- **Folate:** Garbanzo beans, nuts, quinoa, watermelon, and peaches
- **Iron:** Whole grains, nuts, and quinoa
- **Potassium:** Garbanzo beans, nuts, flaxseed, apples, watermelon, and peaches
- **Protein:** Flaxseed, nuts, quinoa, and garbanzo beans

# Discovering the many benefits of whole grains

When it comes to grains, choosing the whole-grain variety is always better. Not only do you get more fiber, but you also get the benefits of having all three parts of the grain: the germ, endosperm, and bran. When a grain is refined, it loses the germ, which is where most of the beneficial nutrients are found, and the bran, which is where the fiber is.

The benefits of eating whole grains are numerous and can include reduced risk of stroke, diabetes, heart disease, and high blood pressure, as well as better weight control. You can find whole grains by reading food labels and looking for the phrase *whole-grain* in front of many common grains.

These foods are always whole grain: Amaranth, barley, buckwheat, corn (including popcorn), millet, oats, quinoa, brown and wild rice, rye, sorghum, teff, whole wheat, spelt, bulgur, cracked wheat, and wheat berries.

The next time you're at the store, look for the whole-grain variety of commonly eaten grains, like whole-wheat bread (and bread products such as bagels, English muffins, pitas, and crackers), whole-grain or corn tortillas, whole-grain pasta and cereals, and brown or wild rice. Also try substituting whole-grain flour in part or in total for the all-purpose, or white, flour in recipes.

# Apple Cinnamon Trail Mix

**Prep time:** 5 min • **Yield:** 4 servings

| *Ingredients* | *Directions* |
|---|---|
| ½ cup dried apples, cut into chunks | *1* In a large bowl, combine all the ingredients. Gently toss them with clean hands or mix them with a spoon. |
| 1 cup Apple Cinnamon Cheerios | |
| ½ cup almonds | *2* Divide the trail mix into 4 equal servings and put each one into an individual snack bag to enjoy later. |
| ½ cup pecan halves | |
| ¼ cup white chocolate chips | |

*Per serving:* Calories 321 (From Fat 206); Fat 23g (Saturated 4); Cholesterol 2mg; Sodium 64mg; Carbohydrate 27g (Dietary Fiber 5g); Protein 7g; Iron 3mg; Calcium 105mg; Folate 77mcg.

*Vary It!* To switch up the flavors in this trail mix, try using plain or another variety of Cheerios and dried berries, mango, pineapple, or other dried fruit.

*Note:* Trail mix can add up in calories very quickly because of the calorie-dense nuts and dried fruits. Enjoy it in small quantities and eat it slowly.

# *Quinoa Nut Mix*

**Prep time:** 10 min • **Cook time:** 33–35 min • **Yield:** 8 servings

| *Ingredients* | *Directions* |
|---|---|
| 1 cup water | *1* Preheat the oven to 350 degrees. Line a large baking sheet with parchment paper. |
| ½ cup quinoa, rinsed | |
| 1 cup almonds | *2* In a small saucepan, heat the water to a boil. Add the quinoa, stir, and return to a boil. Reduce the heat, stir, and cover to let the quinoa simmer for about 8 to 10 minutes, or until the quinoa is slightly undercooked. Fluff with a fork and drain any remaining water. |
| ½ cup cashews | |
| ½ cup pecans | |
| ½ cup walnuts | |
| ¼ cup flaxseed | *3* In a large bowl, mix together the almonds, cashews, pecans, walnuts, flaxseed, and cooked quinoa. |
| 1 egg white | |
| ½ teaspoon cinnamon | *4* In a small bowl, whisk together the egg white, cinnamon, salt, and sugar. Pour the egg white mixture over the nut mixture and stir to coat the nuts and quinoa evenly. |
| ¼ teaspoon salt | |
| 2 tablespoons sugar | |
| | *5* Spread the nut mix evenly on the prepared baking sheet. Bake for 25 minutes, stirring occasionally. |
| | *6* Transfer the parchment paper with the nut mix to a wire rack to cool. When the nut mix is cool to the touch, break it into chunks with your hands. Serving size is about ½ cup. |

*Per serving:* Calories 322 (From Fat 227); Fat 25g (Saturated 0g); Cholesterol 0mg; Sodium 91mg; Carbohydrate 20g (Dietary Fiber 6g); Protein 10g; Iron 3mg; Calcium 76mg; Folate 36mcg.

*Note:* If you're using salted nuts, you don't need to add any salt to the recipe.

*Vary It!* Feel free to mix up the nuts and seeds to include your favorites. Add dried fruit if desired.

# Crunchy Garbanzo Beans

**Prep time:** 10 min  •  **Cook time:** 40 min  •  **Yield:** 4 servings

| *Ingredients* | *Directions* |
|---|---|
| **1 tablespoon olive oil** | *1* Preheat the oven to 400 degrees. Line a large rimmed baking pan with aluminum foil. Spread the olive oil over the foil. |
| **¼ teaspoon salt** | |
| **Dash of pepper** | |
| **¼ cup flour** | *2* In a large resealable plastic bag, add the salt, pepper, flour, rosemary, and garlic powder. Add the beans to the bag, zip it up, and shake it to coat the beans evenly. |
| **1 teaspoon dried rosemary, crushed** | |
| **½ teaspoon garlic powder** | |
| **One 15-ounce can garbanzo beans, drained, rinsed, and patted dry** | *3* Pour the coated beans into a mesh sifter and shake gently to remove the excess flour. Spread the coated beans evenly on the prepared baking pan. Bake for 20 minutes. |
| **2 tablespoons grated Parmesan cheese** | |
| | *4* Remove the beans from the oven and stir them around on the pan. Bake for another 20 minutes. Let the beans cool slightly until they're no longer hot to the touch. |
| | *5* Place the beans in a serving bowl and sprinkle them with Parmesan cheese. Toss the beans to coat them with the cheese. Serving size is about ½ cup. |

*Per serving:* Calories 134 (From Fat 46); Fat 5g (Saturated 1g); Cholesterol 2mg; Sodium 318mg; Carbohydrate 17g (Dietary Fiber 3g); Protein 5g; Iron 1mg; Calcium 62mg; Folate 138mcg.

*Note:* Also called chickpeas, these beans are high in protein and fiber, so they make a healthy, crunchy snack alternative.

*Tip:* Baked garbanzo beans don't stay crunchy for very long, so find friends to share them with while they're fresh. Store leftovers in a tightly covered container in the refrigerator for up to three days.

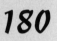

# Truffle-Flavored Popcorn

**Prep time:** 5 min • **Cook time:** About 15 min • **Yield:** 3 servings

| *Ingredients* | *Directions* |
|---|---|
| **1 tablespoon olive oil** | **1** In a stockpot, heat the olive oil over medium heat for 3 to 4 minutes. |
| **⅓ cup popcorn kernels** | |
| **½ teaspoon truffle salt** | **2** Add the popcorn. Cover the pot and slowly move it back and forth on the burner to move the kernels around in the pot and to distribute the oil evenly on the kernels. |
| **2 tablespoons unsalted butter, melted** | |
| **2 tablespoons grated Parmesan cheese** | **3** Heat the popcorn until the popping slows to every few seconds. (It typically takes about 10 minutes for the kernels to reach the right temperature and start popping, but as soon as the popping starts, listen carefully and pull the pot off the heat when the popping slows so that the popcorn doesn't burn.) |
| | **4** Place the popcorn in a large bowl. |
| | **5** Add the truffle salt to the melted butter and stir. Pour the mixture over the popcorn, stirring well to coat the popcorn evenly. Sprinkle the popcorn with the Parmesan cheese and toss to coat evenly. One serving is about 3 cups. |

*Per serving:* Calories 201 (From Fat 128); Fat 14g (Saturated 6g); Cholesterol 23mg; Sodium 447mg; Carbohydrate 16g (Dietary Fiber 3g); Protein 4g; Iron 1mg; Calcium 48mg; Folate 6mcg.

*Note:* I fell in love with truffle oil popcorn at a restaurant as part of a dessert course. Then I went to Italy and fell in love with truffle oil all over again. A little bit goes a long way to give a decadent surge of flavor. If you have truffle oil, you can use 1 tablespoon of that rather than olive oil to pop the kernels. If you like a lot of truffle flavor, use both truffle oil and truffle salt, but feel free to use one or the other if you have both.

*Tip:* Popcorn is a whole grain and is actually quite low in calories if you pop it yourself, using minimal oil and butter.

# Minty Watermelon Salsa

**Prep time:** 15 min • **Yield:** 8 servings

| Ingredients | Directions |
|---|---|
| 2 cups finely chopped watermelon, seeds removed | **1** In a large bowl, combine the watermelon, peach, cucumber, and fresh mint. |
| 1 peach, pitted and diced | |
| ½ cup thinly sliced and diced cucumber | **2** In a small bowl, whisk together the lime juice and sugar. Pour the lime juice mixture over the fruit and stir well. |
| 2 tablespoons chopped fresh mint | |
| ¼ cup fresh lime juice | **3** Serve ⅓ cup of salsa with 1 ounce of whole-grain tortilla chips for dipping. |
| 2 tablespoons sugar | |
| 8 ounces whole-grain tortilla chips | |

*Per serving:* Calories 185 (From Fat 66); Fat 7g (Saturated 1g); Cholesterol 0mg; Sodium 113mg; Carbohydrate 28g (Dietary Fiber 3g); Protein 3g; Iron 1mg; Calcium 29mg; Folate 7mcg.

*Note:* This fruity salsa is a refreshing change to tomato-based salsas. The mint and sweetness of the watermelon and peaches complement each other nicely for an interesting combination.

*Vary It!* Feel free to add red or green onions, chopped fresh cilantro, or other vegetables to switch up the flavors in this recipe. If you like your salsa a bit spicier, add some finely diced jalapeño pepper.

## How to Juice a Lime

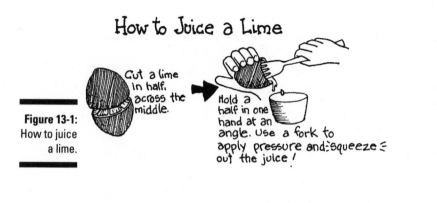

Cut a lime in half, across the middle.

Hold a half in one hand at an angle. Use a fork to apply pressure and squeeze out the juice!

**Figure 13-1:**
How to juice a lime.

# Small Bites for Your Growing Belly: Tapas-Style Meals

One of my favorite restaurants to visit on a date night with my husband or when gathering with girlfriends is a tapas-style place. *Tapas* are small plates (think appetizer-sized) of hot and cold foods that you share with your dining companions. The best part about tapas is that you get to try new dishes without having to commit to only one of them for your meal.

Take advantage of the time before Baby arrives to get together with friends and family and host a tapas night where the entire meal consists of various appetizers. Serve a variety of cold and hot dishes to please your guests' palates. Whenever possible, make what you can ahead of time. (I tell you how long each recipe in this section takes to prepare and cook so that you can plan ahead.)

## Enjoy a flavorful mocktail

Even though alcohol is off the menu when you're pregnant, you can still whip up some mouthwatering nonalcoholic drinks that will complement your tapas spread. Try one or more of the following mocktail ideas:

✔ **Cranberry Twist:** Cran-raspberry juice with sparkling water and a twist of lime

✔ **Frozen Strawberry Lemonade:** Lemon juice, water, frozen strawberries, and sugar blended with ice

✔ **Grape Fizz:** Concord grape juice, blackberry sorbet, and sparkling water

✔ **Mock Champagne:** White grape juice, pineapple juice, and ginger ale

✔ **Orange Pineapple Slush:** Orange juice, pineapple juice, and a splash of lemon juice, blended with ice

✔ **Shirley Temple:** Lemon-lime soda with grenadine and a maraschino cherry

✔ **Virgin Daiquiri:** Frozen strawberries, sweet and sour mix, and a splash of grenadine blended with ice

# Avocado Shrimp Martinis

**Prep time:** 10 min • **Yield:** 6 servings

| *Ingredients* | *Directions* |
|---|---|
| **1 ripe avocado, peeled and diced** | *1* In a small bowl, combine the avocado, tomato, lime juice, salt, red onion, and cilantro. Mix well, slightly mashing the avocado into the rest of the ingredients. |
| **1 tomato, diced** | |
| **Juice of 1 lime** | |
| **½ teaspoon salt** | *2* Pour the mixture into 6 martini glasses (about ⅓ cup per glass). |
| **3 tablespoons chopped red onion** | |
| **2 tablespoons freshly chopped cilantro** | *3* Line the rim of each martini glass with 4 to 5 jumbo shrimp. Dip the shrimp into the avocado mixture to enjoy. |
| **1 pound jumbo shrimp, peeled and deveined, tails still on** | |

*Per serving: Calories 129 (From Fat 46); Fat 5g (Saturated 1g); Cholesterol 147mg; Sodium 366mg; Carbohydrate 5g (Dietary Fiber 3g); Protein 17g; Iron 3mg; Calcium 33mg; Folate 27mcg.*

*Note:* Shrimp is highly perishable. Eat it within 24 hours after you purchase it to be safe.

*Tip:* If the shrimp won't stay on the rim of the martini glasses, cut a small slit in the shrimp.

## How to Pit and Peel an Avocado

 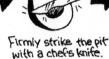

**Figure 13-2:** How to pit and peel an avocado.

Slice avocado in half lengthwise and pull apart.

Firmly strike the pit with a chef's knife.

Lift the pit out with a gentle twist of the knife.

GENTLY scoop out the meat with a spoon.

Chop or slice according to your recipe.

# Fig and Olive Bruschetta

**Prep time:** 15 min, plus marinating time  •  **Cook time:** About 10 min  •  **Yield:** About 12 servings

| Ingredients | Directions |
|---|---|
| ½ cup water | **1** In a small saucepan, heat the water and figs over medium heat. Bring to a boil. Reduce heat and cook for 5 minutes, or until the figs become soft and have absorbed most of the water. Transfer the figs to a medium bowl. |
| 1 cup dried figs, chopped | |
| 2 teaspoons olive oil | |
| ½ teaspoon fresh lemon juice | |
| 1 tablespoon balsamic vinegar | **2** Add the olive oil, lemon juice, vinegar, thyme, oregano, kalamata and black olives, and garlic to the bowl with the figs. Mix well. Refrigerate for several hours to allow the flavors to marinate. |
| ½ teaspoon dried thyme | |
| ½ teaspoon dried oregano | |
| ⅓ cup pitted and chopped kalamata olives | **3** After the figs have been marinating for several hours, preheat the oven to 450 degrees. Slice the baguette diagonally into ½-inch slices. Arrange the bread on a cookie sheet and bake on the top rack for 4 to 5 minutes, or until it's golden and crispy. |
| ⅓ cup chopped black olives | |
| 1 clove garlic, minced | |
| 1 loaf French baguette | **4** Spread each slice of baguette with a thin layer of goat cheese and top with the fig and olive mixture. Add a few pieces of toasted walnuts. Serve two slices per serving. |
| 3 ounces pasteurized goat cheese | |
| ⅓ cup chopped toasted walnuts | |

*Per serving:* Calories 233 (From Fat 86); Fat 10g (Saturated 3g); Cholesterol 6mg; Sodium 302mg; Carbohydrate 34g (Dietary Fiber 4g); Protein 5g; Iron 1mg; Calcium 59mg; Folate 24mcg.

*Note:* The explosion of different flavors in this recipe is wonderful! You get tangy from the goat cheese, salty from the olives, and sweet from the figs.

*Vary It!* If you aren't a fan of goat cheese, use light cream cheese instead.

# Steamed Artichoke with Garlic-Herb Dipping Sauce

**Prep time:** 10 min • **Cook time:** 25–35 min • **Yield:** 4 servings

| Ingredients | Directions |
|---|---|
| Water for boiling<br><br>1 whole raw artichoke<br><br>½ cup light mayonnaise<br><br>2 teaspoons fresh lemon juice<br><br>1 teaspoon minced garlic<br><br>1 teaspoon dried tarragon<br><br>Salt and pepper to taste | **1** Fill a pot with 3 inches of water and bring it to a boil over high heat.<br><br>**2** Remove the outer leaves of the artichoke and trim the stem. Place a steaming rack (or basket) in the pot over the boiling water. Place the artichoke on the rack with the stem side down. Cover and steam for 25 to 35 minutes, or until you can easily remove a petal from the inside of the artichoke. Remove the rack (or basket) from the pan and let the artichoke cool slightly.<br><br>**3** In a small bowl, combine the light mayonnaise, lemon juice, garlic, tarragon, and salt and pepper to taste. Serve the artichoke on a platter with the dipping sauce. |

*Per serving:* Calories 123 (From Fat 91); Fat 10g (Saturated 2g); Cholesterol 10mg; Sodium 279mg; Carbohydrate 7g (Dietary Fiber 2g); Protein 1g; Iron 1mg; Calcium 26mg; Folate 30mcg.

*Note:* Artichokes are one of the best sources of antioxidants, and they're relatively low in calories. I often use canned or jarred artichoke hearts in salads or pasta dishes.

*Tip:* If you don't have a steaming rack or basket for your pot, you can boil the artichoke. Doing so takes about 25 to 35 minutes. If you're short on time, you can microwave the artichoke. Just put it in a bowl with a little water, cover it with plastic wrap, and cook it on high for about 7 to 8 minutes.

*Tip:* To enjoy this recipe, pull each leaf from the artichoke and dip it into the sauce. Gently bite down on the leaf and scrape the "meat" of the artichoke with your teeth. Then discard the empty leaf.

# Sun-Dried Tomato and Ricotta Stuffed Mushrooms

**Prep time:** 15 min • **Cook time:** About 45 min • **Yield:** 5 servings

| Ingredients | Directions |
|---|---|
| ¾ cup water | *1* Preheat the oven to 425 degrees. Line a baking sheet with parchment paper. |
| ¼ cup bulgur wheat | |
| 1 tablespoon olive oil | *2* In a medium saucepan, bring the water to a boil. Add the bulgur wheat, cover the pan, and simmer on medium heat for 20 minutes. Drain the excess water if needed. Set aside. |
| 2 cloves garlic, minced | |
| 1 cup chopped kale | |
| ¼ cup chopped sun-dried tomatoes (not packed in oil) | *3* Heat the olive oil in a large skillet over medium heat. Add the garlic, kale, sun-dried tomatoes, parsley, and oregano and cook until the vegetables are softened, about 5 minutes. Remove from heat. |
| 1 tablespoon chopped fresh parsley | |
| 1 teaspoon dried oregano | |
| ¼ cup ricotta cheese | *4* In a medium bowl, combine the cooked bulgur wheat, vegetables, and ricotta cheese and stir until well mixed. |
| 10 large stuffing mushrooms, washed and patted dry | |
| | *5* Remove the stems from the mushrooms and arrange them, tops down, on the prepared baking sheet. Spoon the vegetable, bulgur, and cheese mixture (a few tablespoons) into each mushroom cap. |
| | *6* Bake the stuffed mushrooms for 20 minutes, or until they're tender and heated through. Serve immediately. |

*Per serving:* Calories 98 (From Fat 43); Fat 5g (Saturated 2g); Cholesterol 6mg; Sodium 76mg; Carbohydrate 11g (Dietary Fiber 3g); Protein 5g; Iron 1mg; Calcium 59mg; Folate 17mcg.

*Note:* Bulgur wheat is a whole grain often used in Mediterranean and Middle Eastern cooking. It's easy to prepare, and you can use it in recipes in place of rice.

*Vary It!* If you're not a fan of ricotta cheese, mix ¼ cup Parmesan cheese with the bulgur wheat and vegetables or top the mushrooms with mozzarella cheese instead (pasteurized, of course).

# Asian-Style Chicken Wings

**Prep time:** 10 min, plus marinating time • **Cook time:** 30–35 min • **Yield:** 4 servings

| Ingredients | Directions |
|---|---|
| 2 tablespoons low-sodium soy sauce | *1* In a small bowl, combine the soy sauce, sesame oil, honey, garlic, ginger, orange juice, orange zest, and five-spice powder. Mix well. |
| 2 tablespoons sesame oil | |
| 2 tablespoons honey | *2* Place the chicken wings in a large resealable plastic bag. Pour the marinade on top. Refrigerate for at least 2 hours, turning the bag over once. |
| 2 cloves garlic, minced | |
| 1 teaspoon minced fresh ginger | *3* After the chicken has marinated, preheat the oven to 425 degrees. Spray a wire cooling rack with non-stick cooking spray and place it on top of a rimmed baking sheet. |
| 2 tablespoons orange juice | |
| 1 teaspoon orange zest | |
| 1 teaspoon Chinese five-spice powder | *4* In a large bowl, combine the breadcrumbs, peanuts, and flour. Mix well. Roll the marinated wings in the breadcrumb mixture to coat them. Place each wing on the prepared wire rack. |
| 1½ pounds chicken wings, tips trimmed | |
| Nonstick cooking spray | |
| 1 cup panko breadcrumbs | *5* Bake the wings for 30 to 35 minutes, or until the wings are golden brown. |
| ¼ cup salted roasted peanuts, finely chopped | |
| ¼ cup all-purpose flour | |

*Per serving:* Calories 297 (From Fat 141); Fat 16g (Saturated 4g); Cholesterol 55mg; Sodium 172mg; Carbohydrate 17g (Dietary Fiber 1g); Protein 21g; Iron 1mg; Calcium 17mg; Folate 45mcg.

*Note:* Wings are traditionally pretty high in fat. But these wings are baked, so they're a much healthier option for when the mood strikes!

*Tip:* Use the marinade to coat boneless, skinless chicken tenders for an Asian-style main dish recipe. Serve with brown rice or rice noodles and stir-fry vegetables.

# Sausage-Stuffed Baked Potato Skins

**Prep time:** 15 min • **Cook time:** About 1 hr 20 min • **Yield:** 6 servings

| Ingredients | Directions |
|---|---|
| Nonstick cooking spray<br><br>3 large russet baking potatoes | **1** Preheat the oven to 375 degrees. Spray a baking sheet with nonstick cooking spray. |
| 1 tablespoon olive oil<br><br>4 cups fresh spinach | **2** Poke holes in the potatoes with a fork and bake the potatoes for 50 to 60 minutes. Allow them to cool for 5 minutes. |
| 1 cup crumbled lean ground sausage without casing<br><br>¼ cup plain breadcrumbs | **3** Handling the potatoes with a hot pad, slice each potato in half and scoop out the insides with a spoon, leaving a ¼-inch-thick shell. |
| 1 teaspoon dried oregano<br><br>¾ cup grated Swiss cheese | **4** In a medium skillet, heat the olive oil and sauté the spinach over medium heat until it's wilted, about 1 to 2 minutes. Transfer the spinach to a large bowl and set aside. |
| Salt and pepper to taste<br><br>2 tablespoons grated Parmesan cheese | **5** In the same skillet, cook the sausage over medium heat until it's lightly browned, about 8 to 10 minutes. Drain any excess oil and blot the sausage with paper towels if necessary. |
| ⅓ cup light sour cream (optional)<br><br>2 tablespoons fresh chives (optional) | **6** Add the sausage to the spinach, along with the breadcrumbs, oregano, Swiss cheese, and salt and pepper to taste. Mix well. |
| | **7** Spoon the sausage mixture into the baked potato skins. Sprinkle them with Parmesan cheese. Bake for 10 minutes, or until the stuffed potato skins are heated through. |
| | **8** Serve half a potato per person with light sour cream and fresh chives (if desired). |

*Per serving:* Calories 279 (From Fat 91); Fat 10g (Saturated 4g); Cholesterol 23mg; Sodium 238mg; Carbohydrate 36g (Dietary Fiber 4g); Protein 12g; Iron 3mg; Calcium 210mg; Folate 72mcg.

*Tip:* Save the insides of the potatoes for mashed potatoes on another day.

# Chicken Lettuce Wraps

**Prep time:** 15 min • **Cook time:** About 15 min • **Yield:** 4 servings

| *Ingredients* | *Directions* |
|---|---|
| 1 tablespoon sesame oil | *1* In a large skillet, heat the sesame oil over medium-high heat. Add the ginger, water chestnuts, and chicken and sauté until the chicken is cooked through, about 10 minutes. |
| 2 teaspoons minced fresh or ground ginger | |
| One 8-ounce can sliced water chestnuts, drained and chopped | *2* Reduce the heat to medium and add the green onions, cabbage, carrots, soy sauce, and teriyaki sauce. Cook until the cabbage is tender, about 2 to 3 minutes more. |
| 1 pound ground chicken breast | |
| 2 green onions, chopped | |
| 1 cup shredded cabbage | *3* Rinse the lettuce leaves and pat them dry with a paper towel. |
| ⅓ cup shredded carrots | |
| 2 tablespoons low-sodium soy sauce | *4* Spoon equal amounts of the chicken mixture onto the center of each lettuce leaf; roll up the leaves and serve. |
| 1 tablespoon teriyaki sauce | |
| 8 leaves of lettuce (Bibb or iceberg) | |

*Per serving:* Calories 204 (From Fat 58); Fat 6g (Saturated 1g); Cholesterol 63mg; Sodium 545mg; Carbohydrate 11g (Dietary Fiber 4g); Protein 25g; Iron 1mg; Calcium 39mg; Folate 39mcg.

*Vary It!* For a vegetarian version, use tofu in place of the chicken.

*Note:* To allow guests to personalize their wraps, serve them with a choice of garnishes, such as sunflower seeds, slivered almonds, chopped peanuts, or dried cranberries.

# White Chicken and Pineapple Flatbread

**Prep time:** 10 min • **Cook time:** 13–15 min • **Yield:** 2 servings

| Ingredients | Directions |
|---|---|
| 1 store-bought whole-wheat flatbread | *1* Preheat the oven to 375 degrees. Place the flatbread directly on the oven rack and bake for 5 minutes. |
| 3 tablespoons prepared Alfredo sauce | |
| ¼ cup chopped pineapple | *2* Spread the Alfredo sauce on top of the hot flatbread. Top with the pineapple, chicken, and mushrooms. Separate the onion slice into rings and place them on the flatbread. Sprinkle the top of the flatbread with the mozzarella cheese. |
| ½ cup shredded, cooked chicken breast | |
| ¼ cup sliced mushrooms | |
| 1 slice onion | *3* Bake for 8 to 10 minutes, or until the flatbread is warmed and the cheese is melted. |
| ¼ cup shredded mozzarella cheese | |
| | *4* Cut the flatbread in half with a pizza cutter and serve immediately. |

*Per serving: Calories 344 (From Fat 119); Fat 13g (Saturated 5g); Cholesterol 50mg; Sodium 511mg; Carbohydrate 35g (Dietary Fiber 6g); Protein 22g; Iron 2mg; Calcium 127mg; Folate 29mcg.*

*Note:* Flatbreads have become really popular in recent years. You can serve them as an appetizer or easily make a meal out of them. Look for whole-grain flatbreads that contain between 100 and 150 calories. I like the Flatout brand.

*Vary It!* For a Mediterranean-style flatbread, use sun-dried tomato pesto in place of the Alfredo sauce, swap pasteurized feta for the mozzarella cheese, and substitute olives for the pineapple.

## How to Trim and Slice Mushrooms

**Figure 13-3:**
How to trim and slice mushrooms.

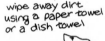
1. wipe away dirt using a paper towel or a dish towel

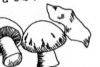

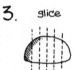
2. Cut off stem

3. slice

# Adding Color (And Nutrients) to Your Plate with Salads

What better way to add a little color to your plate — and squeeze in some servings of fruits and vegetables — than with a nice salad? Choose dark greens and vibrantly colored fruits and vegetables to add a handful of flavor and nutrients to any meal. The key to keeping salads interesting is to combine a variety of flavors to meet your taste palate.

Pregnant women require 2 to 4 (or more!) cups of vegetables per day plus 2 to 3 cups of fruit. If that sounds intimidating, consider that 2 cups of leafy greens is equivalent to 1 cup in terms of serving size. So a nice big salad could net you all your servings of vegetables for the day, and a side salad may get you to one-third (or even one-half) of your requirement. Plus, salads offer a bevy of nutrients. Salad greens and most fruits and veggies provide you with folate, potassium, fiber, and antioxidants. Throw some cheese on your salad and you get calcium; add meat or beans and you get protein and iron (both of which are vital during pregnancy, as I note in Chapter 3).

Try each of this section's nine salad recipes as a main dish or pair them with the following for meals that offer a little more variety:

- ✔ The Mixed Greens with Chicken, Cantaloupe, & Red Grapes Salad works well in a brunch menu with the Broccoli Hash-Brown Quiche in Chapter 12.

- ✔ The Fruity Poppy Seed Salad pairs well with the White Chicken and Pineapple Flatbread in the preceding section.

- ✔ The White Bean and Portobello Salad offers a nice complement to the Spinach, Date, and Blue Cheese Chicken Panini in Chapter 14.

- ✔ The Fresh Mozzarella, Tomato, and Pepper Salad makes a nice starter for Chapter 14's mouth-watering Italian Stuffed Steak Rolls.

- ✔ The Roasted Beet and Pistachio Salad pairs well with a hearty soup like the Souped-Up Split Pea Soup or Black Bean Chili in Chapter 15.

- ✔ If you're feeling Greek, the Deconstructed Greek Salad goes great with the Spanakopita (Greek Spinach Pie) in Chapter 15.

- ✔ The Asian Chicken Spinach Salad is even better when you follow it up with the Mango Coconut Rice Pudding in Chapter 16.

- ✔ The sweetness of the Creamy Grape Salad goes nicely with the crispy Zucchini Patties in Chapter 15.

- ✔ The Cranberry Gelatin Salad works as a sweet side or dessert with the Parmesan-Herb-Crusted Pork Chops in Chapter 14.

# Mixed Greens with Chicken, Cantaloupe, & Red Grapes Salad

**Prep time:** 10 min • **Yield:** 4 servings

| *Ingredients* | *Directions* |
|---|---|
| One 6-ounce bag mixed greens | *1* In a large bowl, combine the greens, chicken, grapes, and cantaloupe. Mix well. |
| 1½ cups chopped cooked rotisserie chicken | |
| 1½ cups red grapes, rinsed | *2* Toss the salad with the ranch dressing to taste. |
| ½ large cantaloupe, peeled, seeded, and chopped | |
| ½ cup light ranch dressing, or to taste | |

*Per serving: Calories 262 (From Fat 103); Fat 12g (Saturated 2g); Cholesterol 55mg; Sodium 612mg; Carbohydrate 24g (Dietary Fiber 3g); Protein 18g; Iron 2mg; Calcium 57mg; Folate 72mcg.*

***Vary It!*** To add some crunch to this salad, sprinkle on some glazed sliced almonds. To boost your calcium, sprinkle on some shredded mozzarella cheese.

***Tip:*** If you're cooking up chicken breasts for dinner, make one or two extra to use in salads like this one the next day.

*Source: Anne Nechkov, professional food stylist and chef*

# Fruity Poppy Seed Salad

**Prep time:** 10 min • **Yield:** 1 serving

| Ingredients | Directions |
|---|---|
| 1 cup spring lettuce | *1* In a large bowl, toss together the lettuce, apple, strawberries, oranges, cranberries, onion, cheese, sunflower seeds, and granola. |
| 1 cup romaine lettuce | |
| ¼ apple, sliced thin | |
| ¼ cup sliced strawberries | *2* Toss the salad with the poppy seed dressing to taste. |
| 2 tablespoons mandarin oranges | |
| 1 tablespoon dried cranberries | |
| 1 tablespoon red onion | |
| 1 tablespoon pasteurized Gorgonzola cheese | |
| 1 tablespoon sunflower seeds | |
| 2 tablespoons granola | |
| 2 tablespoons poppy seed dressing, or to taste | |

*Per serving:* Calories 391 (From Fat 212); Fat 24g (Saturated 3g); Cholesterol 6mg; Sodium 366mg; Carbohydrate 40g (Dietary Fiber 6g); Protein 8g; Iron 2mg; Calcium 104mg; Folate 170mcg.

*Note:* The variety of fruit in this salad brings a welcomed sweet flavor; it's almost like having dessert for lunch!

*Tip:* To make this salad a main dish, add 3 ounces of cooked chicken or tofu or ½ cup of beans or cottage cheese.

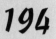

# White Bean and Portobello Salad

**Prep time:** 10 min • **Cook time:** 5–7 min • **Yield:** 1 serving

| Ingredients | Directions |
| --- | --- |

**Ingredients**

Nonstick cooking spray

1 large portobello mushroom cap, sliced into ¼-inch strips

1 teaspoon plus 2 teaspoons balsamic vinegar

2 cups fresh spinach, stems removed

1 slice red onion

⅓ cup canned navy beans, drained and rinsed

¼ cup chopped sun-dried tomatoes (not packed in oil)

2 tablespoons sliced black olives

2 tablespoons shredded Parmesan cheese

1 tablespoon pine nuts

2 teaspoons olive oil

**Directions**

*1* Spray a medium nonstick skillet with cooking spray and heat it over medium heat. Add the mushroom and 1 teaspoon of balsamic vinegar and cook until the mushroom is tender, about 5 to 7 minutes, turning once.

*2* In a large bowl, combine the spinach, onion, beans, tomatoes, olives, cheese, and pine nuts. Toss the salad with 2 teaspoons each of balsamic vinegar and olive oil for the dressing. Place the hot portobello strips on top of the salad.

*Per serving:* Calories 395 (From Fat 175); Fat 19g (Saturated 4g); Cholesterol 8mg; Sodium 791mg; Carbohydrate 39g (Dietary Fiber 10g); Protein 20g; Iron 7mg; Calcium 304mg; Folate 196mcg.

*Note:* I have a slight obsession with beans because they're a high-fiber, plant-based source of protein that also contains plenty of folate, potassium, iron, and other nutrients that are ideal for pregnant women. Try this (and other salad recipes, for that matter) with kidney beans, garbanzo beans, or black beans.

# Fresh Mozzarella, Tomato, and Pepper Salad

**Prep time:** 15 min • **Yield:** 1 serving

| *Ingredients* | *Directions* |
|---|---|
| 2 cups spring lettuce mix | *1* Place the lettuce in a bowl and top it with the tomato, bell pepper, pepperoncini, mozzarella cheese, and fresh basil. |
| 1 plum tomato, sliced | |
| ¼ yellow bell pepper, seeded and sliced | |
| 2 tablespoons sliced pepperoncini | *2* Drizzle the salad with the balsamic vinegar and olive oil. Toss everything together (if desired). |
| Two 2-inch slices fresh, pasteurized mozzarella | |
| 4 leaves fresh basil, chopped | |
| 1 tablespoon balsamic vinegar | |
| 2 teaspoons olive oil | |

*Per serving:* Calories 295 (From Fat 196); Fat 22g (Saturated 9g); Cholesterol 45mg; Sodium 303mg; Carbohydrate 13g (Dietary Fiber 4g); Protein 13g; Iron 3mg; Calcium 404mg; Folate 146mcg.

*Note:* The inspiration behind this salad comes from the traditional Caprese salad with fresh mozzarella, basil, and tomatoes. When you add in pepperoncinis and throw the whole thing onto a base of mixed greens, you get a completely different look and feel for this traditional favorite.

*Tip:* You can also use small bite-sized balls of fresh mozzarella for this recipe. Just make sure the cheese is pasteurized.

# Roasted Beet and Pistachio Salad

**Prep time:** 20 min • **Cook time:** 30–45 min • **Yield:** 4 servings

| Ingredients | Directions |
|---|---|
| Nonstick cooking spray | *1* Preheat the oven to 350 degrees. Spray a baking dish with nonstick cooking spray. Place the beets on the baking sheet and cover with foil. Bake for 30 to 45 minutes, or until the beets are tender when pierced with a fork. Set aside to cool. |
| 4 red beets, trimmed | |
| 2 shallots, chopped | |
| 1 tablespoon chopped fresh thyme | |
| 2 tablespoons olive oil | *2* After the beets have cooled to the touch, remove their outer skin by rubbing them with a paper towel. Slice the beets thinly. |
| 1 tablespoon balsamic vinegar | |
| Salt and pepper to taste | *3* In a large bowl, combine the shallots, thyme, olive oil, balsamic vinegar, and salt and pepper to taste. Add the sliced beets. |
| One 6-ounce package spring mix lettuce | |
| ½ cup crumbled, pasteurized goat cheese | *4* Place the lettuce on individual serving plates and top each serving with one-fourth of the beet mixture, goat cheese, and pistachios. |
| ½ cup shelled pistachios | |

*Per serving:* Calories 240 (From Fat 165); Fat 18g (Saturated 5g); Cholesterol 11mg; Sodium 125mg; Carbohydrate 14g (Dietary Fiber 4g); Protein 8g; Iron 2mg; Calcium 98mg; Folate 101mcg.

*Tip:* For best results, cover and refrigerate the prepared beet mixture for at least 3 hours before serving.

*Note:* This salad is so flavorful that you don't even need additional dressing. However, if you must, drizzle your salad with additional balsamic vinegar and olive oil or a vinaigrette of your choice.

# Deconstructed Greek Salad

**Prep time:** 15 min • **Yield:** 4 servings

| *Ingredients* | *Directions* |
|---|---|
| 3 medium red tomatoes, chopped | *1* In a large bowl, combine the tomatoes, cucumber, onion, green pepper, radishes, olives, and feta cheese cubes. |
| 1 large cucumber, peeled and chopped | |
| ½ small red onion, chopped | *2* In a small bowl, whisk together the olive oil, vinegars, mustard, garlic powder, oregano, basil, crumbled feta cheese, and salt and pepper to taste. |
| 1 green bell pepper, seeds removed and chopped | |
| 8 radishes, chopped | *3* Pour the dressing over the veggies and toss to coat evenly. |
| ½ cup kalamata olives, pitted | |
| ½ cup pasteurized feta cheese cubes | |
| 3 tablespoons olive oil | |
| 2 tablespoons red wine vinegar | |
| 2 tablespoons balsamic vinegar | |
| ½ teaspoon Dijon mustard | |
| ¼ teaspoon garlic powder | |
| ½ teaspoon dried oregano | |
| ½ teaspoon dried basil | |
| 1 tablespoon crumbled, pasteurized feta cheese | |
| Salt and pepper to taste | |

*Per serving:* Calories 244 (From Fat 174); Fat 19g (Saturated 5g); Cholesterol 19mg; Sodium 514mg; Carbohydrate 15g (Dietary Fiber 3g); Protein 5g; Iron 1mg; Calcium 143mg; Folate 48mcg.

*Note:* This salad is a twist on the traditional Greek village salad. Instead of lettuce, this salad consists of large chunks of vegetables combined with feta cheese and olives.

# Asian Chicken Spinach Salad

**Prep time:** 20 min • **Yield:** 2 servings

## Ingredients

4 cups fresh spinach

1 green onion, chopped

⅓ cup shredded carrots

⅓ red bell pepper, sliced

⅓ cup shelled, cooked edamame

⅓ cup mandarin oranges, rinsed and drained

1 tablespoon brown sugar

2 tablespoons low-sodium soy sauce

1 tablespoon sesame oil

2 tablespoons rice vinegar

½ teaspoon Dijon mustard

¼ teaspoon minced fresh ginger

One 8-ounce boneless, skinless chicken breast, cooked and shredded

¼ cup slivered almonds

## Directions

1   In a large bowl, combine the spinach, green onion, carrots, bell pepper, edamame, and oranges.

2   In a small bowl, whisk together the brown sugar, soy sauce, sesame oil, vinegar, mustard, and ginger.

3   Top the salad with the cooked chicken breast, slivered almonds, and soy-sauce-ginger dressing. Toss to coat everything evenly.

*Per serving:* Calories 502 (From Fat 175); Fat 19g (Saturated 3g); Cholesterol 96mg; Sodium 840mg; Carbohydrate 38g (Dietary Fiber 11g); Protein 46g; Iron 5mg; Calcium 189mg; Folate 232mcg.

*Note:* This very colorful, nutrient-rich salad can be a side salad without the chicken or an entree salad with the chicken.

# Creamy Grape Salad

**Prep time:** 15 min • **Yield:** 5 servings

| *Ingredients* | *Directions* |
|---|---|
| 1 cup green grapes, rinsed and sliced in half | *1* In a large bowl, combine the grapes, pineapple, and apple. Drizzle the fruit with the lemon juice and stir. |
| 1 cup red grapes, rinsed and sliced in half | |
| One 15-ounce can pineapple chunks, drained | *2* In a small mixing bowl, beat together the sugar, sour cream, cream cheese, and vanilla. |
| 1 Golden Delicious apple, diced | |
| 1 teaspoon fresh lemon juice | *3* Add the creamed mixture to the fruit and stir with a spoon until the fruit is coated evenly. Sprinkle the chopped pecans on top of the grape salad before serving. |
| ¼ cup sugar | |
| 4 ounces light sour cream | |
| 4 ounces light cream cheese, softened | |
| ½ teaspoon vanilla extract | |
| ¼ cup chopped pecans | |

*Per serving: Calories 245 (From Fat 104); Fat 12g (Saturated 5g); Cholesterol 25mg; Sodium 114mg; Carbohydrate 35g (Dietary Fiber 2g); Protein 4g; Iron 1mg; Calcium 69mg; Folate 10mcg.*

*Note:* This recipe features a couple of slight twists to the traditional Waldorf salad. I'm not a fan of celery, so I leave it out. But you're welcome to add in ½ cup of chopped celery if you prefer. I also use pecans rather than walnuts, but feel free to use your favorite nut.

*Tip:* This salad is rich and creamy enough to serve as a dessert. It's also a great item to bring to a potluck.

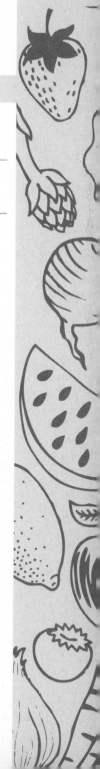

# Cranberry Gelatin Salad

**Prep time:** 10 min, plus refrigerating time • **Cook time:** About 7 min • **Yield:** 8 servings

| Ingredients | Directions |
|---|---|
| 1 cup water | **1** Bring the water to a boil. Add the gelatin mix to the boiling water and stir until all the mix is dissolved. |
| One 3-ounce package cranberry gelatin mix | |
| One 15-ounce can whole cranberry sauce | **2** Mix in the cranberry sauce, apples, and banana. Pour the mixture into a large glass or ceramic dish and refrigerate until formed, about 90 minutes. |
| 1 small Granny Smith apple, diced | |
| 1 small Red Delicious apple, diced | **3** Spread the whipped topping on top of the formed salad and serve cold. |
| 1 large banana, sliced | |
| 1 cup light frozen whipped topping, thawed | |

*Per serving:* Calories 166 (From Fat 11); Fat 1g (Saturated 0g); Cholesterol 0mg; Sodium 36mg; Carbohydrate 39g (Dietary Fiber 2g); Protein 1g; Iron 0mg; Calcium 3mg; Folate 4mcg.

*Note:* This salad is great for a holiday gathering, but because canned cranberry sauce is available year-round, you can enjoy Cranberry Gelatin Salad anytime of the year.

*Tip:* Fruity gelatin salads are a great way to get fresh or canned fruit into a meal. Serve this salad as a side dish or a dessert.

# Chapter 14

# The Land, Sea, and Air: Main Dish Recipes

**Recipes in This Chapter**

▶ Good to the Last Lick Casserole
▶ Beef Empanadas
▶ Beef and Bean Quesadillas
▶ Nana's Moussaka
▶ Indian Lentil Slow Cooker Beef Stew
▶ Italian Stuffed Steak Rolls
▶ Cocoa-Rubbed Grilled Steaks
▶ Spaghetti with Clam Sauce
▶ Mango Avocado Salmon
▶ Pecan-Crusted Tilapia with Pear and Fig Chutney
▶ Thai Scallops with Noodles
▶ Garden Fresh Paella
▶ Super Easy Pulled Pork
▶ Parmesan-Herb-Crusted Pork Chops
▶ Turkey Cheeseburger Chowder
▶ Sauerkraut and Turkey Sausage Pasta Bake
▶ Rosemary Chicken on Asparagus Risotto
▶ Curry Chicken Salad
▶ Crispy Lime Chicken Tenders
▶ Chicken Kabobs
▶ Peachy Chicken Barley Pilaf
▶ Spinach, Date, and Blue Cheese Chicken Panini

🍴 🥄 🍷 🌶 🌿

## In This Chapter

▶ Enjoying lean cuts of beef in a variety of ways
▶ Tempting your palate with an assortment of seafood
▶ Creating delicious ways to savor the white meats: pork, turkey, and chicken

**I**f you're looking for a meal idea that packs a nutrient-dense punch, look no further than meat! Beef, chicken, turkey, pork, and seafood are all packed in nutrition for you and your baby. In fact, some of the most important pregnancy nutrients — namely iron, zinc, and B vitamins — are abundant in animal proteins such as beef, poultry, pork, seafood, and eggs.

The recipes in this chapter are guaranteed to satisfy your tastes for ethnic dishes (think Italian, Asian, Greek, Caribbean, Mexican, Latin, and Indian) as well as those down-home traditional recipes everyone loves — all with a nutrient-rich pregnancy twist, of course. Every recipe included in this chapter has you and your developing baby in mind. Not only do these recipes provide you all the nutrients found in meat, but they also include plenty of whole grains, fruits, and vegetables to further boost their nutritional value.

In addition to the wide mix of flavors you get in this chapter, you find a variety of cooking styles. By the time you finish reading, you'll be baking, broiling, sautéing, slow cooking, and (if you're lucky) convincing your partner to do a little grilling. So get ready to fill up on the delicious proteins that await you in this chapter's recipes.

# Beef, It's What's for Pregnancy

Not many main dishes are as dense in nutrients as beef, which is why it's at the top of the pregnancy must-have food list. It's really too bad beef got a bad rap a few years ago for being high in fat because it's really not as fatty as you may think. Twenty-nine cuts of beef actually meet the U.S. Government's guidelines for lean meat, and the leanest of them all is an eye round roast or steak. This particular cut has just 144 calories and 4 grams of fat (1.4 grams of which are saturated). That's almost as lean as a skinless chicken breast!

Many people shy away from lean cuts of beef because they fear they may not be as moist. If I've just described you, it's time to learn the cooking techniques of braising, roasting, and stewing. A day in the slow cooker makes any cut of lean beef fall apart as soon as you pierce it with a fork. Marinating lean beef can also help to tenderize and moisten it for your eating pleasure.

Whether or not the cut of beef you're working with is lean, always be aware of the following beef-focused food safety guidelines (for more information on food safety, flip to Chapter 10):

- ✔ When you're cutting raw beef, always use a separate cutting board from the one you use for vegetables. After you finish cutting, wash the board and utensils well with hot, soapy water.

- ✔ Cook beef until it reaches an internal temperature of 160 degrees or higher according to a meat thermometer.

- ✔ Trim any visible fat from steak before grilling so that you don't get flare-ups of fire. Fat drips off when heated, which is a good thing because then you don't eat it but a bad thing if the flame shoots up near your face or hands.

The seven beef recipes in this chapter offer you an assortment of different ways to cook beef. The first recipe, Good to the Last Lick Casserole, has been in my family for generations. Life on the farm in Wisconsin meant meat and potatoes, and this casserole was the perfect way to cook a delicious, filling meal and still complete all the daily chores of farm life. The next several recipes take you on an international adventure that ends with a down-home feel thanks to Cocoa-Rubbed Grilled Steak. Yep, you read that right: Chocolate steak!

***Note:*** Several of the recipes in this section call for lean ground beef. Even though the 90 percent lean beef may cost a bit more, leaner beef requires less waste (in the form of grease to drain off), which means more meat for your dollar and more nutrients! The dollars you spend on more nutritious food are well worth the benefits to you and your baby!

# Good to the Last Lick Casserole

**Prep time:** 15 min • **Cook time:** 1 hr 30 min • **Yield:** 4 servings

| *Ingredients* | *Directions* |
|---|---|
| **Nonstick cooking spray** | *1* Preheat the oven to 350 degrees. Spray a 2-quart casserole dish with nonstick cooking spray. |
| **One 10.5-ounce can condensed tomato soup** | |
| **One 8-ounce can tomato sauce** | *2* In a small bowl, mix together the tomato soup, tomato sauce, salt, garlic powder, and oregano. |
| **½ teaspoon salt** | |
| **¼ teaspoon garlic powder** | *3* In a large bowl, mix together ½ of the chopped onion with the potatoes and corn. Stir in ⅔ of the tomato soup mixture. Pour the veggie and tomato soup mixture into the prepared casserole dish. |
| **½ teaspoon dried oregano** | |
| **1 onion, chopped** | |
| **4 medium potatoes, peeled and sliced** | *4* Crumble the raw beef over the vegetable mixture. Top the beef with the remaining onions and the rest of the tomato soup mixture. |
| **2 cups frozen corn, thawed, or 2 cups canned corn, drained** | |
| **1 pound lean ground beef** | *5* Cover the casserole with foil and bake for 1 hour and 30 minutes. Divide into fourths and serve. |

*Per serving: Calories 418 (From Fat 88); Fat 10g (Saturated 3g); Cholesterol 31mg; Sodium 776mg; Carbohydrate 62g (Dietary Fiber 6g); Protein 25g; Iron 4mg; Calcium 37mg; Folate 72mcg.*

***Note:*** Because this casserole cooks for an entire hour and 30 minutes, you don't have to worry about mixing raw beef with your vegetables. Everything will be cooked and safe by the time you get it out of the oven.

*Source: Elaine Kohls, grandmother of author*

# Beef Empanadas

**Prep time:** 20 min • **Cook time:** 37–40 min • **Yield:** 6 servings

| Ingredients | Directions |
|---|---|
| Nonstick cooking spray | **1** Preheat the oven to 375 degrees. Spray a baking sheet with nonstick cooking spray. |
| 1 tablespoon olive oil | |
| 1 onion, chopped | **2** In a medium skillet, heat the olive oil over medium heat. Sauté the onion and bell peppers until they're tender, about 5 minutes. |
| ¼ cup finely chopped green bell pepper | |
| ¼ cup finely chopped red bell pepper | **3** In a separate large skillet, cook the ground beef until it's brown, about 8 minutes. Add the salt, pepper, and paprika and cook for 2 more minutes. Add the cooked onions and peppers, olives, tomato, and raisins and cook until the flavors are well blended, about 10 minutes. Remove the skillet from heat, stir in the hard-boiled egg, and set the mixture aside. |
| ¾ pound lean ground beef | |
| ¼ teaspoon salt | |
| ¼ teaspoon pepper | |
| 2 teaspoons paprika | |
| ¼ cup sliced green olives | |
| 1 small tomato, peeled and chopped | **4** Place ¼ cup of water in a small bowl. Spread the dough for one empanada on a clean counter and roll it out until it's about ½ inch thick. Scoop 1 heaping tablespoon of the beef filling onto the dough, leaving a ¾-inch border of dough. Wet your finger with the water and lightly spread it over the border. Fold the dough over and press the outside edge with a fork to seal. Repeat until you run out of dough and filling. |
| ¼ cup raisins | |
| 1 egg, hard boiled and chopped | |
| ¼ cup plus 1 teaspoon water | |
| One 14-ounce package ready-made frozen empanada dough, thawed | **5** Beat the egg with 1 teaspoon of water. Brush the top of each empanada with the egg mixture. Place the empanadas on the baking sheet and bake for 12 to 15 minutes, or until they're brown on top. Serve immediately. |
| 1 egg | |

*Per serving: Calories 369 (From Fat 144); Fat 16g (Saturated 4g); Cholesterol 86mg; Sodium 489mg; Carbohydrate 44g (Dietary Fiber 3g); Protein 20g; Iron 4mg; Calcium 24mg; Folate 22mcg.*

**Tip:** Look for the Goya brand frozen empanada dough called *discos.* If you can't find frozen empanada dough, you can use pizza dough instead. Just roll out the pizza dough and cut it to the desired size of your empanada (I recommend ½ inch thick and 5 inches in diameter).

*Source: Verna Flemming, friend of author*

# Beef and Bean Quesadillas

**Prep time:** 10 min  •  **Cook time:** 15–20 min  •  **Yield:** 4 servings

| Ingredients | Directions |
|---|---|
| 1 tablespoon canola oil | *1* Preheat the oven to 400 degrees. Line a baking sheet with aluminum foil. |
| 4 ounces flank steak, sliced | |
| ½ cup chopped onion | *2* In a medium skillet, heat the oil over medium heat. Add the flank steak and sauté for 5 minutes, stirring frequently. |
| ½ cup chopped plum tomatoes | |
| ½ cup canned black beans, drained and rinsed | *3* Add the onion and tomatoes and cook for another 5 minutes, stirring frequently. Line a medium bowl with a paper towel. Place the beef and onion mixture on top of the paper towel to remove any excess oil. |
| ½ cup shredded cheddar cheese | |
| 8 small corn tortillas | *4* Place four corn tortillas on the baking sheet. Spoon ¼ of the steak mixture onto each tortilla and top each one with equal amounts of black beans and cheese. Add another corn tortilla to the top of each quesadilla and press down softly. |
| | *5* Bake for 5 to 10 minutes, or until the tortillas are slightly brown. |

*Per serving:* Calories 285 (From Fat 107); Fat 12g (Saturated 4g); Cholesterol 28mg; Sodium 251mg; Carbohydrate 31g (Dietary Fiber 5g); Protein 14g; Iron 2mg; Calcium 209mg; Folate 91mcg.

*Tip:* To prevent the quesadillas from curling up while baking, give the top layer a quick shot of nonstick cooking spray.

*Source: Elisa Zied, RD, and author of Feed Your Family Right! (John Wiley & Sons, Inc.) and Nutrition at Your Fingertips (Alpha)*

# Nana's Moussaka

**Prep time:** 15 min, plus standing time • **Cook time:** About 1 hr 45 min • **Yield:** 8 servings

| *Ingredients* | *Directions* |
|---|---|
| 1 large eggplant<br><br>Dash plus ¼ teaspoon plus ¼ teaspoon salt<br><br>1 tablespoon plus 1 tablespoon plus ¼ cup olive oil<br><br>1 onion, diced<br><br>1 pound lean ground beef<br><br>2 ripe tomatoes, diced<br><br>¼ teaspoon plus ¼ teaspoon pepper<br><br>¼ cup flour<br><br>4 cups lowfat milk<br><br>2 eggs, beaten<br><br>2 teaspoons ground cinnamon<br><br>½ teaspoon ground nutmeg | **1** Preheat the oven to 350 degrees. Slice the eggplant into 1-inch-thick slices. Sprinkle the eggplant with a dash of salt and place it in a colander; let it stand for 30 minutes.<br><br>**2** Coat an 11-x-17-inch baking sheet with 1 tablespoon of olive oil. Layer the eggplant slices on the pan and bake for 20 minutes. Set aside.<br><br>**3** In a large skillet, heat 1 tablespoon of olive oil over medium heat. Sauté the onion until it's tender, about 5 minutes. Add the ground beef and cook until it's browned, about 8 minutes, stirring frequently. Add the tomatoes, ¼ teaspoon of salt, and ¼ teaspoon of pepper and let everything simmer on low for about 5 minutes.<br><br>**4** To prepare the béchamel sauce for the moussaka, heat ¼ cup of olive oil in a medium saucepan over medium heat. Add the flour and cook until the mixture turns a golden color, about 5 minutes. Add the milk and increase the heat to medium-high, stirring constantly to prevent lumps. Bring the mixture to a gentle boil and boil until the sauce has thickened, about 20 minutes.<br><br>**5** Reduce the heat for the sauce to low. Add about ¼ cup of the sauce to the beaten eggs and stir well. Add the egg mixture to the remaining sauce in the pan, stirring constantly. Add the cinnamon, nutmeg, and the rest of the salt and pepper. Continue to stir for 1 more minute.<br><br>**6** To assemble the moussaka, lay the baked eggplant in the bottom of a 2-quart baking dish. Cover it with the beef mixture. Slowly pour the béchamel sauce on top and bake uncovered for 1 hour. |

*Per serving:* Calories 271 (From Fat 152); Fat 17g (Saturated 4g); Cholesterol 74mg; Sodium 204mg; Carbohydrate 15g (Dietary Fiber 2g); Protein 16g; Iron 2mg; Calcium 173mg; Folate 37mcg.

*Source: Evie Lyras, friend of author*

# Indian Lentil Slow Cooker Beef Stew

**Prep time:** 15 min • **Cook time:** 8 hr • **Yield:** 8 servings

| *Ingredients* | *Directions* |
|---|---|
| 1 medium onion, chopped | *1* In a 4- or 6-quart slow cooker, mix together the onion, cauliflower, zucchini, bell pepper, mushrooms, tomatoes, and lentils. Place the beef on top. Add the beef broth, garlic, salt, curry powder, ginger, salt, and nutmeg. Stir everything together. |
| 1 cup bite-sized cauliflower florets | |
| 2 medium zucchini, chopped | |
| 1 red bell pepper, seeded and chopped | |
| One 8-ounce package button mushrooms, sliced | *2* Cover the slow cooker tightly and heat on low for 8 hours. |
| One 14-ounce can no-salt-added diced tomatoes, undrained | |
| 1 cup uncooked lentils, rinsed and picked over | |
| 2 pounds lean chuck or round stew meat, cubed | |
| Three 14-ounce cans low-sodium beef broth | |
| 2 cloves garlic, minced | |
| ½ teaspoon salt | |
| 1 teaspoon curry powder | |
| ½ teaspoon ground ginger | |
| ¼ teaspoon salt | |
| ½ teaspoon ground nutmeg | |

*Per serving:* Calories 293 (From Fat 76); Fat 8g (Saturated 3g); Cholesterol 71mg; Sodium 636mg; Carbohydrate 22g (Dietary Fiber 8g); Protein 33g; Iron 6mg; Calcium 45mg; Folate 160mcg.

*Note:* Even though you may be tempted, don't lift the lid of the slow cooker! Doing so could increase the stew's cooking time by 20 to 30 minutes. Let the stew cook for 8 hours and uncover it when you're ready to serve. (If you don't want to wait 8 hours, increase the heat to the high setting and cook for 4 to 5 hours.)

*Note:* To "pick over" lentils, simply run your hands through the lentils, looking for small stones or debris that may have gotten mixed in during harvesting. Discard anything that doesn't look edible.

*Vary It!* If you aren't fond of Indian spices, leave out the curry, ginger, and nutmeg and use oregano instead.

*Source: Adapted from The Healthy Beef Cookbook by the American Dietetic Association (ADA), the National Cattleman's Beef Association, Richard Chamberlain, and Betsy Hornick, ©2006 (American Dietetic Association and American Cattleman's Beef Association), with permission of John Wiley & Sons, Inc.*

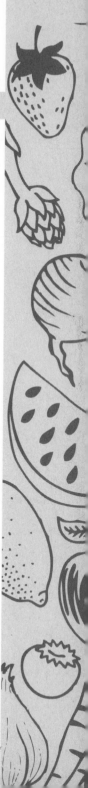

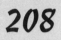

# *Italian Stuffed Steak Rolls*

**Prep time:** 20 min • **Cook time:** About 2 hr 8 min • **Yield:** 4 servings

| *Ingredients* | *Directions* |
|---|---|
| One 10-ounce package frozen spinach, thawed | *1* Preheat the oven to 350 degrees. |
| 2 tablespoons pepperoncini peppers, diced | *2* Squeeze the spinach to remove as much of the excess water as possible. Place it in a medium bowl. Add the peppers, garlic, oregano, red onion, Parmesan cheese, breadcrumbs, and mozzarella cheese. Mix everything together with a fork until it's well blended. |
| 2 cloves garlic, minced | |
| 1 teaspoon dried oregano | |
| 2 tablespoons red onion, chopped | |
| ¼ cup Parmesan cheese | *3* Slice the round steak into four pieces (about 2-x-4 inches each) and pound each piece with a meat tenderizer until they're ½ inch thin. Top each piece of steak with ¼ of the spinach mixture. Roll up each steak and tie it with a clean butcher's string. |
| ¼ cup plain breadcrumbs | |
| ¼ cup shredded mozzarella cheese | |
| 1 pound top round steak | *4* In a large nonstick skillet, heat the oil over medium heat. Add the rolls to the skillet and cook them until they're brown, about 2 minutes on each side, turning them carefully so that all four sides are browned. |
| 1 tablespoon olive oil | |
| One 28-ounce jar marinara sauce | *5* Pour the marinara sauce into the bottom of a 2-quart oven-safe casserole dish. Carefully place each roll into the sauce. |
| | *6* Cover the dish and bake for 2 hours. Remove the rolls from the dish, untie and discard the string, and place each roll on a serving plate. Top with the marinara sauce and serve. |

*Per serving:* Calories 414 (From Fat 174); Fat 19g (Saturated 6g); Cholesterol 74mg; Sodium 1,167mg; Carbohydrate 26g (Dietary Fiber 6g); Protein 34g; Iron 6mg; Calcium 253mg; Folate 122mcg.

*Note:* To reduce the sodium in this dish, look for reduced-sodium cheese and marinara sauce.

# Cocoa-Rubbed Grilled Steaks

**Prep time:** 5 min, plus refrigerating time • **Cook time:** 12–14 min • **Yield:** 2 servings

| Ingredients | Directions |
|---|---|
| 1 teaspoon sea salt | *1* Preheat the grill or grill pan to medium heat. |
| ¼ teaspoon unsweetened cocoa powder | |
| 2 tablespoons ground cinnamon | *2* In a small bowl, mix together the sea salt, cocoa powder, cinnamon, pepper, cumin, brown sugar, chili powder, garlic powder, and onion powder; stir until well combined. |
| 1 teaspoon pepper | |
| 1 teaspoon ground cumin | *3* Rub 2 tablespoons of the mixture onto each side of the steaks. Refrigerate the steaks for 10 minutes to allow the rub to soak into the meat. |
| 1 teaspoon dark-brown sugar | |
| ½ teaspoon chili powder | |
| 1 teaspoon garlic powder | *4* Place the steaks on the preheated grill and cook until they're medium-well or well-done, about 6 to 7 minutes on each side, depending on the steaks' thickness. |
| ¼ teaspoon onion powder | |
| Two 6-ounce boneless sirloin steaks | |

*Per serving:* Calories 233 (From Fat 79); Fat 9g (Saturated 3g); Cholesterol 94mg; Sodium 651mg; Carbohydrate 5g (Dietary Fiber 2g); Protein 33g; Iron 5mg; Calcium 64mg; Folate 12mcg.

*Note:* If you're using an uncovered charcoal grill, the steaks may take 7 to 9 minutes on each side. If you're using a gas grill, the steaks may take between 6 and 7 minutes per side.

*Tip:* Serve this dish with frozen microwaved veggies and a 90-second packet of brown rice for a stress-free dinner.

*Tip:* The less you handle the steaks, the more tender they'll be. Use tongs to turn the steaks on the grill to retain tenderness and flavor.

# *Fishing for Something Different for Dinner: Seafood Dishes*

Not only is seafood okay to eat when you're pregnant, but it's a welcomed part of your diet. The term *seafood* includes fish, shrimp, scallops, clams, lobster, and more. In general, seafood has numerous benefits, not the least of which is that most of it is very low in fat, which means it's also low in calories (unless, of course, you feel compelled to deep-fry it or dip it into a vat of butter). The fat it *does* have is the good kind — omega-3 fatty acids. The DHA and EPA that make up these omega-3 fatty acids are found mostly in fatty fish, such as salmon, herring, tuna, and sardines. (Turn to Chapter 3 to find out all about the benefits these essential fats offer you and your baby and to examine a list of the fish that are highest in omega-3s.)

One of the things I like about seafood is that it's simple and clean in taste. Just a squeeze of lemon and a dash of herbs can go a long way to give it flavor. Throw in some tempting toppings, such as avocado mango salsa or pear and fig chutney, and you soon realize that you really don't have to batter and deep-fry your fish to create a delicious, satisfying meal.

Although seafood has a simple taste, it has an undeserved reputation for being difficult to cook. However, it's actually quite easy to prepare with the right instructions. The biggest thing with seafood is to practice good food safety:

- ✔ Watch out for fish with a high mercury content. These fish include swordfish, tilefish, and king mackerel. Being extra vigilant is especially important during pregnancy because mercury can stay in your system for a long time and may affect nervous system development in your baby. (For the lowdown on which fish are best to eat during pregnancy, turn to Chapters 3 and 9.)

- ✔ Cook fish until it reaches an internal temperature of 145 degrees to prevent food-borne illness.

- ✔ Steer clear of raw or undercooked fish, including oysters, while you're expecting because they can contain harmful bacteria. If you're a sushi lover, go for California rolls (cooked crabstick) or any cooked fish in your rolls.

The five seafood recipes in this chapter give you a nice variety of seafood as well as whole grains, fruits, and veggies. You get clams in the Spaghetti with Clam Sauce and two different fish options in the Mango Avocado Salmon and the Pecan-Crusted Tilapia with Pear and Fig Chutney. I bring in a little Thai influence with the Thai Scallops with Noodles. (What can I say? I'm a sucker for anything with peanut sauce.) Finally, enjoy shrimp with lots of veggies and brown rice in the Garden Fresh Paella.

# Spaghetti with Clam Sauce

**Prep time:** 10 min • **Cook time:** About 25 min • **Yield:** 4 servings

| *Ingredients* | *Directions* |
|---|---|
| **Four 6.5-ounce cans chopped clams** | *1* Drain the cans of clams, reserving ¼ cup of the clam juice. |
| **¼ cup olive oil** | |
| **3 cloves garlic, chopped** | *2* In a medium saucepan, mix together the olive oil, garlic, and onion. Sauté over medium heat until the garlic and onion are soft, about 5 minutes. Add the oregano, pepper, grape juice, reserved clam juice, and mushrooms. Simmer covered until the mushrooms are soft, about 5 minutes. |
| **½ onion, chopped** | |
| **¼ teaspoon dried oregano** | |
| **¼ teaspoon pepper** | |
| **¼ cup white grape juice** | *3* Add the clams, butter, and parsley flakes. Bring the mixture to a boil; then reduce the heat and simmer covered for 3 to 5 minutes. |
| **2 cups button mushrooms** | |
| **2 tablespoons butter** | |
| **2 tablespoons dried parsley flakes** | *4* Fill a large saucepan with water and bring to a boil. Add the spaghetti and cook, stirring frequently, until it's *al dente* (firm but not hard), about 9 to 10 minutes. Drain and transfer the spaghetti to a serving bowl. |
| **Water** | |
| **8 ounces dry whole-grain spaghetti** | |
| **4 tablespoons grated Parmesan cheese** | *5* Pour the clam sauce over the spaghetti and sprinkle with 1 tablespoon of Parmesan cheese per serving. |

*Per serving:* Calories 516 (From Fat 196); Fat 22g (Saturated 7g); Cholesterol 71mg; Sodium 969mg; Carbohydrate 48g (Dietary Fiber 8g); Protein 35g; Iron 7mg; Calcium 114mg; Folate 18mcg.

*Tip:* This recipe originally called for white wine, but I substituted white grape juice considering it's best not to cook with alcohol while pregnant. If you're preparing this dish while pregnant and don't like the sweet flavor, feel free to use reduced-sodium chicken broth rather than grape juice. If you're making this recipe in a nonpregnant state, feel free to swap the grape juice for white wine!

*Note:* This dish is slightly high in sodium, so cut out the Parmesan cheese to reduce the sodium content.

*Source: Anne van den Berg, friend of author and mother of six*

# Mango Avocado Salmon

**Prep time:** 10 min • **Cook time:** 12–15 min • **Yield:** 4 servings

## Ingredients

2 small ripe avocados, peeled, cored, and diced

1 mango, peeled, cored, and diced

2 teaspoons lime juice

2 tablespoons plus 2 tablespoons olive oil

Four 6-ounce salmon fillets

1 lime, cut in half

Salt and pepper to taste

## Directions

**1** Preheat the broiler on high. Line an oven-safe baking pan with foil.

**2** Combine the avocados and mango with the lime juice and 2 tablespoons of olive oil. Toss to coat everything evenly and set aside.

**3** Rinse the salmon fillets, pat them dry with a paper towel, and place them skin side down on the prepared baking pan. Squeeze the lime over the fillets, drizzle them with the remaining 2 tablespoons of olive oil, and season them with salt and pepper to taste.

**4** Place the fish in the oven and broil until the fish browns on top, about 12 to 15 minutes.

**5** Transfer the salmon to a serving plate, top it with the mango avocado compote, and serve.

*Per serving:* Calories 522 (From Fat 315); Fat 35g (Saturated 5g); Cholesterol 97mg; Sodium 136mg; Carbohydrate 15g (Dietary Fiber 5g); Protein 39g; Iron 3mg; Calcium 40mg; Folate 72mcg.

*Note:* Keep the salmon at least 6 to 8 inches from the broiler so the fish doesn't burn on top and remain undercooked on the bottom.

*Tip:* Serve the salmon with whole-grain couscous and a side of sautéed spinach to round out this meal.

*Source: Tina Ruggiero, MS, RD, LD, and coauthor of The Best Homemade Baby Food on the Planet (Fair Winds Press)*

# Pecan-Crusted Tilapia with Pear and Fig Chutney

**Prep time:** 15 min • **Cook time:** 11 min • **Yield:** 4 servings

| Ingredients | Directions |
|---|---|
| **1 pear, peeled, cored, and sliced** | **1** In a small saucepan over medium heat, combine the pear, figs, vinegar, brown sugar, and ginger. Cover and allow the mixture to simmer, stirring frequently, until the pears have softened, about 5 minutes. Remove from heat and set aside. |
| **½ cup chopped, dried figs** | |
| **¼ cup apple cider vinegar** | |
| **1 tablespoon brown sugar** | |
| **⅛ teaspoon minced fresh ginger** | **2** Sprinkle the tilapia with the lemon juice and salt and pepper to taste. |
| **Four 6-ounce tilapia fillets** | **3** In a small bowl, mix together the breadcrumbs, pecans, and garlic powder. In a separate bowl, beat together the eggs and water. |
| **2 tablespoons lemon juice** | |
| **Salt and pepper to taste** | |
| **½ cup plain breadcrumbs** | **4** Sprinkle both sides of each fillet with the flour, dip the fillet into the egg mixture, and dredge it in the pecan and breadcrumb mixture. |
| **3 tablespoons finely chopped pecans** | |
| **¼ cup garlic powder** | **5** In a large skillet, heat the olive oil over medium-high heat. Cook the fillets for 3 minutes on each side. |
| **2 eggs** | |
| **2 tablespoons water** | **6** Top each fillet with ¼ of the pear and fig chutney. |
| **3 tablespoons whole-wheat flour** | |
| **2 tablespoons olive oil** | |

*Per serving: Calories 402 (From Fat 128); Fat 14g (Saturated 3g); Cholesterol 126mg; Sodium 148mg; Carbohydrate 34g (Dietary Fiber 5g); Protein 38g; Iron 3mg; Calcium 82mg; Folate 29mcg.*

*Note:* By pan-sautéing the fish and breading it, you'll get a nice crispy fish without all the fat of deep-frying. You know the fish is done when it flakes easily when you poke it with a fork.

*Tip:* Serve this dish with wild or brown rice and freshly steamed green beans for a complete meal.

*Vary It!* Use apples, cranberries, peaches, or apricots in place of the pear and figs to suit your taste. And if you want more pecan flavor, add some pecans to the chutney, too!

# Thai Scallops with Noodles

**Prep time:** 15 min, plus marinating time • **Cook time:** 10–12 min • **Yield:** 4 servings

| Ingredients | Directions |
|---|---|
| **1 lime, cut in half** | **1** Use a citrus zester or vegetable peeler to remove the zest of half of the lime and put it in a small bowl. Squeeze the juice from both halves of the lime into the same bowl. Add the orange marmalade, red pepper flakes, soy sauce, and garlic. Stir everything together. |
| **2 tablespoons orange marmalade** | |
| **¼ teaspoon crushed red pepper flakes** | |
| **¼ cup reduced-sodium soy sauce** | **2** Place the scallops in a large resealable bag. Add the lime and orange marmalade mixture to the bag and toss gently to cover the scallops evenly. Lay the bag flat in the refrigerator for 15 minutes so the scallops can marinate. |
| **1 clove garlic, minced** | |
| **1 pound scallops** | |
| **1 tablespoon sesame oil** | **3** In a wok or large sauté pan, heat the sesame oil over medium-high heat. Add the scallops and marinade and cook for 2 to 3 minutes per side, or until the scallops are sufficiently steamed. Transfer the scallops to a bowl and cover to keep warm. |
| **½ cup chopped onion** | |
| **1 cup bite-sized broccoli florets** | |
| **½ cup sliced carrots** | |
| **1 cup sugar snap peas** | **4** Add the onion, broccoli, and carrots to the hot pan and cook until they're tender-crisp, about 5 minutes. Add the sugar snap peas and cook for 1 more minute. |
| **8 ounces rice noodles, cooked to package directions** | |
| **½ cup prepared Asian-style peanut sauce** | **5** Add the cooked rice noodles, scallops, and peanut sauce to the skillet and stir until hot. Transfer everything to a serving dish and top with the chopped peanuts. |
| **¼ cup peanuts, chopped** | |

*Per serving:* Calories 566 (From Fat 193); Fat 21g (Saturated 4g); Cholesterol 27mg; Sodium 1,633mg; Carbohydrate 68g (Dietary Fiber 5g); Protein 27g; Iron 2mg; Calcium 84mg; Folate 71mcg.

*Tip:* To reduce the sodium in this dish, use less soy sauce and peanut sauce.

*Vary It!* Instead of scallops, use shrimp, chicken, or tofu. You can also swap the recommended vegetables with your favorites.

# Garden Fresh Paella

**Prep time:** 15 min • **Cook time:** About 30 min • **Yield:** 6 servings

| *Ingredients* | *Directions* |
|---|---|
| 1 tablespoon plus 1 tablespoon olive oil | *1* In a large skillet, heat 1 tablespoon of olive oil over medium heat. Add the onion, garlic, bell pepper, and zucchini. Cook for 3 to 4 minutes, stirring frequently. Add the turkey sausage and uncooked rice and cook for 2 to 3 minutes. |
| 1 onion, chopped | |
| 2 cloves garlic, chopped | |
| 1 red bell pepper, seeded and chopped | |
| 2 zucchini, quartered and sliced | *2* Stir in the vegetable broth, thyme, and saffron. Bring the mixture to a boil and simmer for 15 minutes uncovered, stirring occasionally. |
| 4 ounces lean turkey sausage, sliced | *3* In a separate large skillet, heat 1 tablespoon of olive oil over medium heat. Add the shrimp and cook until pink, about 2 to 3 minutes on each side. |
| One 14-ounce package quick-cooking brown rice | |
| 3 cups vegetable broth | *4* Add the tomatoes, peas, and cooked shrimp to the rice and vegetable mixture and continue to stir and cook for another 3 to 4 minutes. Add the lemon juice. |
| ½ teaspoon dried thyme | |
| ¼ teaspoon dried saffron | |
| 24 large shrimp, peeled, deveined, and tails removed | *5* Transfer the shrimp, rice, and veggie mixture to a serving dish and sprinkle with parsley before serving. |
| 3 tomatoes, seeded and chopped | |
| ½ cup frozen peas, thawed | |
| 2 tablespoons lemon juice | |
| ½ cup chopped fresh parsley | |

*Per serving:* Calories 399 (From Fat 82); Fat 9g (Saturated 1g); Cholesterol 54mg; Sodium 427mg; Carbohydrate 65g (Dietary Fiber 7g); Protein 16g; Iron 4mg; Calcium 85mg; Folate 60mcg.

*Tip:* If the dish is too sticky for you, or if you like your paella a bit soupier, add another cup of vegetable broth.

*Vary It!* Saffron can be pricy, so feel free to leave it out or substitute turmeric instead.

*Note:* This is an excellent one-dish meal: You get your whole grains, vegetables, and protein all in one!

# Embracing the Many White Meats

When it comes to white meat, what's not to like? You get an inexpensive source of high-quality protein that doesn't cost you much in terms of fat and calories, especially if you take the skin off of poultry. White meat generally comes in three varieties:

✔ **Pork:** Although pork is sometimes pink (think ham), it's a meat that most certainly deserves its few minutes of fame in a pregnancy diet. Many cuts of pork are lean and packed with protein, iron, zinc, and numerous B vitamins. This section features two pork-focused recipes: my flavorful Super Easy Pulled Pork and a delectable Parmesan-Herb-Crusted Pork Chop with sage and thyme.

Just be careful to always cook pork to an internal temperature of 160 degrees.

✔ **Turkey:** When most people think of turkey, they think of only one day and one way to make it: the Thanksgiving roast turkey. But this particular white meat is far more versatile. You can buy it ground as either ground turkey or ground turkey breast. (I recommend choosing ground turkey breast over ground turkey whenever possible because it's much lower in fat. Just be aware that it can dry out because it's so lean, so use it in recipes that have vegetables or sauces or throw it in a soup, like in the Turkey Cheeseburger Chowder I include in this section.) You can also buy turkey in sausage form; for a tasty dish involving turkey sausage, check out the Sauerkraut and Turkey Sausage Pasta Bake later in this section or the Garden Fresh Paella in the preceding section.

Always make sure you cook turkey to an internal temperature of 165 degrees.

✔ **Chicken:** People love chicken because its mild flavor makes it an extremely versatile ingredient they can use in all kinds of recipes. You can pair it with just about anything, which I certainly do in this section's six chicken recipes. White meat skinless chicken is about as lean as you can get as far as animal proteins go. Its lean nature makes it a good partner for marinades because it really picks up the flavors.

Always cook chicken well to eliminate the risk of salmonella; *well* means an internal temperature of at least 165 degrees. One good way to know when chicken is fully cooked is when the juices run clear. But of course the best and only way to know for sure is to take its temperature with a meat thermometer.

# Super Easy Pulled Pork

**Prep time:** 5 min • **Cook time:** 7 hr • **Yield:** 8 servings

| Ingredients | Directions |
|---|---|
| Nonstick cooking spray | *1* Spray a 4- to 6-quart slow cooker with nonstick cooking spray. |
| 2 pounds pork shoulder or pork loin | |
| ½ teaspoon salt | *2* Rub the pork with the salt, pepper, onion, and garlic. Place the pork in the slow cooker. Pour the root beer over the pork. |
| ½ teaspoon pepper | |
| 2 tablespoons dried minced onion | *3* Cover the slow cooker tightly and cook on low for 7 hours. Remove the pork from the slow cooker and discard the remaining liquid. |
| 2 cloves garlic, minced | |
| One 12-ounce can root beer | |
| One 12-ounce bottle prepared barbecue sauce | *4* Shred the pork with a fork. Pour the barbecue sauce over the shredded pork and stir to coat the pork evenly. Serve on whole-grain buns. |
| 8 whole-grain hamburger buns | |

*Per serving:* Calories 305 (From Fat 108); Fat 12g (Saturated 4g); Cholesterol 66mg; Sodium 413mg; Carbohydrate 28g (Dietary Fiber 4g); Protein 22g; Iron 2mg; Calcium 67mg; Folate 17mcg.

*Tip:* For enhanced flavor, shred the pork after 6 hours, add the barbecue sauce to the pork in the slow cooker, and continue to heat the pork for another hour.

*Note:* Serve with cole slaw for a complete meal!

# Parmesan-Herb-Crusted Pork Chops

**Prep time:** 10 min • **Cook time:** 40–50 min • **Yield:** 2 servings

| *Ingredients* | *Directions* |
|---|---|
| **Nonstick cooking spray** | *1* Preheat the oven to 400 degrees. Coat a large baking sheet with nonstick cooking spray. |
| **¼ teaspoon salt** | |
| **⅛ teaspoon pepper** | *2* In a small bowl, mix together the salt, pepper, sage, and thyme. Rub the mixture on the outside of the pork chops. |
| **1 teaspoon dried sage** | |
| **½ teaspoon dried thyme** | |
| **Two 8-ounce bone-in pork chops** | *3* Place the Parmesan cheese, beaten egg, and bread-crumbs in three separate shallow bowls. |
| **½ cup grated Parmesan cheese** | *4* Press each side of each pork chop into the Parmesan cheese so that it sticks to the meat. Dredge each chop in the egg, coating each side. Then dip it into the breadcrumbs, pressing the crumbs onto the chop. Place the pork chops on the prepared baking sheet. |
| **1 egg, lightly beaten** | |
| **½ cup plain breadcrumbs** | |
| **2 tablespoons olive oil** | |
| **2 cloves garlic, chopped** | *5* Bake until the pork chops have reached the proper temperature, about 40 to 50 minutes. |

*Per serving:* Calories 480 (From Fat 255); Fat 28g (Saturated 8g); Cholesterol 159mg; Sodium 670mg; Carbohydrate 12g (Dietary Fiber 1g); Protein 42g; Iron 3mg; Calcium 209mg; Folate 27mcg.

*Tip:* Serve with roasted root vegetables like sweet potatoes, carrots, parsnips, turnips, or beets.

# Turkey Cheeseburger Chowder

**Prep time:** 10 min  •  **Cook time:** About 40 min  •  **Yield:** 4 servings

| *Ingredients* | *Directions* |
|---|---|
| 3 potatoes, peeled and cut into 1-inch cubes | *1*  In a large pot, combine the potatoes, carrot, onion, broth, garlic, and pepper. Bring the mixture to a boil. Reduce the heat and simmer until the potatoes are tender, about 15 minutes. |
| 1 small carrot, grated | |
| 1 small onion, chopped | |
| 1½ cups low-sodium chicken or vegetable broth | *2*  In a large skillet, heat the oil over medium heat. Add the ground turkey and cook it until it's no longer pink, about 8 minutes, stirring frequently. |
| 2 cloves garlic, minced | |
| ⅛ teaspoon pepper | *3*  Add the turkey to the potato-broth soup. Stir in 2 cups of milk and cook for another 5 minutes. |
| 1 tablespoon canola oil | |
| 1 pound ground turkey breast | *4*  In a small bowl, combine the remaining ½ cup of milk with the flour and mix until smooth. Gradually stir the flour-milk mixture into the soup. |
| 2 cups plus ½ cup lowfat milk | |
| 3 tablespoons all-purpose flour | |
| 6 ounces Velveeta 2% Milk Pasteurized Cheese | *5*  Bring the soup to a boil and stir. Reduce the heat and simmer until the soup has thickened, about 10 minutes. Stir in the cheese and continue to heat the soup until the cheese is melted, stirring constantly. Remove the soup from heat and serve 1½ cup per serving. |

*Per serving:* Calories 429 (From Fat 94); Fat 11g (Saturated 5g); Cholesterol 98mg; Sodium 1,041mg; Carbohydrate 39g (Dietary Fiber 2g); Protein 44g; Iron 2mg; Calcium 459mg; Folate 37mcg.

*Tip:* To reduce the sodium in this recipe, cut the amount of cheese used in half.

*Vary It!* This recipe calls for ground turkey breast, but you can substitute lean ground beef if you prefer.

*Source: Tami Kohls, aunt of author*

# Sauerkraut and Turkey Sausage Pasta Bake

**Prep time:** 10 min • **Cook time:** About 45 min • **Yield:** 6 servings

| Ingredients | Directions |
|---|---|
| Nonstick cooking spray<br><br>1 tablespoon olive oil | *1* Preheat the oven to 350 degrees. Coat a 2-quart glass or ceramic baking dish with nonstick cooking spray. |
| 1 onion, chopped<br><br>1 green bell pepper, seeded and chopped<br><br>1 cup mushrooms, sliced | *2* In a large skillet, heat the olive oil over medium heat. Add the onion, bell pepper, and mushrooms and cook until all the veggies are tender, about 5 minutes. Set aside. |
| Water<br><br>12 ounces dry whole-grain bow-tie pasta | *3* Fill a large pot with water and bring it to a boil over high heat. Add the pasta and cook until it's al dente, about 12 to 15 minutes, stirring frequently. |
| Four 3-ounce lean turkey sausages<br><br>One 16-ounce can chopped tomatoes, no salt added | *4* In a medium skillet, cook the sausages over medium heat for about 15 minutes, turning frequently. Slice the sausages diagonally into bite-sized pieces. |
| 1 cup sauerkraut<br><br>¼ cup shredded cheddar cheese | *5* In a large bowl, mix together the pasta, sautéed vegetables, sausage, tomatoes, and sauerkraut. Pour the mixture into the prepared baking dish. Sprinkle the cheese over the top of the casserole. |
| | *6* Bake the casserole uncovered for 20 minutes. |

*Per serving: Calories 368 (From Fat 98); Fat 11g (Saturated 4g); Cholesterol 38mg; Sodium 569mg; Carbohydrate 52g (Dietary Fiber 8g); Protein 20g; Iron 4mg; Calcium 84mg; Folate 51mcg.*

*Vary It!* If you're not a fan of sauerkraut, simply leave it out! Note, though, that you may need to add a pinch of salt to the recipe if you take out the kraut.

# Rosemary Chicken on Asparagus Risotto

**Prep time:** 10 min, plus marinating time • **Cook time:** About 45 min • **Yield:** 4 servings

| *Ingredients* | *Directions* |
|---|---|
| **4 split boneless, skinless chicken breasts** | *1* Place the chicken breasts in a deep bowl. Pour the vinegar over the chicken and refrigerate for 30 minutes so the chicken can marinate. |
| **½ cup balsamic vinegar** | |
| **1 tablespoon olive oil** | *2* In a large saucepan, heat the olive oil over medium heat. Add the asparagus and heat until it's tender-crisp, about 4 minutes. Remove the asparagus from the pan and set aside. |
| **½ pound fresh asparagus spears, trimmed and cut into bite-sized pieces** | |
| **¼ cup chopped onion** | *3* In the hot saucepan, add the onion and cook until it's tender, about 2 to 3 minutes. Add the uncooked rice and sauté for 2 to 3 minutes, stirring frequently. |
| **⅔ cup Arborio rice** | |
| **3 cups low-sodium vegetable broth** | *4* Add 1 cup of the vegetable broth and increase the heat to medium-high. Cook uncovered, stirring frequently for 5 minutes. Add 1 more cup of broth, stirring frequently for 5 to 10 minutes. Add the third cup of broth, stirring frequently and cooking until the broth is absorbed, about 15 to 20 more minutes. |
| **1 tablespoon dried rosemary** | |
| **⅓ cup fat-free half-and-half** | |
| **2 tablespoons grated Parmesan cheese** | |
| **¼ teaspoon salt** | *5* Preheat the broiler. Remove the chicken from the vinegar and place it on a broiler pan. Sprinkle half of the rosemary over the chicken. Broil for 5 to 6 minutes on one side. Turn the chicken over and sprinkle the other side with the remaining rosemary. Broil for another 5 to 6 minutes. |
| **⅛ teaspoon pepper** | |
| | *6* When the rice mixture has absorbed the broth and has a creamy consistency, remove it from the heat and stir in the asparagus, half-and-half, cheese, salt, and pepper. Transfer it to a serving platter and place the chicken on top. |

*Per serving: Calories 388 (From Fat 78); Fat 9g (Saturated 2g); Cholesterol 75mg; Sodium 630mg; Carbohydrate 42g (Dietary Fiber 2g); Protein 34g; Iron 2mg; Calcium 120mg; Folate 51mcg.*

*Source (chicken recipe): Keri Gans, MS, RD, CDN, nutrition consultant, speaker, and author of The Small Change Diet (Simon & Schuster)*

# Curry Chicken Salad

**Prep time:** 15 min  •  **Yield:** 6 servings

| Ingredients | Directions |
|---|---|
| ½ **cup light mayonnaise** | *1* In a small bowl, whisk together the mayonnaise, Greek yogurt, and curry powder. Add salt and pepper to taste. Set aside. |
| ½ **cup plain lowfat Greek yogurt** | |
| 1 **tablespoon curry powder** | *2* In a large bowl, combine the chicken, apple, celery, onion, and grapes. |
| **Salt and pepper to taste** | |
| 4 **cups diced cooked chicken breast** | *3* Add the mayo-yogurt mixture and mix until everything is well coated. |
| 1 **Granny Smith apple, cored and diced** | |
| ½ **cup diced celery** | *4* Serve a scoop of chicken salad on each lettuce leaf. Top with the chopped walnuts. |
| ¼ **cup finely chopped red onion** | |
| 1 **cup red seedless grapes, sliced in half** | |
| 6 **large lettuce leaves, washed and dried** | |
| ½ **cup toasted walnuts, roughly chopped** | |

*Per serving:* Calories 343 (From Fat 156); Fat 17g (Saturated 3g); Cholesterol 89mg; Sodium 246mg; Carbohydrate 14g (Dietary Fiber 2g); Protein 33g; Iron 2mg; Calcium 66mg; Folate 32mcg.

*Tip:* For the best taste, make the chicken salad ahead of time and let it chill for 4 hours before serving.

*Vary It!* Pecans work just as well in this recipe if you prefer them over walnuts.

*Source: Evie Lyras, friend of author*

# Crispy Lime Chicken Tenders

**Prep time:** 10 min, plus marinating time  •  **Cook time:** 20–25 min  •  **Yield:** 4 servings

| Ingredients | Directions |
|---|---|
| 1 lime, cut in half | **1** Use a citrus zester or vegetable peeler to remove the zest of half of the lime. Place the zest in a small bowl. Squeeze the juice from both halves of the lime into the same bowl. |
| 1 tablespoon honey | |
| 3 tablespoons olive oil | |
| 2 cloves garlic, minced | **2** Add the honey, olive oil, and garlic to the bowl; whisk everything together. |
| 1 pound raw chicken tenders | |
| Nonstick cooking spray | **3** Place the chicken tenders in a resealable plastic bag. Pour the marinade over the chicken and seal the bag. Lay the bag flat in the refrigerator and marinate for at least 1 hour. |
| ½ teaspoon chili powder | |
| 2 tablespoons dried cilantro | |
| 1 cup panko breadcrumbs | |
| ½ cup plain breadcrumbs | **4** Preheat the oven to 400 degrees. Coat a baking sheet with nonstick cooking spray. |
| | **5** Combine the chili powder, cilantro, and both types of breadcrumbs and spread them out on a plate or shallow bowl. |
| | **6** Remove the chicken from the marinade and discard any extra marinade. Coat the tenders with the breadcrumb mixture and place them on the prepared baking sheet. |
| | **7** Bake the chicken for 20 to 25 minutes, turning once. Turn on the broiler for the last 3 minutes to crisp the chicken. |

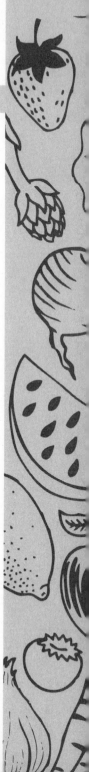

*Per serving: Calories 191 (From Fat 51); Fat 6g (Saturated 1g); Cholesterol 63mg; Sodium 115mg; Carbohydrate 9g (Dietary Fiber 1g); Protein 24g; Iron 1mg; Calcium 22mg; Folate 9mcg.*

**Tip:** If you have time, marinate the chicken for 2 to 4 hours. The longer you marinate, the more flavorful your meal!

**Note:** Serve these tenders with sweet potato fries and another vegetable of your choice. Or if you love salads, put the chicken tenders on top of a bed of greens and serve with your favorite dressing for a crispy chicken salad.

# Chicken Kabobs

**Prep time:** 20 min, plus marinating time • **Cook time:** About 10 min • **Yield:** 4 servings

| *Ingredients* | *Directions* |
|---|---|
| 2 lemons, sliced in half | *1* Squeeze the juice from the lemons into a small bowl, reserving the used halves. Add the olive oil, garlic powder, rosemary, salt, pepper, and parsley to the bowl. Whisk everything together. |
| ½ cup olive oil | |
| 1 teaspoon garlic powder | |
| 1 teaspoon dried rosemary | *2* Place the chicken in a large resealable bag. Place the tomatoes, bell peppers, onions, and mushrooms in a separate bag (use two bags if needed). |
| 1 teaspoon salt | |
| 1 teaspoon pepper | |
| ¼ cup fresh parsley | *3* Divide the marinade evenly between the bags of chicken and vegetables. Add one of the lemon halves to each bag. Lay the bags flat in the refrigerator and marinate for at least 1 hour. |
| 1 pound boneless, skinless chicken breast, cubed | |
| 2 cups grape tomatoes | |
| 1 red bell pepper, seeded and cut into 1-inch pieces | *4* Spray the grill with nonstick cooking spray and preheat to medium-high heat. |
| 1 green bell pepper, seeded and cut into 1-inch pieces | *5* Remove the vegetables from the marinade and discard the lemons. Pour the extra marinade in a small bowl; set aside. Pierce the veggies onto metal skewers and set the skewers on a baking sheet. |
| 1 cup pearl onions, peeled | |
| 8 ounces whole button mushrooms | |
| Nonstick cooking spray | *6* Remove the chicken from the marinade, discarding the extra marinade. Pierce the chicken on metal skewers and set them on a baking sheet. |
| | *7* Grill the chicken until it's well-done, about 7 to 8 minutes, and the veggies until they're crisp-tender, about 10 minutes. Turn the skewers frequently to avoid burning and brush the chicken and veggies with the leftover vegetable marinade while cooking. Remove the chicken and veggies from the skewers and place them on a serving dish. |

***Per serving:*** *Calories 316 (From Fat 149); Fat 17g (Saturated 3g); Cholesterol 63mg; Sodium 642mg; Carbohydrate 16g (Dietary Fiber 3g); Protein 26g; Iron 2mg; Calcium 34mg; Folate 45mcg.*

***Note:*** Serve these tasty kabobs with herbed or wild rice for a complete meal.

# Peachy Chicken Barley Pilaf

**Prep time:** 10 min  •  **Cook time:** About 20 min  •  **Yield:** 4 servings

| *Ingredients* | *Directions* |
|---|---|
| 2 cups water | *1* In a medium saucepan, bring the water and salt to a boil over medium-high heat. Add the barley and stir. Reduce the heat to low, cover, and simmer for 10 to 12 minutes, or until all the liquid is absorbed. Remove from heat and let stand for 10 minutes. |
| ½ teaspoon salt | |
| 1 cup quick-cooking barley | |
| 1 tablespoon olive oil | |
| 2 boneless, skinless chicken breasts, cut into bite-sized chunks | *2* In a large skillet, heat the olive oil over medium heat. Add the chicken and cook until it's browned, about 7 to 8 minutes, stirring frequently. |
| ¼ cup lime juice | *3* In a small bowl, whisk together the lime juice and white vinegar. In a large bowl, mix together the peaches and pomegranate seeds. Pour the lime juice mixture over the fruit and stir to coat everything evenly. |
| ¼ cup white balsamic vinegar | |
| 1 cup frozen sliced peaches, thawed | |
| ⅓ cup pomegranate seeds | |
| ⅓ cup chopped fresh parsley | *4* Add the barley and chicken to the fruit and stir gently. Sprinkle in the parsley, stir to combine, and serve immediately. |

*Per serving:* Calories 359 (From Fat 51); Fat 6g (Saturated 1g); Cholesterol 37mg; Sodium 338mg; Carbohydrate 60g (Dietary Fiber 9g); Protein 19g; Iron 2mg; Calcium 36mg; Folate 25mcg.

*Note:* This is a wonderful dish for enjoying in the late fall and winter, when not a lot of produce is in season. Pomegranates are in season at this time, and you can find frozen peaches any time of year.

*Tip:* You can find ready-to-use pomegranate seeds in the produce section of most supermarkets. To save money, you can seed the pomegranate yourself, but note that doing so adds time to the recipe.

*Tip:* You can eat this leftover the next day as a cold barley salad.

# Spinach, Date, and Blue Cheese Chicken Panini

**Prep time:** 5 min • **Cook time:** About 10 min • **Yield:** 1 serving

| Ingredients | Directions |
|---|---|
| 2 slices crusty white sandwich bread | **1** Place a medium skillet over medium heat. Spread one side of each slice of bread with the margarine. Place one bread slice, margarine side down, in the skillet. |
| 1 tablespoon trans-fat-free margarine spread | |
| ½ cup fresh, washed, and dried spinach, stems removed | **2** Microwave the spinach for 30 seconds to wilt it. Microwave the chicken until it's steaming hot, about 30 to 45 seconds. |
| 3 ounces thinly sliced reduced-sodium deli chicken breast | **3** Add the chicken, spinach, and date to the bread slice in the skillet. |
| 1 fresh Medjool date, pit removed and sliced | **4** Spread mayonnaise on the side of the remaining piece of bread without margarine. |
| 1 tablespoon light mayonnaise | **5** Add the blue cheese to the sandwich in the skillet and top with the second piece of bread, mayonnaise side down. |
| 1 tablespoon crumbled pasteurized blue cheese | **6** Use the bottom of another heavy skillet to press down the sandwich. Cook until the bottom slice of bread is browned, about 4 minutes. Flip the sandwich and press it down with the heavy skillet. Cook until that side of the bread is browned, about another 4 minutes. |

*Per serving:* Calories 588 (From Fat 230); Fat 26g (Saturated 9g); Cholesterol 50mg; Sodium 882mg; Carbohydrate 72g (Dietary Fiber 7g); Protein 22g; Iron 3mg; Calcium 110mg; Folate 97mcg.

*Note:* This recipe calls for deli-style chicken. To be safe, heat all deli meat until it's steaming to reduce the risk of listeria contamination. Doing so is simple in this recipe because you can stick the deli meat in the microwave and transfer it immediately to the hot panini to keep it hot.

*Tip:* If you have a panini press you can use it in place of the skillets I use here.

# Chapter 15

# Plants, Please! Meatless Side and Main Dishes

**Recipes in This Chapter**

- ↻ Tomato Bulgur Soup
- ↻ Broccoli Cheese Soup
- ↻ Souped-Up Split Pea Soup
- ↻ Black Bean Chili
- ↻ Ratatouille with Cannellini Beans
- ↻ Quinoa Tabbouleh with Garbanzo Beans
- ↻ Sloppy Lentil Joes
- ↻ Giant Beans with Spinach and Feta
- ↻ Tofu Vegetable Stir-Fry
- ↻ Sesame Noodle Salad
- ↻ Baked Ziti with Tofu
- ↻ Wheat Berry Edamame with Dried Fruit
- ↻ Steamed Broccoli with Mustard Sauce and Cashews
- ↻ Zucchini Patties
- ↻ Spanakopita (Greek Spinach Pie)
- ↻ Sweet Potato Hash
- ↻ Vegetable Lasagna
- ↻ Homemade Gnocchi with Pesto
- ↻ Broccoli, Beans, and Feta Pasta
- ↻ Roasted Eggplant, Olive, and Goat Cheese Homemade Pizza

🌂🍶🦐🥢❀🥕

## In This Chapter

▶ Preparing soups that warm and fill your belly

▶ Discovering how beans and soy make delicious, protein-packed alternatives to meat

▶ Whipping up some tasty veggie dishes

▶ Incorporating nutritious ways to eat pasta and pizza

*P*eople eat from two main categories: plants and animals. Along with making other healthy lifestyle choices, eating balanced diets based on plant foods may help prevent many of the chronic conditions that affect Americans, including heart disease, diabetes, and certain cancers. Focusing on plant-based foods while you're pregnant allows you to get whole grains, fruits, vegetables, nuts, and beans that provide the essential nutrients and fiber you and your baby need.

Just because plant-based diets may be better for you doesn't mean you need to become a vegetarian during or after your pregnancy. For our purposes, *plant-based* simply means that most of your plate contains grains, fruits, vegetables, nuts, and seeds. The rest of your plate's contents can come from animals — meats, eggs, and dairy.

Actually, pregnancy isn't the best time to make a major life change by becoming a vegetarian. If you want to reduce your meat intake, make sure you replace that meat with plant-based proteins, such as legumes (beans), soy, nuts, and seeds.

This chapter includes 20 tempting plant-based recipes. Each one can be a meal all by itself, or you can pair one of these meatless recipes with your favorite animal source of protein.

# Filling Up on Soups and Chilis

Soups are an excellent way to get your vegetables! Most soups have at least some kind of vegetable, whether they're broth based with just a bit of carrots and celery or vegetable based with pureed black beans or tomatoes. Unless they're cream-of-something, most soups are fairly low in fat, too.

Even though soups sometimes take a while to cook, they're generally easy to prepare. You toss a few ingredients into a pot, shut the lid, and let it simmer while you go and relax. Soon the house fills up with the aromas of delicious, filling soup.

To make sure you have plenty of room for all the broth and other ingredients that go into homemade soups, I recommend using either a stockpot or a Dutch oven, like the ones shown in Figure 15-1, whenever you prepare soups.

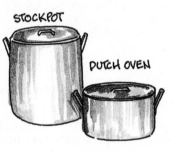

**Figure 15-1:**
A stockpot (left) and Dutch oven (right).

This section gives you four different vegetarian soup options. Have a bowl all by itself or try these ideas for creating a balanced meal:

- **Tomato Bulgur Soup:** The bulgur and beans in this tomato-based soup give it a hearty texture that's quite filling. Add a side salad to get even more veggie power from the meal.

- **Broccoli Cheese Soup:** The rich flavor of this cheese-based soup goes well with a light side salad and slice of whole-grain bread.

- **Souped-Up Split Pea Soup:** Split pea soup is hearty and goes well with some crusty bread, which you can use to scoop it up.

- **Black Bean Chili:** The beans that make up the base of this chili provide fiber and protein, which makes this soup meal-worthy, not just a starter. Pair it with a simple fruit salad.

# Tomato Bulgur Soup

**Prep time:** 10 min • **Cook time:** About 30 min • **Yield:** 6 servings

| Ingredients | Directions |
|---|---|
| ½ cup plus 3½ cups low-sodium vegetable broth | **1** In a stockpot, heat ½ cup of vegetable broth on high heat until it's boiling, about 10 minutes. |
| 2 cloves garlic, finely chopped | |
| 1 small yellow onion, finely chopped | **2** Add the garlic, onion, and cumin. Cook for 5 minutes, or until the onions are clear. |
| 1 teaspoon cumin | |
| 1 cup uncooked bulgur | **3** Stir in the bulgur, remaining vegetable broth, diced tomatoes, and cannellini beans. Bring the mixture to a boil. Reduce the heat to low and cover for 10 minutes. |
| One 14-ounce can no-salt-added diced tomatoes | |
| One 15-ounce can cannellini beans, rinsed and drained | **4** Add the basil and spinach and stir. Add salt and pepper (if desired). Cover for another 5 minutes, or until the bulgur is tender and the spinach is wilted. Serve 2 cups per serving. |
| 2 fresh basil leaves, chopped | |
| 4 cups fresh spinach | |
| Salt and pepper to taste | |

*Per serving:* Calories 159 (From Fat 9); Fat 1g (Saturated 0g); Cholesterol 0mg; Sodium 412mg; Carbohydrate 33g (Dietary Fiber 9g); Protein 7g; Iron 2mg; Calcium 73mg; Folate 77mcg.

*Note:* If you end up with leftovers, the soup will probably be thicker the next day as the bulgur continues to absorb liquid. Add milk or water as needed to get the soup back to the desired consistency.

*Source: Allison Marco, MS, RD*

# Broccoli Cheese Soup

**Prep time:** 15 min • **Cook time:** 30–35 min • **Yield:** 10 servings

| Ingredients | Directions |
|---|---|
| **One 10-ounce package frozen chopped broccoli** | **1** In a Dutch oven, combine the broccoli, potatoes, rice, and water. Heat the broccoli mixture over medium heat and simmer for 25 to 30 minutes. |
| **2 medium white potatoes, peeled and cubed** | |
| **⅓ cup uncooked whole-grain rice** | **2** In a small skillet, heat the butter over medium heat. Add the onions and sauté them until they're clear, about 5 minutes. |
| **4 cups water** | |
| **1 tablespoon butter** | **3** Add the onions, carrots, celery soup, tomatoes, and cheeses to the Dutch oven. Add the Worcestershire sauce and salt and pepper to taste. Stir in the parsley. Continue to cook until the soup mixture is hot but not boiling, about 5 minutes. Stir frequently to prevent the cheese from sticking to the bottom. |
| **1 cup chopped sweet onions** | |
| **1 cup grated carrots** | |
| **Two 10.75-ounce cans 98% fat-free cream of celery soup** | |
| **One 10-ounce can Rotel tomatoes, undrained** | **4** Remove from heat. Serve 1½ cups per serving and add a heaping tablespoon of sour cream to each cup, stirring right before serving. |
| **1½ cups cubed Velveeta 2% Milk Pasteurized Cheese** | |
| **½ cup shredded Lorraine Swiss cheese** | |
| **½ cup shredded sharp cheddar cheese** | |
| **½ cup grated Parmesan cheese** | |
| **1 teaspoon Worcestershire sauce** | |
| **Salt and pepper to taste** | |
| **½ cup chopped parsley** | |
| **½ cup light sour cream** | |

*Per serving:* Calories 265 (From Fat 93); Fat 10g (Saturated 6g); Cholesterol 31mg; Sodium 1,243mg; Carbohydrate 30g (Dietary Fiber 3g); Protein 15g; Iron 1mg; Calcium 401mg; Folate 34mcg.

*Tip:* To reduce the sodium in this dish, cut back on the amount of cheese and use no-salt-added canned tomatoes and low-sodium soup.

*Source: Ruth Hey, BSN, MEd, CPEN, and RN at Arnold Palmer Hospital for Children*

# Souped-Up Split Pea Soup

**Prep time:** 10 min • **Cook time:** About 50 min • **Yield:** 8 servings

| *Ingredients* | *Directions* |
|---|---|
| ½ pound green split peas | *1* Rinse the split peas in a colander and sort through them to pick out any rocks or debris. |
| ½ pound yellow split peas | |
| One 48-ounce container low-sodium vegetable broth | *2* Pour the vegetable broth into a stockpot. Add the peas and winter squash and heat the mixture over high heat for 5 minutes, stirring frequently. |
| One 12-ounce box frozen winter squash, thawed | |
| 1 small onion, chopped | *3* Add the chopped onion, carrots, garlic, and salt and pepper to taste to the pot. |
| ½ cup chopped carrots | |
| 3 cloves garlic, chopped | *4* Reduce the heat to medium-low. Cover and simmer for 45 minutes, or until the peas are soft, stirring frequently. Serve 1½ cups per serving. |
| Salt and pepper to taste | |

**Per serving:** *Calories 253 (From Fat 6); Fat 1g (Saturated 0g); Cholesterol 0mg; Sodium 341mg; Carbohydrate 48g (Dietary Fiber 6g); Protein 16g; Iron 3mg; Calcium 43mg; Folate 103mcg.*

**Tip:** Some people like to puree split pea soup for a creamier texture. If you're one of them, simply use an immersion blender or pour the soup into a regular blender in small batches and blend until smooth. If you're using a regular blender, simply return the soup to the pot to get it back to the desired serving temperature.

**Vary It!** You can use chicken broth if you aren't vegetarian and want a bit of chicken flavor.

*Source: Bonnie Taub-Dix, author of Read It Before You Eat It (Plume)*

# Black Bean Chili

**Prep time:** 10 min • **Cook time:** 40–50 min • **Yield:** 6 servings

| Ingredients | Directions |
|---|---|
| 1 tablespoon olive oil | *1* In a Dutch oven, heat the olive oil over medium heat. Add the onion, bell pepper, cumin, and garlic and sauté until the veggies are tender, about 5 minutes. |
| 1 medium sweet onion, chopped | |
| 1 red bell pepper, seeded and chopped | *2* Add the tomatoes, oregano, chili powder, and salt. Cook for 10 minutes. |
| 1 tablespoon ground cumin | |
| 4 cloves garlic, chopped | *3* Add the black beans and vegetable broth and cook for 20 to 30 minutes. |
| One 15-ounce can no-salt-added diced tomatoes, undrained | |
| 1 teaspoon dried oregano | *4* Add the cilantro and cook for 5 minutes. Remove the soup from heat and serve, sprinkling lime juice on top (if desired). Serve 1½ cups per serving. |
| 1 tablespoon chili powder | |
| ½ teaspoon salt | |
| Two 14-ounce cans black beans, undrained | |
| One 15-ounce can reduced-sodium vegetable broth | |
| 2 tablespoons chopped fresh cilantro | |
| 2 tablespoons lime juice (optional) | |

*Per serving:* Calories 178 (From Fat 36); Fat 4g (Saturated 0g); Cholesterol 0mg; Sodium 617mg; Carbohydrate 27g (Dietary Fiber 10g); Protein 9g; Iron 4mg; Calcium 82mg; Folate 150mcg.

**Tip:** Add a dollop of light sour cream to your bowl if you like your chili a bit creamier.

*Source: Stacey Sullivan, friend of author and mother of three*

# Creative and Tasty Bean- and Soy-Based Alternatives to Meat

Whether you call them *legumes* or *beans,* this group of vegetables offers lots of benefits. Nutritionally, these starchy, plant-based proteins are superstars because they're high in fiber (up to 13 grams per cup!), have the *amino acids* (building blocks of protein) you need, are loaded in potassium, magnesium, iron, and more, and are super high in antioxidants. In fact, some studies show that red beans have more antioxidants in them than either spinach or blueberries. (If you're worried about the side effects of beans, the magical fruit, head to Chapter 6 for tips on how to reduce gas.)

Perhaps you've avoided beans in the past because of the whole soaking overnight thing. Never fear! Canned beans are just as healthy as the dried kind, and you don't have to soak them or cook them for hours. Simply break out your can opener and dinner is minutes — not hours — away. To reduce the sodium in canned beans by about one-third, drain and rinse the beans before adding them to your favorite recipe.

One particular type of bean — the soybean — is one of very few plant-based foods known as a *complete protein,* meaning that it has all the essential amino acids your body needs. No wonder soybeans are a natural meat replacement! Soy comes in many forms: tofu, edamame (green soybean), tempeh, soy nuts, soy milk, and the numerous meat alternatives, like veggie burgers, that fill today's grocery aisles.

This section features several bean-based recipes, including four different soy-based recipes. Two of these soy-based recipes use tofu and two use edamame.

- ✔ **Tofu:** Tofu has a naturally bland flavor, which is why it picks up flavors so easily. Extra-firm tofu is good for stir-frying, whereas silken tofu is perfect in smoothies or desserts in place of heavy cream or cream cheese. You can find plain tofu in your grocery store's produce aisle. To track down various flavors of marinated tofu ready to break out of the package and add to your favorite dishes, head to a health-food store.

- ✔ **Edamame:** Most people know edamame just as an appetizer found in the pod (don't eat the pod; it isn't edible!) at their favorite sushi place, but shelled edamame can make a welcome addition to salads, soups, and casseroles. You find it in the frozen food aisle or vacuum packed in the produce section.

# Ratatouille with Cannellini Beans

**Prep time:** 20 min, plus standing time • **Cook time:** 30 min • **Yield:** 8 servings

| Ingredients | Directions |
|---|---|
| 1 medium eggplant, cut into chunks | **1** Place the eggplant in a colander. Sprinkle it with salt and let it sit for 15 minutes. |
| ½ teaspoon salt | |
| 1 tablespoon olive oil | **2** In a large cast-iron skillet or a stockpot, heat the olive oil over medium heat. Add the onion, garlic, and bell peppers and cook for 5 minutes. |
| 1 small yellow onion, chopped | |
| 3 cloves garlic, chopped | |
| 1 red bell pepper, seeded and chopped | **3** Add the eggplant to the skillet and cook for another 5 minutes, stirring frequently to prevent the eggplant from sticking to the bottom. |
| 1 green bell pepper, seeded and chopped | |
| ½ cup chopped sun-dried tomatoes (not packed in oil) | **4** Add the sun-dried tomatoes, zucchini, mushrooms, marinara sauce, beans, fennel, thyme, and basil. Sprinkle with salt and pepper to taste. Reduce the heat to low and simmer for 20 minutes, stirring occasionally. Serve 2 cups per serving. |
| 1 zucchini, cut into chunks | |
| 1 cup sliced raw mushrooms | |
| One 24-ounce jar prepared marinara sauce | |
| One 15-ounce can cannellini beans, drained and rinsed | |
| 1 teaspoon dried fennel | |
| 1 teaspoon dried thyme | |
| 1 teaspoon dried basil | |
| Salt and pepper to taste | |

*Per serving:* Calories 131 (From Fat 36); Fat 4g (Saturated 1g); Cholesterol 0mg; Sodium 546mg; Carbohydrate 20g (Dietary Fiber 5g); Protein 5g; Iron 2mg; Calcium 61mg; Folate 53mcg.

*Tip:* Serve this ratatouille with a nice crusty piece of whole-grain bread or pour it over a bed of whole-grain pasta or brown rice for a well-balanced meal.

*Vary It!* I sometimes add fresh spinach right before the ratatouille is done simmering. Feel free to sprinkle it with shredded pasteurized Parmesan or Asiago cheese for a little extra flavor.

# Quinoa Tabbouleh with Garbanzo Beans

**Prep time:** 15 min, plus standing time • **Cook time:** About 15 min • **Yield:** 4 servings

| *Ingredients* | *Directions* |
|---|---|
| 2 cups water | **1** In a medium saucepan, bring the water to a boil. Stir in the quinoa and salt. Reduce the heat to low, cover the pan, and simmer for about 15 minutes. Set aside and allow the quinoa to cool to room temperature. Drain any extra water remaining. |
| 1 cup red quinoa, dry | |
| ¼ teaspoon salt | |
| ¼ cup olive oil | |
| ¼ cup lemon juice | **2** In a large bowl, combine the olive oil, lemon juice, pepper, tomatoes, cucumber, olives, green onions, garbanzo beans, parsley, and mint. Stir in the cooled quinoa and serve 1½ cups at room temperature. |
| ¼ teaspoon pepper | |
| 1½ cups quartered cherry or grape tomatoes | |
| 1 cucumber, seeded and diced | |
| ½ cup sliced black olives | |
| 3 green onions, chopped | |
| One 15-ounce can garbanzo beans, rinsed and drained | |
| ¾ cup chopped fresh parsley | |
| ¼ cup chopped fresh mint leaves | |

*Per serving:* Calories 401 (From Fat 171); Fat 19g (Saturated 2g); Cholesterol 0mg; Sodium 445mg; Carbohydrate 50g (Dietary Fiber 9g); Protein 12g; Iron 9mg; Calcium 139mg; Folate 120mcg.

*Vary It!* Use white, black, or tri-color quinoa. The only real difference is the color of your meal. Add chopped chicken or tofu to boost the protein content.

**Figure 15-2:** Uncooked quinoa (left) and cooked quinoa (right).

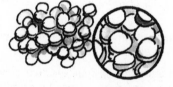
UNCOOKED QUINOA

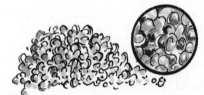
COOKED QUINOA

# Sloppy Lentil Joes

**Prep time:** 20 min • **Cook time:** About 45 min • **Yield:** 6 servings

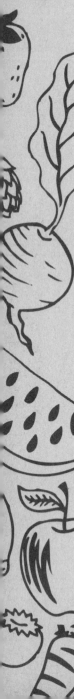

| Ingredients | Directions |
|---|---|
| 1½ cups lentils | **1** Rinse the lentils and pick through them to remove any stones or debris. |
| 1 tablespoon olive oil | |
| 1 yellow onion, chopped | **2** In a large pot, heat the olive oil over medium-high heat. Sauté the onion, bell pepper, carrot, and celery for about 5 minutes, or until the veggies are tender. |
| 1 yellow bell pepper, seeded and chopped | |
| 1 carrot, shredded | |
| 1 stalk celery, thinly chopped | **3** Add the chili powder, tomatoes, water, vinegar, lentils, brown mustard, Bragg Liquid Aminos or Worcestershire sauce, brown sugar, garlic, and bay leaf and bring the mixture to a boil. Reduce the heat to low and simmer for 40 minutes, or until the lentils are tender. Remove the bay leaf. Serve 1 cup per serving. |
| 1 tablespoon chili powder | |
| One 15-ounce can crushed tomatoes, undrained | |
| 2½ cups water | |
| ¼ cup red wine vinegar | |
| 1 tablespoon brown mustard | |
| 1 tablespoon Bragg Liquid Aminos or Worcestershire sauce | |
| 1 tablespoon brown sugar | |
| 1 clove garlic, minced | |
| 1 bay leaf | |

*Per serving:* Calories 249 (From Fat 30); Fat 2g (Saturated 0g); Cholesterol 0mg; Sodium 477mg; Carbohydrate 42g (Dietary Fiber 13g); Protein 15g; Iron 6mg; Calcium 51mg; Folate 262mcg.

*Tip:* Serve the lentil mixture over crusty whole-grain bread in an open-face style for a whole new take on the sloppy Joe. You can also serve it over brown rice.

*Note:* If you have time, you can make this recipe in a slow cooker. After you sauté the vegetables, just add everything to the slow cooker and cook on low for 4 to 6 hours, or until the lentils are tender.

# Giant Beans with Spinach and Feta

**Prep time:** 10 min  •  **Cook time:** 35 min  •  **Yield:** 6 servings

| *Ingredients* | *Directions* |
|---|---|
| 1 tablespoon plus 1 tablespoon olive oil | *1* Preheat the oven to 350 degrees. |
| 1 yellow onion, chopped | *2* In a medium skillet, heat 1 tablespoon of olive oil over medium heat. Add the onions, garlic, and spinach and cook until tender, about 5 minutes. |
| 2 cloves garlic, chopped | |
| 4 cups fresh spinach, stems trimmed | |
| Two 15-ounce cans giant butter beans, drained and rinsed | *3* In a large bowl, mix together the butter beans, dill, pepper, parsley, tomatoes, and lemon juice. Stir in the cooked onions, garlic, and spinach, and stir gently with a spoon. Add the feta cheese and stir until combined. |
| 1 teaspoon dried dill | |
| ¼ teaspoon pepper | |
| ¼ cup chopped fresh parsley | |
| 1 cup canned diced tomatoes, undrained | *4* Transfer the mixture to a 2-quart baking dish. Top with the breadcrumbs and the remaining olive oil. Bake for 30 minutes and then serve 1 cup per serving. |
| ¼ cup lemon juice | |
| 1 cup crumbled, pasteurized feta cheese | |
| ¼ cup plain breadcrumbs | |

*Per serving:* Calories 203 (From Fat 92); Fat 10g (Saturated 4g); Cholesterol 22mg; Sodium 589mg; Carbohydrate 24g (Dietary Fiber 6g); Protein 10g; Iron 3mg; Calcium 201mg; Folate 117mcg.

*Note:* If you can't find canned giant butter beans, use canned baby butter beans. Or try using the dry variety of giant butter beans. Simply cook the dry beans according to the package directions and continue with the rest of this recipe.

*Tip:* Serve this as a main dish with brown rice or pasta or on the side of chicken or fish.

# Tofu Vegetable Stir-Fry

**Prep time:** 20 min • **Cook time:** About 15 min • **Yield:** 4 servings

| Ingredients | Directions |
|---|---|
| One 14-ounce package extra-firm tofu, drained | **1** Sandwich the tofu on a plate between paper towels and press down slightly. Discard the top towel. Take another paper towel and place it on top of the tofu and put a plate on top of the paper towel. Let it sit for 15 minutes. Remove the towels from the tofu and cut the tofu into bite-sized pieces. |
| 1 teaspoon plus 1 tablespoon sesame oil | |
| 1 clove garlic, minced | |
| ½ teaspoon minced fresh ginger | **2** In a small saucepan, heat 1 teaspoon of sesame oil and the garlic and ginger over medium heat. Add the broth, soy sauce, brown sugar, and Tabasco sauce (if desired). Heat just to a boil. |
| ½ cup vegetable broth | |
| 2 tablespoons low-sodium soy sauce | |
| 2 tablespoons brown sugar | **3** In a small bowl, dissolve the cornstarch in the vinegar. Whisk the cornstarch mixture into the sauce you made in Step 2. Heat at a full boil until the sauce thickens, about 2 to 3 minutes. Remove from heat. |
| 3 dashes Tabasco sauce (optional) | |
| 2 teaspoons cornstarch | |
| 2 teaspoons rice wine vinegar | **4** In a wok or large skillet, heat 1 tablespoon of sesame oil over medium-high heat. Add the broccoli, cauliflower, and carrots. Stir-fry for 3 minutes. Add the bok choy and water chestnuts and stir-fry for 2 more minutes. Add the sugar snap peas and tofu and cook for an additional 2 to 3 minutes. |
| 2 cups chopped broccoli florets | |
| 1 cup chopped cauliflower | |
| 1 cup sliced carrots | |
| 1 cup sliced bok choy (Chinese cabbage) | **5** Add the sauce you made in Steps 2 and 3 to the tofu-veggie mixture and stir to coat everything evenly. Serve 2 cups of the stir-fry over ¾ cup of brown rice. |
| ½ cup canned sliced water chestnuts, drained | |
| 1½ cups sugar snap peas | |
| 3 cups prepared brown rice | |

*Per serving:* Calories 410 (From Fat 112); Fat 12g (Saturated 2g); Cholesterol 0mg; Sodium 431mg; Carbohydrate 57g (Dietary Fiber 8g); Protein 18g; Iron 4mg; Calcium 200mg; Folate 100mcg.

*Vary It!* Use whatever vegetables you like in this stir-fry. Other options include asparagus, onions, bell peppers, and shiitake or button mushrooms. You can also add peanuts or cashews for added flavor.

# Sesame Noodle Salad

**Prep time:** 10 min • **Cook time:** About 10 min • **Yield:** 4 servings

| Ingredients | Directions |
|---|---|
| 6 ounces whole-grain linguini pasta | *1* Cook the linguini according to the package directions and drain. |
| 2 tablespoons lime juice | |
| 2 tablespoons sesame oil | *2* In a small bowl, whisk together the lime juice, sesame oil, soy sauce, honey, and ginger to create the dressing. |
| 1 tablespoon low-sodium soy sauce | |
| 1 tablespoon honey | |
| 1 teaspoon grated fresh ginger | *3* In a large serving bowl, toss together the drained pasta, cabbage, carrots, edamame, green onions, and sesame seeds. Add the dressing and toss to coat everything evenly. |
| 2 cups thinly shredded red cabbage | |
| 2 cups shredded carrots | |
| 2 cups frozen shelled edamame, thawed | *4* Serve at room temperature (2 cups per serving). |
| ¾ cup chopped green onions | |
| 4 tablespoons sesame seeds | |

*Per serving: Calories 419 (From Fat 142); Fat 16g (Saturated 2g); Cholesterol 0mg; Sodium 215mg; Carbohydrate 55g (Dietary Fiber 12g); Protein 18g; Iron 4mg; Calcium 127mg; Folate 222mcg.*

*Source: Dawn Jackson Blatner, RD, and author of The Flexitarian Diet (McGraw-Hill)*

# Baked Ziti with Tofu

**Prep time:** 20 min • **Cook time:** About 1 hr • **Yield:** 10 servings

| *Ingredients* | *Directions* |
|---|---|
| Nonstick cooking spray<br><br>One 14-ounce package extra-firm tofu, drained | *1* Preheat the oven to 425 degrees. Spray a 9-x-13-inch glass baking dish with nonstick cooking spray. |
| 1 pound whole-grain ziti pasta<br><br>1 tablespoon olive oil<br><br>1 small onion, chopped | *2* Sandwich the tofu on a plate between paper towels and press down slightly. Discard the top towel. Take another paper towel and place it on top of the tofu and put a plate on top of the paper towel. Let it sit for 15 minutes. |
| 1 red bell pepper, seeded and chopped | *3* Cook the ziti according to the package directions. Drain and set aside. |
| 2 teaspoons chopped garlic<br><br>¼ teaspoon ground nutmeg<br><br>½ cup chopped fresh parsley<br><br>1 teaspoon dried oregano | *4* In a medium skillet, heat the olive oil over medium heat. Add the onion, bell pepper, and garlic. Sauté until the veggies are soft, about 5 minutes, stirring frequently. Set aside. |
| 1 teaspoon dried basil<br><br>12 ounces part-skim shredded mozzarella cheese, divided | *5* In a large bowl, crumble the tofu with your hands until the texture resembles that of cottage cheese. Add the nutmeg, parsley, oregano, and basil to the tofu and mix gently. Stir in half of the mozzarella cheese. |
| Two 24-ounce jars marinara sauce<br><br>¼ cup grated Parmesan cheese | *6* Add the cooked pasta and vegetable mixture to the cheese and tofu mixture; stir well. Add the marinara sauce and stir until well combined. |
| | *7* Transfer the pasta mixture to the prepared baking dish. Sprinkle the top of the pasta with the Parmesan cheese and the remaining mozzarella cheese. |
| | *8* Bake uncovered for 35 to 45 minutes, or until the cheese is melted and lightly browned. Serve 2 cups of pasta per serving. |

*Per serving:* Calories 389 (From Fat 121); Fat 13g (Saturated 5g); Cholesterol 21mg; Sodium 766mg; Carbohydrate 49g (Dietary Fiber 7g); Protein 2g; Iron 4mg; Calcium 349mg; Folate 62mcg.

# Wheat Berry Edamame with Dried Fruit

**Prep time:** 15 min, plus standing time • **Cook time:** 60 min • **Yield:** 6 servings

| Ingredients | Directions |
|---|---|
| 3 cups water | **1** In a medium saucepan, bring the water and salt to a boil over medium-high heat. Add the wheat berries. Reduce the heat to low, cover, and simmer for 60 minutes, or until the wheat berries are soft. Drain the excess water and allow the wheat berries to cool to room temperature. |
| ½ teaspoon salt | |
| 1½ cups wheat berries, uncooked | |
| 1 cup cooked and shelled edamame | **2** In a medium bowl, combine the edamame, apricots, and dates. |
| 1 cup quartered dried apricots | |
| 1 cup pitted and diced Medjool dates | **3** In a small bowl, whisk together the pomegranate juice, olive oil, and vinegar. |
| ½ cup 100% pomegranate juice | |
| 2 tablespoons olive oil | **4** Combine the wheat berries with the edamame mixture. Gently fold in the feta cheese and toasted pecans. Drizzle the mixture with the pomegranate dressing and toss to coat everything evenly. Serve 1½ cups per serving at room temperature. |
| 1½ tablespoons white balsamic vinegar | |
| 1 cup crumbled, pasteurized feta cheese | |
| ¾ cup chopped, toasted pecans | |

*Per serving:* Calories 563 (From Fat 205); Fat 23g (Saturated 5g); Cholesterol 22mg; Sodium 488mg; Carbohydrate 83g (Dietary Fiber 13g); Protein 14g; Iron 5mg; Calcium 173mg; Folate 88mcg.

*Note:* Wheat berries can also be sold as whole wheat kernels. Some packages tell you to soak them overnight in water. You don't have to do so as long as you cook them well, but you certainly can soak them if you want to. Because wheat berries take so long to cook, make up a larger batch and use them in another recipe later in the week. They keep plain in your fridge for several days.

*Note:* Dates are an often-forgotten fruit! They're good plain, but they also go well in salads, pasta dishes, and casseroles.

# Embracing Vegetables

If you're like most people, you're not getting the recommended amounts of vegetables (or fruits) each day. Maybe one of the reasons is because produce goes bad in your crisper drawer before you get a chance to eat it. Maybe you think frozen or canned vegetables aren't as healthy as getting them fresh. Think again! Studies have found that frozen and canned vegetables are just as nutritious as — and sometimes more nutritious than — their fresh counterparts.

Produce that's picked to be canned or frozen is picked at its peak of ripeness and nutritional value. The longer a food stays on the vine or tree or in the soil, the more nutrients it absorbs. I'm not sure where the nutrients go, but studies have found that fresh produce can lose up to 75 percent of its vitamin C when stored longer than seven days, even if it's refrigerated after harvesting.

Of course, you should still make fresh veggies part of your diet. To get the most out of your fresh produce in terms of nutrients and taste, purchase it as close after harvest as possible and eat it sooner rather than later. Farmers' markets have become popular because they offer fresh, ripe produce that you can take home and use that day. To lock in nutrients, steam or microwave your produce instead of boiling it.

The bottom line is that all produce is a winner, particularly during pregnancy, thanks to the abundance of folate, fiber, magnesium, and vitamins C and A found in vegetables. To help you incorporate plenty of veggies in your diet, I include four vegetable-focused recipes in this section. You can enjoy each one as a main course or as a side dish. The decision is yours.

## Locking in the good stuff: Freezing and canning

Although fresh produce is always a good choice, don't overlook frozen and canned varieties of your favorite fruits and veggies. The first step in the freezing process is *blanching* the produce (exposing it briefly to hot water or steam) to kill bacteria and stop the enzymes that cause it to go bad. The blanching process locks in the nutrients, and the frozen state acts as the preservative. While frozen, bacteria are dormant and can't cause spoiling.

Vegetables that wind up in a can are sealed in so there's no spoilage. Sodium is often added to canned vegetables, but the amount is less than you may think and usually not more than what people typically add when cooking with fresh produce. Look for low-sodium varieties of canned vegetables if you're concerned about sodium and drain and rinse the veggies because you can reduce about 40 percent of the sodium by doing so.

# Steamed Broccoli with Mustard Sauce and Cashews

**Prep time:** 10 min  •  **Cook time:** About 7 min  •  **Yield:** 4 servings

| Ingredients | Directions |
|---|---|
| 1 head broccoli, cut into spears<br><br>1 tablespoon olive oil<br><br>2 green onions, finely chopped<br><br>2 cloves garlic, minced<br><br>1 tablespoon water<br><br>1 tablespoon Dijon mustard<br><br>2½ tablespoons white vinegar<br><br>2 tablespoons honey<br><br>Salt and pepper to taste<br><br>½ cup cashews, chopped | *1* Steam the broccoli using a steamer basket in a covered saucepan over boiling water for about 6 minutes. Drain and set aside in a medium serving bowl.<br><br>*2* In a medium skillet, heat the olive oil over medium heat. Add the green onions and garlic and sauté for 1 minute.<br><br>*3* In a small bowl, whisk together the water, mustard, white vinegar, honey, and salt and pepper to taste. Add the sautéed onions and garlic to the wet ingredients.<br><br>*4* Drizzle the sauce over the broccoli and stir to coat. Top with the cashews. |

*Per serving:* Calories 178 (From Fat 105); Fat 12g (Saturated 2g); Cholesterol 0mg; Sodium 158mg; Carbohydrate 17g (Dietary Fiber 2g); Protein 5g; Iron 2mg; Calcium 41mg; Folate 31mcg.

*Vary It!* Use cauliflower rather than broccoli or do a mixture of both! Instead of cashews, try chopped peanuts or pecans.

*Tip:* If you don't have fresh broccoli available, use frozen and microwave it for 3 minutes. Then follow Steps 2 through 4 to prepare the sauce and the nuts.

*Tip:* You can also use the sauce in this recipe as a marinade or salad dressing. Or you can use it to add a bit of flavor to any plain steamed vegetable.

# Zucchini Patties

**Prep time:** 10 min • **Cook time:** 16–20 min • **Yield:** 4 servings

| Ingredients | Directions |
|---|---|
| 1 medium zucchini, unpeeled<br><br>¼ cup diced sweet onion<br><br>¼ cup diced red bell pepper<br><br>2 tablespoons chopped sun-dried tomatoes (not packed in oil)<br><br>3 tablespoons whole-wheat flour<br><br>¼ teaspoon garlic powder<br><br>¼ teaspoon salt<br><br>¼ teaspoon salt-free seasoning mix of your choice<br><br>1 teaspoon minced fresh thyme<br><br>2 eggs, lightly beaten<br><br>1 cup shredded cheddar cheese<br><br>1 tablespoon canola oil | *1* Use a hand-held grater to shred the zucchini into a medium bowl. Mix in the onion, bell pepper, and sun-dried tomatoes.<br><br>*2* In a small bowl, mix together the flour, garlic powder, salt, seasoning mix, and thyme. Add the dry seasoning mix to the vegetables. Mix in the beaten eggs and cheese.<br><br>*3* Heat the oil on a nonstick griddle over medium heat. Drop about ¼ cup of the mixture on the griddle for each patty and flatten gently with a spatula so it can cook thoroughly. Cook the patties for about 4 to 5 minutes on each side. The patties are done when the centers are cooked through.<br><br>*4* Repeat Step 3 for the rest of the mixture. Serve two patties per serving. |

*Per serving: Calories 222 (From Fat 141); Fat 16g (Saturated 7g); Cholesterol 136mg; Sodium 356mg; Carbohydrate 9g (Dietary Fiber 2g); Protein 12g; Iron 2mg; Calcium 239mg; Folate 33mcg.*

**Note:** Some people call these patties zucchini pancakes. Anything that resembles a pancake causes my father to put syrup on it, which drives my mom crazy. But these are savory pancakes, not sweet ones. No syrup necessary! (You're welcome to put a pat of butter on each patty or dip bite-sized pieces into a dill yogurt dip.)

*Source: Jean Timpel, mother of author*

# Spanakopita (Greek Spinach Pie)

**Prep time:** 30 min • **Cook time:** About 1 hr • **Yield:** 6 servings

| *Ingredients* | *Directions* |
|---|---|
| **Nonstick cooking spray** | *1* Preheat the oven to 350 degrees. Spray a 9-x-9-inch square baking pan with nonstick cooking spray. |
| **1 tablespoon plus ¼ cup olive oil** | |
| **2 cloves garlic, minced** | *2* In a large skillet, heat 1 tablespoon of olive oil over medium heat. Add the garlic and onion and sauté for 3 minutes. Add the spinach and parsley and sauté until the spinach cooks down, about 1 minute. Remove from heat, drain any excess liquid, and set aside to allow the mixture to cool. |
| **1 large onion, chopped** | |
| **Two 10-ounce packages fresh spinach, stems removed and chopped** | |
| **¼ cup chopped fresh parsley** | *3* In a large bowl, mix together the beaten eggs, ricotta cheese, and feta cheese. Add the dill, nutmeg, and oregano. Stir the egg and cheese mixture into the spinach mixture. |
| **2 eggs, lightly beaten** | |
| **½ cup ricotta cheese** | |
| **1½ cups crumbled, pasteurized feta cheese** | *4* Lay five sheets of phyllo dough in the baking pan so that they cover the entire bottom of the pan. Brush the top of each sheet lightly with olive oil. |
| **⅓ cup chopped fresh dill** | |
| **¼ teaspoon ground nutmeg** | *5* Fill the phyllo-lined pan with the spinach mixture and fold any overhanging dough over the spinach filling. |
| **1 teaspoon dried oregano** | |
| **10 sheets frozen phyllo dough, completely thawed** | *6* Brush the top of the dough and mixture with olive oil and layer the remaining five sheets of phyllo dough on top of the filling, making sure to brush each sheet with oil. |
| | *7* Tuck any overhanging dough into the pan to seal the pie. Bake for 45 to 60 minutes, or until the top turns golden brown. |

*Per serving:* Calories 385 (From Fat 219); Fat 24g (Saturated 9g); Cholesterol 115mg; Sodium 793mg; Carbohydrate 30g (Dietary Fiber 6g); Protein 14g; Iron 5mg; Calcium 318mg; Folate 164mcg.

*Tip:* To save on time, try using frozen spinach rather than fresh. Just thaw it in the microwave and squeeze out the excess water before using it. You can also use 2 tablespoons of dried dill if you don't have fresh.

# Sweet Potato Hash

**Prep time:** 10 min  •  **Cook time:** 25 min  •  **Yield:** 4 servings

| Ingredients | Directions |
|---|---|
| 1 tablespoon olive oil | **1** In a large skillet, heat the olive oil over medium heat. Add the sweet potatoes, cinnamon, nutmeg, and cloves. Cook for 10 minutes and then add the apple pieces. Cook until the potatoes are tender when poked with a fork, about 10 minutes. |
| 2 large sweet potatoes, diced | |
| 1 teaspoon ground cinnamon | |
| ½ teaspoon ground nutmeg | |
| ¼ teaspoon ground cloves | **2** Add the raisins and cook until the potatoes and apples have begun to crisp around the edges, about 5 minutes. Add the chives. Serve immediately. |
| 1 Granny Smith apple, diced | |
| ¼ cup golden raisins | |
| 2 tablespoons coarsely chopped chives | |

*Per serving:* Calories 179 (From Fat 34); Fat 4g (Saturated 1g); Cholesterol 0mg; Sodium 12mg; Carbohydrate 36g (Dietary Fiber 5g); Protein 2g; Iron 1mg; Calcium 42mg; Folate 24mcg.

*Note:* This sweet potato hash makes a great side dish for pork or chicken entrees.

---

## Relying on prewashed greens for convenience

The modern focus on convenience makes preparing fresh salads as easy as making any other meal (maybe even easier!). The prewashed bags of greens available at most grocery stores require nothing more than tearing open the bag, giving the greens a quick rinse, and pouring them into a salad bowl.

*Remember:* Even though the greens are prewashed, give them another rinse to be extra cautious about the pesky bacteria that can contaminate fresh greens; find out more about potentially harmful bacteria in Chapter 4.

If you also purchase precut fruits and veggies, crumbled or shredded cheese, and premade dressing, you can literally have a salad ready in 3 minutes or less.

# Serving Up Pasta and Pizza

Who doesn't love to eat pasta and pizza in one form or another? Although the Italians are known for both, many cultures have adopted their own versions of noodles and the famous pizza pie.

Pizza often gets a bad rap, but I think it's actually quite the nutritional gem. The crust provides carbs and important B vitamins (like folate, which is crucial during pregnancy), the pizza sauce provides lycopene among other nutrients, and the cheese provides calcium, protein, and vitamin D.

To make your pizza a bit healthier, follow these guidelines:

- ✔ Choose whole-grain crust when available.

- ✔ Skip the greasy toppings like pepperoni and sausage. Choose Canadian bacon or white-meat chicken if you want meat.

- ✔ Load up on veggies and get creative with super-healthy veggies like spinach, eggplant, zucchini, broccoli, asparagus, and more!

- ✔ Order your pizza with half the normal amount of cheese. Most pizza places are happy to honor your request.

- ✔ Make your own pizza instead of ordering it from a restaurant. Making your own pizza allows you to control what you put on it.

I share a yummy pizza recipe, as well as a few pasta dishes, in this section.

## Tomatoes: The savory fruit

Technically, tomatoes are a fruit, but many people think of them as a vegetable because they aren't as sweet as most fruits and you eat them in savory foods. Whatever you decide to call them, make sure you call them to dinner or lunch or even breakfast! Why? Because tomatoes contain a phytonutrient called *lycopene,* which has been shown to help prevent heart disease and certain cancers, specifically breast, pancreatic, and colon.

Ketchup is one way to get in your daily dose of tomato. In fact, the U.S. Department of Agriculture actually considers this condiment a vegetable. Research shows that your body absorbs lycopene better when it's heated and combined with a bit of fat. So eat your ketchup with a fat-containing food (like a lean burger) or have marinara sauce with a bit of oil in it. Now I'm not saying french fries dipped in ketchup are the most nutritious food on the planet, but that ketchup may not be so bad after all!

If ketchup isn't your thing, look for other ways to get your tomatoes: sun-dried tomatoes, tomato juice, tomato sauce, or just plain sliced tomatoes.

# Vegetable Lasagna

**Prep time:** 25 min, plus standing time • **Cook time:** About 1 hr • **Yield:** 8 servings

## Ingredients

One 10-ounce box frozen chopped spinach

1 tablespoon olive oil

1 small onion, chopped

2 cloves garlic, chopped

1 red bell pepper, seeded and diced

1 medium zucchini, thinly sliced

8 ounces button mushrooms, sliced

One 15-ounce container lowfat ricotta cheese

One 16-ounce container lowfat pasteurized cottage cheese

1 egg, lightly beaten

1 tablespoon salt-free Italian herb seasoning

8 ounces part-skim mozzarella cheese, shredded and divided

½ cup grated Parmesan cheese, divided

Two 26-ounce jars marinara sauce

8 ounces lasagna noodles, cooked and drained

## Directions

*1* Preheat the oven to 350 degrees. Defrost the spinach in the microwave and squeeze out the excess water.

*2* In a large skillet, heat the olive oil over medium heat. Sauté the onion, garlic, bell pepper, zucchini, and mushrooms until tender, about 4 to 5 minutes. Set aside.

*3* In a medium bowl, mix together the ricotta cheese, cottage cheese, egg, and Italian seasoning. Mix in the spinach and half of the mozzarella and Parmesan cheeses.

*4* Spread a thin layer of pasta sauce in the bottom of a 9-x-13-inch glass baking dish. Place one layer of lasagna noodles (about 5 noodles) on top of the sauce. Spread ⅓ of the spinach-cheese mixture on top of the noodles. Sprinkle ⅓ of the pepper and zucchini mixture on top of the cheese. Spread 1 cup of pasta sauce over the vegetables. Repeat these layers twice more. Add a final layer of noodles and top with the remaining sauce.

*5* Cover the dish with foil and bake for 45 minutes. Uncover and sprinkle the remaining Parmesan cheese and mozzarella cheese on top. Bake for 10 to 15 more minutes, or until the cheese is melted. Let stand for 10 minutes before cutting and serving.

*Per serving:* Calories 445 (From Fat 146); Fat 16g (Saturated 7g); Cholesterol 66mg; Sodium 1,379mg; Carbohydrate 46g (Dietary Fiber 6g); Protein 31g; Iron 4mg; Calcium 482mg; Folate 142mcg.

*Note:* This recipe uses part cottage cheese rather than all ricotta cheese, which allows you to use less mozzarella cheese. The result is a reduced amount of fat and calories and an increased amount of protein. (Ricotta cheese doesn't require the word *pasteurized* on the label because the heat treatment used during curd formation meets the heat requirements for pasteurization and makes it safe to eat. You'll see the word *pasteurized* on cottage cheese packages, though.)

# Homemade Gnocchi with Pesto

**Prep time:** 30 min  •  **Cook time:** About 20 min  •  **Yield:** 6 servings

| Ingredients | Directions |
|---|---|
| **2 large white baking potatoes** | *1* Poke several holes in the potatoes with a fork. Microwave them on high for 6 minutes. Wear an oven mitt and turn the potatoes over. Microwave them for another 5 to 6 minutes, or until they're tender when squeezed. Allow the potatoes to cool enough to hold them without burning your hands. Peel the potatoes. |
| **3 cloves garlic** | |
| **¼ cup pine nuts** | |
| **¼ cup chopped walnuts** | |
| **2 cups fresh basil leaves** | |
| **½ teaspoon plus ½ teaspoon salt** | *2* In a food processor, combine the garlic, pine nuts, and walnuts. Blend until they have a pastelike consistency. Add the basil, ½ teaspoon of salt, pepper, ⅓ cup of olive oil, and Parmesan cheese and blend just until combined. |
| **¼ teaspoon pepper** | |
| **⅓ cup plus 1 tablespoon olive oil** | *3* In a medium pot, bring the water to a boil over high heat. Add the remaining salt to the water. |
| **¼ cup shredded Parmesan cheese** | *4* Use a hand mixer or potato masher to mash the peeled potatoes until there are no lumps and the texture is light and fluffy. Stir in the egg yolks. Add 1½ cups of the flour and stir until it forms dough. |
| **5 cups water** | |
| **2 egg yolks, lightly beaten** | |
| **2 cups all-purpose flour** | *5* Transfer the dough to a floured surface. Add enough of the remaining flour so that it isn't sticky. Cut the dough into four sections. Gently roll each section into a long rope. Cut the rope into bite-sized pieces. |
| **¼ cup pasteurized Gorgonzola crumbles, for garnish** | |
| | *6* In a large skillet, heat 1 tablespoon of olive oil over medium heat. |
| | *7* Add the gnocchi to the boiling water, putting only half in at a time. When the gnocchi float to the top (after about 3 to 5 minutes), take them out and put them in the hot skillet. As the gnocchi brown, remove them from the skillet and place them in a large serving bowl. Pour the pesto over the gnocchi and toss to coat. Sprinkle with the crumbled Gorgonzola. |

*Per serving:* Calories 457 (From Fat 225); Fat 25g (Saturated 5g); Cholesterol 78mg; Sodium 326mg; Carbohydrate 48g (Dietary Fiber 4g); Protein 11g; Iron 4mg; Calcium 119mg; Folate 113mcg.

# Broccoli, Beans, and Feta Pasta

**Prep time:** 5 min • **Cook time:** About 20 min • **Yield:** 4 servings

| *Ingredients* | *Directions* |
|---|---|
| 6 cups water | *1* In a large saucepan, bring the water to a boil over high heat. Add the cavatappi pasta and cook for 8 to 10 minutes, or until it's *al dente* (firm but not hard). Drain and set aside. |
| 6 ounces whole-grain cavatappi pasta | |
| 2 cups broccoli florets | |
| 1 tablespoon olive oil | *2* In a large pot, steam the broccoli in a steamer basket over 1 cup of boiling water over medium-high heat for 4 to 5 minutes, or until tender-crisp. Set the broccoli aside and reserve 2 tablespoons of the water the broccoli was cooked in. |
| 4 cloves garlic, chopped | |
| 1 cup canned cannellini beans, drained and rinsed | |
| 1 tablespoon dried Italian seasoning | *3* In a large skillet, heat the olive oil over medium heat. Add the garlic and sauté for 1 minute. Add the steamed broccoli, the 2 tablespoons of reserved water, the beans, and the Italian seasoning. Stir for about 3 minutes. |
| ¼ cup crumbled, pasteurized feta cheese | |
| | *4* Reduce the heat to low and add the cooked pasta and feta cheese. Stir for about 2 minutes. Serve immediately. |

**Per serving:** *Calories 270 (From Fat 58); Fat 6g (Saturated 2g); Cholesterol 8mg; Sodium 225mg; Carbohydrate 45g (Dietary Fiber 8g); Protein 12g; Iron 3mg; Calcium 128mg; Folate 117mcg.*

***Vary It!*** Add roasted or sun-dried tomatoes or mix in a marinara sauce if you want that traditional tomato taste in your pasta dish. You can also use penne or any other pasta that you find.

*Source: Keri Gans, MS, RD, CDN, nutrition consultant, speaker, and author of The Small Change Diet (Simon & Schuster)*

# Roasted Eggplant, Olive, and Goat Cheese Homemade Pizza

**Prep time:** 30 min, plus standing time • **Cook time:** 30–35 min • **Yield:** 6 servings

| *Ingredients* | *Directions* |
|---|---|
| 1 package prepared pizza dough | *1* Preheat the oven to 400 degrees. Let the pizza dough stand at room temperature. Place the eggplant in a colander and sprinkle it with salt. Let it sit for 15 minutes. |
| ½ unpeeled eggplant, sliced | |
| Dash of salt | |
| Nonstick cooking spray | *2* Spray a large baking sheet with nonstick cooking spray. Brush both sides of the eggplant slices with the olive oil and place them on the baking sheet. Bake for 12 to 15 minutes, turning once. Let the eggplant cool but keep the oven on. |
| 1 tablespoon olive oil | |
| 2 tablespoons flour | |
| ½ cup pizza sauce | |
| ½ cup fresh spinach, stems removed and torn into pieces | *3* Spray a cookie sheet or pizza pan with nonstick cooking spray. Dust the counter with the flour and use a floured rolling pin to roll out the pizza dough to the desired thickness (about ¼ inch if you like thin crust). Place the dough on the prepared cookie sheet or pizza pan. Spread with pizza sauce. |
| 2 tablespoons chopped sun-dried tomatoes (not packed in oil) | |
| 2 tablespoons sliced black olives | |
| 2 tablespoons sliced green olives | *4* Dice the cooled eggplant. Top the pizza with the eggplant, spinach, sun-dried tomatoes, black and green olives, and pine nuts. Sprinkle with the mozzarella cheese and goat cheese. |
| 2 tablespoons pine nuts | |
| 1 cup shredded part-skim mozzarella cheese | *5* Bake for 18 to 20 minutes, or until the cheese is melted. Let stand for a few minutes before cutting. |
| ½ cup crumbled, pasteurized goat cheese | |

*Per serving:* Calories 334 (From Fat 85); Fat 9g (Saturated 4g); Cholesterol 15mg; Sodium 595mg; Carbohydrate 43g (Dietary Fiber 3g); Protein 15g; Iron 1mg; Calcium 154mg; Folate 55mcg.

*Note:* For a smoky eggplant taste, place the eggplant slices on a medium-hot grill and cook for 4 minutes on each side.

*Tip:* If you can find it, opt for whole-wheat pizza dough to get more fiber and added nutrients.

# Chapter 16

# How Sweet It Is: Dessert Recipes

## In This Chapter

▶ Creating smooth and creamy recipes that are packed with good nutrition

▶ Enjoying chocolate without the guilt

▶ Sweetening your dessert plate with the refreshing taste of fruit

### Recipes in This Chapter

↻ Mixed Berry Frozen Yogurt

↻ Kiwi Custard Pie

↻ Banana Mini Trifle

↻ Mango Coconut Rice Pudding

↻ Fudgy Peppermint Black Bean Brownies

↻ Dark Chocolate Cherry Pistachio Bark

↻ Chocolate Lover's Sippable Sundae

↻ Peanut Butter Chocolate Chip Pie

↻ Chocolate Butterscotch Chip Bundt Cake

↻ Fruit Cookie Pizza

↻ Pineapple Spice Loaf with Cream Cheese Frosting

↻ Lemon Raspberry Cupcakes

↻ Apple Cinnamon Crêpes

↻ White Chocolate Berry Oatmeal Cookies

🍴 🥄 ↻ 🍴 ✴ 🌿

*T*he best advice I can give you when it comes to eating dessert (a favorite hobby of mine, I might add) is to be fully present in what you're doing at that exact moment. Dessert is too good and too high in calories to eat in front of the TV or while you're doing or thinking of something else. Sit down with your dessert of choice and enjoy every bite. Take small bites, close your eyes, and savor the flavor. If you do this, you'll be surprised by how *little* dessert you really need to truly satisfy your sweet tooth.

This chapter features three main types of desserts: smooth and creamy treats, chocolate wonders, and fruity favorites. Most of these recipes are good-for-you dessert options that have a significant amount of nutritional value. However, I just want to put the disclaimer out there that not every recipe in this chapter is a nutritional powerhouse. After all, sometimes you just need a little bit of sweet pleasure. My hope is that these desserts will nourish as well as satisfy your sweet cravings during your pregnancy. (No matter what your cravings are telling you, I guarantee you can find something in this chapter to satisfy 'em.)

# *Whipping Up Smooth and Creamy Treats*

Did you know that you crave textures as well as tastes? Sometimes you know you want something sweet, but after going through a cookie and a few bites of cake, you still aren't satisfied and find yourself searching for more. That may be because even though the cookie and cake were sweet, they didn't satisfy the creamy texture you were craving. Ice cream, pudding, mousse, and custard provide you with the creamy goodness that hits the spot.

All too often, *creamy* means exactly that: cream! Most creamy concoctions call for heavy whipping cream, which is extremely high not only in calories but also in artery-clogging saturated fat. Definitely not the best thing for you and your baby. Instead of using heavy cream, the recipes in this section use either reduced-fat (2%) or lowfat (1%) milk. Milk provides nourishing nutrients like calcium and protein with less impact on your overall caloric budget and your arteries. You can play around with substituting reduced-fat milk, evaporated skim milk, or fat-free half and half in many of your favorite creamy recipes.

Not only do the following four recipes satisfy your "creamy tooth," but they're also packed with nutrition! Here's a sneak peek of some of the nutrients and corresponding foods you'll find in these recipes:

- ✔ **Antioxidants:** Berries, bananas, mango, and kiwi
- ✔ **Calcium:** Milk and yogurt
- ✔ **Fiber:** Berries, bananas, mango, kiwi, and brown rice
- ✔ **Folate:** Berries, bananas, mango, and kiwi
- ✔ **Potassium:** Berries, bananas, mango, and kiwi
- ✔ **Protein:** Milk, yogurt, and brown rice

## Enjoying ice cream the healthy way

Store-bought ice creams are one easy way to satisfy your cravings for creamy goodness. Following are some tricks for enjoying these treats without overloading on empty calories and fat:

- ✔ Look for reduced-fat or fat-free ice cream or frozen yogurt in your favorite flavors.

- ✔ Practice portion control by scooping a half-cup serving into a small serving bowl and walking away from the container.

- ✔ Give yourself a limit by purchasing individually wrapped ice cream treats on a stick or in sandwich form. When the wrapper is empty, you know you're finished!

# Mixed Berry Frozen Yogurt

**Prep time:** 10 min • **Freeze time:** 2 hr • **Yield:** 6 servings

| Ingredients | Directions |
|---|---|
| 1 cup frozen strawberries<br><br>1 cup frozen blueberries<br><br>1 cup frozen raspberries<br><br>1 cup plain lowfat Greek yogurt<br><br>¼ cup powdered sugar<br><br>Nonstick cooking spray<br><br>6 fresh whole strawberries<br><br>6 mint sprigs (optional) | *1* Place the frozen berries, yogurt, and powdered sugar into a food processor or blender. Mix until the fruit is well mixed but still a bit chunky.<br><br>*2* Lightly coat 6 individual ramekins with nonstick cooking spray. Divide the berry mixture among the 6 ramekins. Cover each dish with plastic wrap and place it in the freezer. Freeze for 2 hours, or until the mixture is firm.<br><br>*3* Unmold the frozen yogurt by running a hot knife around the edge of each ramekin and quickly dipping it in hot water. Invert each ramekin over a small plate and shake gently to get the yogurt to slide out.<br><br>*4* Garnish each serving with a whole strawberry and a mint sprig (if desired). Serve immediately. |

*Per serving:* Calories 85 (From Fat 10); Fat 1g (Saturated 1g); Cholesterol 3mg; Sodium 12mg; Carbohydrate 16g (Dietary Fiber 3g); Protein 4g; Iron 1mg; Calcium 56mg; Folate 16mcg.

*Vary It!* Instead of berries, try this recipe with your favorite fruit combination. Think peaches, pineapple, bananas, mango, papaya . . . the possibilities are as great as the fruit you can find!

*Tip:* Feel free to enjoy the frozen yogurt right from the ramekin if you're in a rush for something sweet and creamy!

*Note:* If you don't have individual ramekins on hand, simply pour the berry mixture into a medium glass bowl, cover, and freeze. When the yogurt's frozen, scoop it out using an ice cream scoop.

*Source: Tina Ruggiero, MS, RD, LD, and coauthor of The Best Homemade Baby Food on the Planet (Fair Winds Press)*

# Kiwi Custard Pie

**Prep time:** 10 min • **Cook time:** About 55 min • **Yield:** 8 servings

| Ingredients | Directions |
|---|---|
| 1 premade frozen pie shell | *1* Allow the frozen pie shell to thaw for 15 minutes at room temperature. Preheat the oven to the temperature indicated on the pie shell package and bake until the shell is just barely browned, about 15 minutes. |
| 4 eggs | |
| 1 cup reduced-fat milk | |
| ¾ cup sugar | *2* In a large bowl, use an electric mixer to mix together the eggs, milk, sugar, and vanilla until well blended. |
| 1½ teaspoons vanilla | |
| 5 ripe kiwi fruit, peeled and sliced | *3* Arrange the kiwi slices neatly in the pie shell. Pour the filling mixture over the kiwi. Bake for about 40 minutes, or until the filling is golden and set. Serve warm and store any leftovers covered in the refrigerator. |

*Per serving:* Calories 234 (From Fat 75); Fat 8g (Saturated 3g); Cholesterol 108mg; Sodium 153mg; Carbohydrate 36g (Dietary Fiber 2g); Protein 5g; Iron 1mg; Calcium 66mg; Folate 38mcg.

*Vary It!* I like this pie best when it's warm, but if you're a cold-pie lover, try it chilled. You can also use a premade graham cracker crust in place of the traditional pie crust.

*Tip:* Check the pie after 30 minutes of baking time to see if the crust is browning. If it is, you may want to cover the edges with some foil to make sure it doesn't overbrown.

*Source: Anne Nechkov, professional food stylist and chef*

# Banana Mini Trifle

**Prep time:** 15 min, plus refrigerating time • **Yield:** 8 servings

| Ingredients | Directions |
|---|---|
| One 3.4-ounce package cheesecake-flavored instant pudding mix | *1* Empty the dry pudding mix into a large bowl. Add the milk and use an electric mixer to slowly combine the dry mix and milk. |
| 1½ cups lowfat milk | |
| 4 ounces light frozen whipped topping, thawed | *2* Fold in the whipped topping. Refrigerate the mixture for 5 minutes. |
| 24 vanilla wafer cookies | *3* Use a food processor to crush the vanilla wafer cookies, leaving small chunks of cookie. |
| 2 bananas, thinly sliced | |
| ½ cup mini chocolate chips | *4* In individual glass dishes, layer the ingredients one on top of another, starting with the crushed cookies, then the pudding, then the slices of banana, and finally the mini chocolate chips. Repeat once. |
| | *5* Finish off each serving with a small sprinkle of cookie chunks and chocolate chips. Serve immediately. |

*Per serving:* Calories 231 (From Fat 69); Fat 8g (Saturated 4g); Cholesterol 2mg; Sodium 237mg; Carbohydrate 38g (Dietary Fiber 1g); Protein 3g; Iron 1mg; Calcium 66mg; Folate 13mcg.

*Vary It!* If you're not much of a cheesecake fan, feel free to use vanilla or banana-flavored pudding instead. Also, add a layer or two of coconut flakes for a fun twist.

*Tip:* Wine glasses make great individual serving dishes for this yummy trifle.

# Mango Coconut Rice Pudding

**Prep time:** 10 min • **Cook time:** 1 hr 35 min • **Yield:** 6 servings

| Ingredients | Directions |
|---|---|
| **Nonstick cooking spray** | **1** Preheat the oven to 325 degrees. Coat an 8-x-8-inch baking dish with nonstick cooking spray. |
| **2 cups water** | |
| **⅛ teaspoon salt** | **2** In a medium saucepan, bring the water and salt to a boil. Add the rice. Return the water to a boil and then reduce the heat to low. Cover and simmer until the rice is tender and the liquid has been absorbed, about 50 minutes. |
| **1 cup uncooked medium-grain brown rice** | |
| **1½ cups lowfat milk** | |
| **1 egg** | |
| **⅓ cup sugar** | **3** In a large bowl, stir together the cooked rice, milk, egg, sugar, coconut extract, cinnamon, nutmeg, and dried mango. |
| **½ teaspoon coconut extract** | |
| **¼ teaspoon cinnamon** | |
| **⅛ teaspoon nutmeg** | **4** Pour the rice mixture into the prepared dish and cover with foil. Bake for 30 minutes. Remove the dish from the oven and sprinkle the dried coconut on top. Bake uncovered for another 15 minutes. Serve warm. |
| **½ cup chopped, dried mango** | |
| **⅓ cup dried, sweetened coconut flakes** | |

*Per serving:* Calories 164 (From Fat 23); Fat 3g (Saturated 2g); Cholesterol 2mg; Sodium 101mg; Carbohydrate 33g (Dietary Fiber 1g); Protein 3g; Iron 1mg; Calcium 82mg; Folate 20mcg.

*Tip:* To save time, use instant brown rice. For Step 2, simply cook the rice as directed on the package. Then follow the rest of the directions.

*Vary It!* Instead of mango and coconut, use pineapple or raisins or experiment with dried cranberries or blueberries. You can also swap vanilla extract for the coconut extract.

# Pregnancy Must-Have: Chocolate!

Sometimes a girl just *needs* chocolate. Then she gets pregnant. For some women, the cravings for chocolate intensify. Chocolate contains quite a few calories thanks to all the fat and sugar, but it's not all bad for you.

One study found that pregnant women who ate the equivalent of one dark chocolate candy bar per day had an almost 70 percent reduced chance of having preeclampsia. Why? Because dark chocolate has several nutrients that make it at least somewhat nutritious:

- ✔ **Theobromine:** This *alkaloid* (a naturally occurring chemical compound) gives the cocoa bean its bitter taste, but research shows that it also assists in blood pressure control and relaxes the smooth muscle around the blood vessels so that they dilate more easily.

- ✔ **Flavonoids:** These plant-based, naturally occurring chemicals offer several health benefits, including antioxidant activity. Dark chocolate specifically contains the flavonoid epicatechin, which reduces the risk of blood clots.

- ✔ **Magnesium:** This mineral is linked to lowering blood pressure.

Perhaps you're wondering whether chocolate has to be dark for you not to feel guilty about eating it. Dark chocolate has more cocoa in it, so it generally has higher levels of the good stuff. Milk chocolate has less, and white chocolate has none. (White chocolate is actually just sugar and fat; it doesn't contain any cocoa, which means it doesn't contain any of the healthy ingredients I mention in the preceding list.)

Although chocolate has its positives, it's not something you should eat with reckless abandon — even if your cravings are telling, make that *commanding*, you to do so. The reality is that chocolate still contains a lot of calories, and it tastes so good that it's hard to stop eating after you start. Also, chocolate can give pregnant women heartburn. Given these facts, try to indulge wisely and use at least a bit of moderation when eating chocolate. I can't give you hard and fast numbers of how much chocolate you can eat in a day because those numbers depend on what else you're eating. If you're pretty darn healthy and are minding your calories everywhere else, you can eat about an ounce of chocolate every day (that's equivalent to six Hershey kisses).

This section has five chocolate recipes to satisfy your strongest chocolate cravings. When you're craving chocolate and ice cream, go for the Chocolate Lover's Sippable Sundae. It's decadent but the portion is still manageable. The Peanut Butter Chocolate Chip Pie is out of this world, and a little goes a long way to satisfy. Don't be afraid to enjoy your chocolate; just be sure to do so in moderation!

# Fudgy Peppermint Black Bean Brownies

**Prep time:** 10 min • **Cook time:** 30 min • **Yield:** 16 servings

| Ingredients | Directions |
|---|---|
| Nonstick cooking spray<br><br>One 15-ounce can black beans, drained and rinsed<br><br>3 eggs<br><br>3 tablespoons canola oil<br><br>½ cup unsweetened cocoa powder<br><br>⅛ teaspoon salt<br><br>½ teaspoon peppermint extract<br><br>¾ cup sugar<br><br>½ cup semisweet chocolate chunks<br><br>¼ cup ground peppermint candies | **1** Preheat the oven to 350 degrees. Spray an 8-x-8-inch baking pan with nonstick cooking spray.<br><br>**2** In a blender or food processor, puree the black beans, eggs, oil, cocoa powder, salt, peppermint extract, and sugar until smooth. Fold in the chocolate chunks.<br><br>**3** Pour the batter into the prepared pan and bake uncovered for 25 minutes.<br><br>**4** Remove the brownies from the oven and sprinkle the ground peppermint candies on top. Bake for another 5 minutes, or until the edges start to pull away from the pan.<br><br>**5** Cut the brownies while they're still warm before the candy topping has a chance to cool completely and harden. |

*Per serving:* Calories 130 (From Fat 47); Fat 5g (Saturated 2g); Cholesterol 0mg; Sodium 62mg; Carbohydrate 18g (Dietary Fiber 2g); Protein 2g; Iron 1mg; Calcium 12mg; Folate 17mcg.

*Note:* If you don't spill the (black) beans about your secret ingredient, I promise no one will ever know they're in there.

*Tip:* I like to use ground candy canes or round peppermints for this recipe.

*Vary It!* Not a fan of peppermint? Exchange vanilla extract for the peppermint kind and drizzle raspberry preserves on top in place of the candies (just swirl the preserves into the batter with a knife prior to baking). You can also use white chocolate chips in place of the chocolate chunks.

# Dark Chocolate Cherry Pistachio Bark

**Prep time:** 15 min, plus refrigerating time • **Yield:** 24 servings

| *Ingredients* | *Directions* |
|---|---|
| **1 pound dark chocolate** | *1* Line a large baking sheet with parchment paper. |
| **¼ cup coarsely chopped, unsalted, roasted almonds** | *2* In a large microwave-safe bowl, break up the chocolate with your hands. Microwave the dark chocolate on high until it's completely melted (up to 2 minutes), stirring every 30 seconds. |
| **½ cup coarsely chopped shelled pistachios** | |
| **¾ cup coarsely chopped dried cherries** | *3* Stir the almonds, pistachios, and cherries into the melted chocolate. |
| | *4* Spread the mixture onto the prepared pan and refrigerate until the bark is set, about 30 minutes. |
| | *5* Break the chocolate into 1-ounce pieces and serve. |

*Per serving:* Calories 141 (From Fat 74); Fat 8g (Saturated 4g); Cholesterol 1mg; Sodium 1mg; Carbohydrate 15g (Dietary Fiber 3g); Protein 2g; Iron 1mg; Calcium 9mg; Folate 2mcg.

***Vary It!*** Use cashews rather than pistachios, blueberries rather than cherries, or milk chocolate rather than dark.

***Note:*** Thanks to the red color of the cherries and the green color of the pistachios, this recipe may become a new favorite treat for your holiday parties.

CHOPPING NUTS

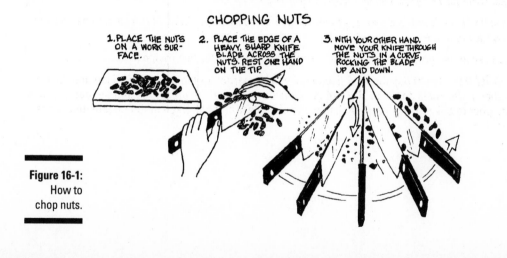

1. PLACE THE NUTS ON A WORK SURFACE.

2. PLACE THE EDGE OF A HEAVY, SHARP KNIFE BLADE ACROSS THE NUTS. REST ONE HAND ON THE TIP.

3. WITH YOUR OTHER HAND, MOVE YOUR KNIFE THROUGH THE NUTS IN A CURVE, ROCKING THE BLADE UP AND DOWN.

**Figure 16-1:**
How to
chop nuts.

# Chocolate Lover's Sippable Sundae

**Prep time:** 10 min • **Yield:** 2 servings

| *Ingredients* | *Directions* |
|---|---|
| 1 cup chocolate lowfat frozen yogurt | *1* In a blender, blend the frozen yogurt and milk until smooth. |
| ¼ cup lowfat milk | |
| 4 tablespoons hot fudge, warmed and divided | *2* Pour half of the yogurt mixture into two 8-ounce glasses. Drizzle 1 tablespoon of hot fudge over each shake. Top the two shakes with ⅛ cup of the cookie pieces. |
| ¼ cup crumbled chocolate sandwich cookies, divided | |
| 2 tablespoons light whipped topping (spray can or tub) | *3* Divide the other half of the yogurt mixture evenly between the two shakes on top of the cookie layer. Top each shake with another tablespoon of hot fudge. |
| 2 maraschino cherries | |
| | *4* Sprinkle the rest of the cookie pieces on top of the fudge in each glass. Add 1 tablespoon of whipped topping on top. Place one cherry on top of each glass. Enjoy with a straw. |

*Per serving:* Calories 346 (From Fat 77); Fat 9g (Saturated 4g); Cholesterol 7mg; Sodium 334mg; Carbohydrate 62g (Dietary Fiber 3g); Protein 9g; Iron 2mg; Calcium 218mg; Folate 25mcg.

*Note:* This recipe doesn't have an overwhelming amount of nutritional value, but when you're craving ice cream and chocolate, it's guaranteed to hit the spot!

*Vary It!* Add a banana to the shake mixture and use strawberries in the layers in place of the cookie pieces to make a strawberry-banana chocolate split sundae!

# *Peanut Butter Chocolate Chip Pie*

**Prep time:** 10 min, plus refrigerating time • **Yield:** 8 servings

| *Ingredients* | *Directions* |
|---|---|
| **One 8-ounce package ⅓-reduced-fat pasteurized cream cheese, softened** | *1* In a large mixing bowl, use an electric mixer to cream together the cream cheese, peanut butter, and sugar. Fold in the whipped topping. |
| **½ cup peanut butter** | |
| **½ cup sugar** | *2* Pour the pie filling into the cookie crust and spread evenly. |
| **One 8-ounce container light frozen whipped topping, thawed** | |
| **Prepared chocolate cookie pie crust** | *3* Decorate the outside edge of the pie with mini chocolate chips. Refrigerate for 30 minutes or more before serving. |
| **½ cup mini chocolate chips** | |

*Per serving: Calories 473 (From Fat 269); Fat 30g (Saturated 13g); Cholesterol 22mg; Sodium 377mg; Carbohydrate 45g (Dietary Fiber 2g); Protein 9g; Iron 2mg; Calcium 39mg; Folate 30mcg.*

*Note:* It doesn't matter whether you use creamy or crunchy peanut butter, so pick whichever one you like better.

*Tip:* This pie is so decadent and delicious that you can get away with cutting the slices smaller than ⅛ of the pie. A little goes a long way to satisfy!

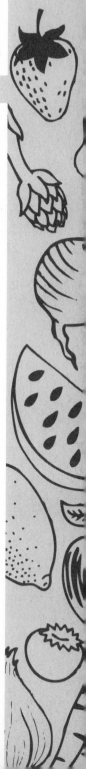

# Chocolate Butterscotch Chip Bundt Cake

**Prep time:** 15 min, plus cooling time • **Cook time:** 45–50 min • **Yield:** 16 servings

| Ingredients | Directions |
|---|---|
| Nonstick cooking spray | *1* Preheat the oven to 350 degrees. Spray a Bundt pan with nonstick cooking spray. |
| 1¼ cups sugar | |
| 2 eggs | *2* In a small mixing bowl, use an electric mixer to mix together the sugar, eggs, and oil. Add 1½ cups of milk, the lemon juice, and the vanilla extract slowly and mix well. |
| ¼ cup canola oil | |
| 1½ cups plus 2 tablespoons lowfat milk | |
| 1 tablespoon lemon juice | *3* In a large mixing bowl, mix together the flours, cocoa powder, baking powder, baking soda, and salt. Pour the liquid mixture over the dry mixture and mix until everything is moistened and blended. Stir in ½ cup of butterscotch chips with a spoon. |
| 2 teaspoons vanilla extract | |
| 1½ cups whole-wheat flour | |
| 1 cup all-purpose flour | |
| ½ cup unsweetened cocoa powder | *4* Pour the batter into the prepared Bundt pan. Bake for 45 to 50 minutes. |
| 2 teaspoons baking powder | |
| 1½ teaspoons baking soda | *5* Remove the pan from the oven, set it on a wire rack, and allow the cake to cool for 10 minutes. Turn the partially cooled cake upside down over a serving plate and gently shake the pan to get the cake out. Allow the cake to cool completely. |
| ½ teaspoon salt | |
| 1 cup butterscotch chips, divided | |
| | *6* Prepare the butterscotch glaze by melting the remaining ½ cup of butterscotch chips and 2 tablespoons of milk in a small microwave-safe bowl for 45 seconds, or until melted. Drizzle the glaze over the top of the cake. |

*Per serving:* Calories 216 (From Fat 65); Fat 7g (Saturated 3g); Cholesterol 25mg; Sodium 240mg; Carbohydrate 35g (Dietary Fiber 2g); Protein 4g; Iron 1mg; Calcium 50mg; Folate 20mcg.

*Vary It!* Don't love butterscotch? Make this a triple-chocolate cake by using chocolate chips in place of the butterscotch chips for both the cake and the glaze.

# Diving into the Refreshing, Sweet Taste of Fruit

As I'm sure you already know, what you're supposed to eat and what you want to eat aren't always the same thing. Because you *need* nutrient-rich foods but may often *want* something sweet when you're pregnant, fruity dishes, particularly fruit desserts, are the perfect solution.

Fruit contains natural sugars that give it that sweet taste, so you don't have to add a ton of sugar to make a gratifying dessert. And the best part about including fresh, frozen, or dried fruit in your sweet treats is that you get a handful of extra vitamins, minerals, and fiber for you and your baby. So when creamy or chocolate desserts seem a little too rich for your tastes, focus on refreshing fruit desserts instead.

Not only is fruit flavorful, but it's also colorful! Fruit adds color to your table, and with that color comes a bevy of nutrients:

- ✔ Orange and yellow fruits are high in *antioxidants,* such as beta carotene and vitamin C, which improve immunity and protect cells. Try to eat plenty of oranges, tangerines, cantaloupe, mango, lemon, papaya, pineapple, pumpkin, and apricots.

- ✔ Blue and purple fruits contain the phytonutrients *anthocyanins,* which help with memory. Be sure to eat your share of grapes (raisins), plums (prunes), blackberries, blueberries, and dates.

- ✔ Green fruits contain chlorophyll and are high in essential nutrients such as folate and carotenoids, which help improve vision. Healthful green fruits include kiwi and honeydew.

- ✔ Red fruits contain the heart-healthy compounds lycopene and anthocyanins. Eat apples, strawberries, raspberries, cherries, watermelon, pomegranate, and red grapefruit for heart health.

This section has five fruity and delicious recipes that are sure to refresh; they're no slouch in the nutrition department either. When you dig into these dishes, you'll get some whole grains (courtesy of oats and whole-wheat flour), lots of fiber (thanks to the wide variety of fruits), and, of course, folate galore!

If you're looking for a burst of sunshine on your dessert plate, check out the Lemon Raspberry Cupcakes. They're sweet, tart, and creamy all in one. For a colorful party plate, make the Fruit Cookie Pizza and have fun artfully arranging the fruit. You're sure to impress your guests!

# Fruit Cookie Pizza

**Prep time:** 20 min • **Cook time:** 12–15 min • **Yield:** 12 servings

| Ingredients | Directions |
|---|---|
| Nonstick cooking spray | **1** Preheat the oven to 350 degrees. Spray a 10-inch pizza pan with nonstick cooking spray. |
| One 18-ounce package refrigerated sugar cookie dough | **2** Spread the cookie dough on the bottom of the pizza pan to create the crust. Bake for 12 to 15 minutes, or until golden brown. Set the crust aside to cool. |
| One 8-ounce package ⅓-reduced-fat pasteurized cream cheese, softened | |
| ½ cup sugar | **3** In a large bowl, use an electric mixer to beat together the cream cheese, sugar, vanilla extract, and orange zest. |
| 1 teaspoon vanilla extract | |
| 1 tablespoon orange zest | |
| 2½ cups sliced fresh strawberries | **4** Transfer the cooled cookie crust to a serving platter and spread the cream cheese mixture on top of it. |
| 1 cup peeled and sliced kiwi fruit | **5** Arrange the strawberries, kiwi, and blueberries on top of the crust, gently pressing them into the cream cheese mixture so that they stay in place. Use a pizza cutter to cut the fruit pizza into 12 slices. |
| 1 cup blueberries | |

*Per serving: Calories 315 (From Fat 131); Fat 15g (Saturated 5g); Cholesterol 28mg; Sodium 276mg; Carbohydrate 43g (Dietary Fiber 2g); Protein 4g; Iron 1mg; Calcium 63mg; Folate 37mcg.*

***Tip:*** You may have to let the cookie dough sit out for a few minutes before it's soft enough to press into the pan. But for food safety reasons, don't allow it to sit out for more than 1 hour.

***Vary It!*** Use raspberries, peaches, cherries, bananas, pineapple, mango — whatever kind of fruit you love or is in season. (If you opt for bananas, toss 'em in lemon juice so they don't brown and ruin the look of your pizza.)

# Pineapple Spice Loaf with Cream Cheese Frosting

**Prep time:** 20 min, plus cooling time • **Cook time:** 60 min • **Yield:** 16 servings

| *Ingredients* | *Directions* |
|---|---|
| **Nonstick cooking spray** | *1* Preheat the oven to 325 degrees. Coat a loaf pan with nonstick cooking spray. |
| **2 eggs** | |
| **1 cup sugar** | |
| **1 teaspoon plus ½ teaspoon vanilla extract** | *2* In a small bowl, use an electric mixer to beat the eggs, sugar, 1 teaspoon of vanilla, and oil. Mix in the applesauce, carrots, and pineapple. |
| **2 tablespoons canola oil** | |
| **½ cup unsweetened applesauce** | |
| **½ cup finely shredded carrots** | *3* In a large bowl, combine the flours, baking soda, salt, cinnamon, allspice, and nutmeg. Add the wet mixture to the dry mixture and mix with an electric mixer until moistened. |
| **½ cup canned, crushed pineapple, drained** | |
| **¾ cup whole-wheat flour** | |
| **¾ cup all-purpose flour** | *4* Pour the batter into the prepared loaf pan. Bake for 60 minutes, or until a toothpick inserted into the center comes out clean. Cool the loaf in the pan on a wire rack for at least 1 hour. |
| **½ teaspoon baking soda** | |
| **½ teaspoon salt** | |
| **½ teaspoon cinnamon** | *5* To prepare the frosting, beat together the cream cheese, butter, ½ teaspoon of vanilla, and powdered sugar. Spread the icing on top of the cooled loaf. |
| **½ teaspoon allspice** | |
| **½ teaspoon nutmeg** | |
| **4 ounces ⅓-reduced-fat pasteurized cream cheese, softened** | |
| **1 tablespoon butter, softened** | |
| **1 cup powdered sugar** | |

**Per serving:** *Calories 179 (From Fat 45); Fat 5g (Saturated 2g); Cholesterol 34mg; Sodium 150mg; Carbohydrate 31g (Dietary Fiber 1g); Protein 3g; Iron 1mg; Calcium 15mg; Folate 17mcg.*

**Tip:** To turn this recipe into a breakfast bread rather than a dessert, simply leave off the cream cheese frosting.

**Vary It!** If you like nuts in your bread, add ½ cup of chopped pecans or walnuts to the batter before baking.

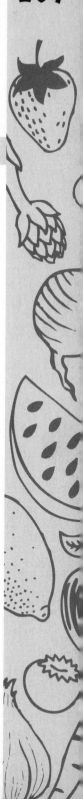

# Lemon Raspberry Cupcakes

**Prep time:** 40 min, plus cooling time  •  **Cook time:** 20 min  •  **Yield:** 12 servings

| *Ingredients* | *Directions* |
|---|---|
| ½ cup plus 2 tablespoons butter, softened | **1** Preheat the oven to 350 degrees. Line a 12-cup muffin pan with paper liners. |
| 1 cup plus ¼ cup sugar | |
| 1 tablespoon lemon zest | **2** In a large bowl, use an electric mixer to cream ½ cup of butter and 1 cup of sugar. Add the lemon zest, eggs, and buttermilk and mix well. |
| 2 eggs | |
| ½ cup buttermilk | **3** In a separate bowl, mix together the flour, salt, and baking soda. Slowly add the dry ingredients to the wet ingredients and mix until just moistened. |
| 1¼ cups all-purpose flour | |
| ¼ teaspoon salt | |
| ¼ teaspoon baking soda | **4** Spoon the batter into the muffin cups, filling each cup ⅔ of the way full. Spoon ½ teaspoon of raspberry preserves on top of each cupcake, making sure to keep the preserves in the center of each muffin cup. |
| 3 tablespoons plus 2 tablespoons raspberry preserves | |
| ½ cup lemon juice | **5** Bake for 20 minutes, or until a toothpick inserted into a cupcake comes out clean. Cool the cupcakes in the pan on a wire rack for 5 minutes and then remove them from the pan. |
| 4 ounces ⅓-reduced-fat pasteurized cream cheese, softened | |
| 1 teaspoon vanilla extract | **6** In a medium bowl, whisk together the lemon juice and the remaining ¼ cup of sugar. With a toothpick, poke small holes in the top of the warm cupcakes. Using a pastry brush, brush the lemon syrup onto the cupcakes. |
| ½ cup powdered sugar | |
| 4 ounces light frozen whipped topping, thawed | **7** To prepare the frosting, use an electric mixer to cream 2 tablespoons of butter and the cream cheese until smooth. Beat in the remaining 2 tablespoons of preserves and the vanilla extract. Slowly add the powdered sugar and beat until smooth. Fold in the whipped topping. Spread the frosting on top of the cooled cupcakes. |

*Per serving: Calories 318 (From Fat 124); Fat 14g (Saturated 9g); Cholesterol 69mg; Sodium 136mg; Carbohydrate 45g (Dietary Fiber 0g); Protein 4g; Iron 1mg; Calcium 29mg; Folate 33mcg.*

**Tip:** If you don't have buttermilk, mix 1 cup of reduced-fat milk with 1 tablespoon of lemon juice or white vinegar. Let the mixture stand for 5 to 10 minutes before using it.

*Source: Kristina LaRue, RD*

# Apple Cinnamon Crêpes

**Prep time:** 10 min • **Cook time:** About 10 min • **Yield:** 2 servings

| *Ingredients* | *Directions* |
|---|---|
| 1 teaspoon butter | ***1*** Melt the butter in a medium skillet. Add the apple, cinnamon, nutmeg, and powdered sugar. Cook until the apple pieces are soft, about 3 to 4 minutes. |
| 1 apple, peeled and finely chopped | |
| Dash of cinnamon | |
| Dash of nutmeg | ***2*** In a medium bowl, whisk together the egg, melted butter, milk, water, salt, sugar, and vanilla. Gradually stir in both flours. |
| 1 tablespoon powdered sugar | |
| 1 egg, lightly beaten | |
| 1 tablespoon butter, melted | ***3*** Heat a 12-inch nonstick skillet over medium heat. Spray the skillet with nonstick cooking spray. |
| ¼ cup lowfat milk | |
| ¼ cup water | ***4*** Pour half of the batter into the hot skillet. Tilt the pan to make sure the batter coats the surface of the pan in a very thin layer. |
| ⅛ teaspoon salt | |
| 1 teaspoon sugar | ***5*** Cook for about 2 minutes, or until the bottom is slightly browned. Loosen the crêpe with a spatula, flip it, and cook it on the other side for 1 minute. Remove the crêpe from the pan and set it on a covered plate to keep it warm. |
| ⅛ teaspoon vanilla | |
| ¼ cup whole-wheat flour | |
| ¼ cup all-purpose flour | |
| Nonstick cooking spray | ***6*** Repeat Steps 4 and 5 to make the other crêpe. |
| | ***7*** Spoon half of the apple mixture into each crêpe and gently roll it up. Serve immediately. |

*Per serving:* Calories 311 (From Fat 135); Fat 15g (Saturated 8g); Cholesterol 138mg; Sodium 195mg; Carbohydrate 38g (Dietary Fiber 4g); Protein 8g; Iron 2mg; Calcium 65mg; Folate 47mcg.

*Vary It!* Instead of using apple cinnamon filling, fill your crêpes with some chocolate hazelnut spread, a sliced banana, and a sprinkle of coconut.

# White Chocolate Berry Oatmeal Cookies

**Prep time:** 15 min • **Cook time:** 24–30 min • **Yield:** 24 servings

| Ingredients | Directions |
|---|---|
| 6 tablespoons butter, softened | **1** Preheat the oven to 350 degrees. Cover two cookie sheets with parchment paper. |
| ¾ cup packed brown sugar | |
| 1 egg | **2** In a large bowl, use an electric mixer to beat together the butter and brown sugar. Add the egg and almond extract and mix well. |
| 1 teaspoon almond extract | |
| 1½ cups rolled oats | |
| ⅓ cup whole-wheat flour | **3** In a separate bowl, use a spoon to mix together the oats, both kinds of flour, baking soda, and salt. |
| ⅓ cup all-purpose flour | |
| 1 teaspoon baking soda | **4** Slowly add the dry ingredients to the wet ingredients and mix until moistened. Add the blueberries, cherries, and chocolate chips and mix until the fruit and chocolate chips are just blended in. |
| ½ teaspoon salt | |
| ½ cup dried blueberries | |
| ½ cup dried cherries | |
| ½ cup white chocolate chips | **5** Use a tablespoon to drop the cookie dough onto the baking sheets, leaving 2 inches between each cookie. |
| | **6** Bake each batch of cookies for 12 to 15 minutes, or until the cookies are browned on top. Cool the cookies on the pans for a few minutes and then transfer them to a wire rack to cool completely. |

*Per serving:* Calories 126 (From Fat 41); Fat 5g (Saturated 3g); Cholesterol 17mg; Sodium 111mg; Carbohydrate 20g (Dietary Fiber 1g); Protein 2g; Iron 1mg; Calcium 20mg; Folate 6mcg.

*Vary It!* Use dark chocolate chips in place of the white chocolate chips, take out the blueberries, and double the amount of dried tart cherries for a chocolate-covered cherry cookie.

*Tip:* If you're in a time pinch, you can bake both cookie sheets at the same time. Just try to fit both cookie sheets on the same oven rack.

# Chapter 17

# Cook It Fast: Speedy Recipes Ready in 10 Minutes or Less

### Recipes in This Chapter

- Decaf Mocha Smoothie
- Dill and Chive Veggie Dip
- Honey Orange Grapefruit Salad
- Three-Bean Artichoke Salad
- ▶ Chicken Hummus Pita
- Havarti Pear Grilled Cheese on Pumpernickel
- Sesame Asparagus
- Sautéed Summer Fruit over Ice Cream
- Ricotta Parfait
- Grilled Bananas

🍴🥒🍅🌶🥕

## In This Chapter

▶ Incorporating convenience foods that can save you time while still nourishing you and your baby

▶ Enjoying delicious, flavorful dishes that are fast and easy to prepare

*W*ith the hectic pace of life today, carving out the time to cook a balanced meal can be tough. Toss pregnancy into the mix and you have an added dimension — you're busy *and* tired *and* your feet may be swollen. All the more reason not to spend hours on your feet in the kitchen.

When you're feeling tired and want to spend as little time cooking as possible, quick and simple meals sound pretty good! Hence, I've devoted this entire chapter to recipes that require very easy, quick preparation. You can have them on the table in 10 minutes or less. I've tried to include a variety of recipes to meet your need for speed — speedy recipes that is! Most of them use some kind of convenience food to make your life easier, and all of them supply nutrients that you and your growing baby need. Whatever time of day you're in a hurry — breakfast, lunch, dinner, snack time, or dessert — you're sure to find the perfect quick (and delicious!) recipe in this chapter.

# *Relying on Convenience Foods*

One of the first rules of quick cooking is relying on *convenience foods,* as in foods that have been prepared and designed for ease of use and consumption. Convenience foods have gotten a bit of a bad reputation because some people believe that convenience automatically equals unhealthiness, but that's just not true. Sure, some convenience foods have a good deal of fat, sugar, or salt added, but this section proves that convenience can mean not only quick and delicious but also healthy and nutritious.

You likely have to pay a bit more for convenience foods, but if they save you time and reduce your (and your baby's!) stress level, the extra cost is well worth it.

Following is a whole list of options for cutting out preparation time while still maintaining the nutritional value of your food:

- ✔ **Precut fruits and vegetables:** Studies have shown that people are more likely to eat fruit when it's already cut up and ready to go than when they have to cut it up themselves. As for veggies? A lot of fresh veggies now come in a bag that goes straight into the microwave for steaming. Check out the Honey Orange Grapefruit Salad to experience the joys of precut produce for yourself; it calls for canned or jarred grapefruit that's presectioned so there's no mess.

- ✔ **Precut and pureed spices:** You've likely been using chopped garlic for a while, but have you seen the fresh purees of basil, oregano, ginger, lemongrass, and the like? When you don't want to buy fresh herbs and waste the leftovers, look for these tubes of herbs, which will keep for much longer and still give you the taste of fresh in your recipe. For a recipe that takes advantage of these prepared spice wonders, check out the Dill and Chive Veggie Dip recipe, which uses jarred, minced garlic.

- ✔ **Prechopped and ground nuts and seeds:** Don't have time to chop your walnuts, pecans, or flaxseed? You can buy them prechopped. Give pre-ground flaxseed a try in the Decaf Mocha Smoothie recipe.

- ✔ **Bottled lemon and lime juice:** The little bottles of lemon and lime juice are so easy to store and use that I don't buy fresh lemons or limes anymore unless I need the zest or want the actual wedges. For a yummy dish that uses bottled lemon juice, try the Three-Bean Artichoke Salad.

- ✔ **Frozen and canned vegetables:** Don't forget about the convenience of simply sticking a bag of frozen veggies in the microwave or popping open a can and draining it. Canned beans and stewed tomatoes are two staples that I always have in my cabinet. The Three-Bean Artichoke Salad recipe uses three different cans of vegetables: two cans of beans and one can of artichokes.

✔ **Prepared hummus:** You could make your own hummus, but why would you, given the incredible variety of flavored hummus available? Try out the super-easy, super-fast Chicken Hummus Pita recipe by using the prepared hummus of your choice.

✔ **Precooked, presliced, and preportioned meats:** These can range from canned chicken and tuna to roasted chicken at the grocery store to frozen meatballs to precooked refrigerated meat ready to add to a recipe. If you buy meats when they're warm (like hot rotisserie chicken), just be sure to reheat them to the safe temperatures listed in Chapter 10, based on the type of meats you've purchased. Check out the Chicken Hummus Pita for a tasty way to use this convenience food.

# Making the most of your microwave

Not only is your microwave a tool for fast cooking, but it's also often a healthier way to cook. Here are some of my favorite ways to use a microwave:

✔ **Boil water.** Especially when you need just a small amount, boiling water in the microwave is super easy. For larger batches, start boiling the water in the microwave and then transfer it to a pan.

✔ **Melt foods.** You can quickly melt margarine, chocolate, and pretty much anything else in the microwave. Be sure to melt the food in batches and stir it in between so you don't overcook and burn it.

✔ **Defrost frozen foods.** Skip dangerous countertop defrosting in favor of using the safer (and faster!) defrost setting on your microwave.

✔ **Prepare frozen meals.** You can't beat the convenience of a meal ready in three to five minutes.

✔ **Make grains.** One of my secret weapons for dinner is microwaveable packets of brown rice or (my favorite) quinoa/wild rice blend.

Just open the top of the package and stick it in the microwave for 90 seconds. If that's too convenient for you, you can also cook instant rice or couscous in about 5 minutes.

✔ **Precook potatoes.** If I want my baked potato to have a crispy peel but don't have the time to bake it all the way, I precook it in the microwave for 5 to 6 minutes and then just use the oven for 10 minutes to finish it off and crisp it up. (Just don't forget to poke holes in the potato before popping it in the microwave.) As for quartered potatoes that are destined for the skillet, I often microwave them for a few minutes to soften them before throwing them in the skillet; doing so really speeds up the cooking process.

✔ **Steam vegetables.** Instead of boiling or steaming veggies on the stove, add a touch of water to the bottom of a microwave-safe bowl and add your fresh, frozen, or canned veggies of choice. Then microwave them.

✔ **Make breakfast.** Oatmeal, quinoa, cream of wheat, hot chocolate, coffee, tea — all these breakfast staples can be prepared in the microwave in seconds.

# Decaf Mocha Smoothie

**Prep time:** 5 min • **Yield:** 1 serving

| Ingredients | Directions |
|---|---|
| 1½ **cups ice** | **1** In a blender, combine all the ingredients. Blend until smooth. |
| ½ **cup strong decaf coffee, chilled** | |
| ½ **cup lowfat milk** | **2** Pour the smoothie mixture into a tall glass and enjoy. |
| 1 **tablespoon chocolate syrup** | |
| 1 **tablespoon sugar** | |
| 1 **tablespoon unsweetened cocoa powder** | |
| 1 **tablespoon ground flaxseed** | |
| ¼ **cup plain nonfat Greek yogurt** | |
| 1 **small banana** | |

*Per serving:* Calories 328 (From Fat 49); Fat 6g (Saturated 2g); Cholesterol 5mg; Sodium 100mg; Carbohydrate 62g (Dietary Fiber 7g); Protein 13g; Iron 2mg; Calcium 222mg; Folate 50mcg.

*Vary It!* If you're a peanut butter lover, add a tablespoon of creamy peanut butter before blending.

*Note:* If you're missing your coffee or high-calorie blended coffee drinks, this one is sure to satisfy! The banana boosts the nutritional content and you get your coffee fix!

# Dill and Chive Veggie Dip

**Prep time:** 5 min, plus refrigerating time • **Yield:** 6 servings

| *Ingredients* | *Directions* |
|---|---|
| **1 cup plain nonfat Greek yogurt** | *1* In a small bowl, combine all the ingredients. Stir until well blended. |
| **¼ cup light mayonnaise** | |
| **1 tablespoon dried dill** | *2* Refrigerate for 2 hours before serving to allow the flavors to blend. |
| **¼ teaspoon seasoning salt** | |
| **2 tablespoons chopped fresh chives** | |
| **1 teaspoon preminced garlic** | |
| **Pepper to taste** | |

*Per serving:* Calories 56 (From Fat 30); Fat 3g (Saturated 1g); Cholesterol 4mg; Sodium 122mg; Carbohydrate 3g (Dietary Fiber 0g); Protein 4g; Iron 0mg; Calcium 36mg; Folate 1mcg.

*Tip:* If you're in a hurry, you can serve this dip immediately after making it. It tastes just fine even if you don't let the flavors blend in the fridge for 2 hours.

*Note:* Serve this dip with an assortment of raw carrots, broccoli, red peppers, cauliflower, celery, grape tomatoes, and more for dipping.

*Note:* Never keep perishable dips like this at room temperature for longer than 2 hours. After 2 hours are up, throw out the dip. Don't reuse any dip that's been sitting out.

# Honey Orange Grapefruit Salad

**Prep time:** 10 min • **Yield:** 4 servings

| *Ingredients* | *Directions* |
|---|---|
| One 15-ounce can mandarin oranges in juice, drained | *1* In a medium bowl, mix together the oranges, grapefruit, banana, and kiwi. |
| One 15-ounce can red grapefruit sections in light syrup, drained | *2* Drizzle the fruit mixture with the honey and sprinkle the mint on top. Toss the fruit gently to cover everything evenly and serve immediately. |
| 1 large banana, sliced | |
| 1 kiwi, peeled and sliced | |
| 1 tablespoon honey | |
| 2 tablespoons chopped fresh mint | |

*Per serving:* Calories 130 (From Fat 4); Fat 0g (Saturated 0g); Cholesterol 0mg; Sodium 6mg; Carbohydrate 33g (Dietary Fiber 2g); Protein 2g; Iron 1mg; Calcium 33mg; Folate 25mcg.

*Note:* You can also use jarred grapefruit sections, which you find in the refrigerated produce section. The jarred grapefruit is typically packaged in juice rather than syrup, which means less sugar.

*Vary It!* Use mangos, peaches, pears, and berries in this salad in place of, or in addition to, some of the fruit listed.

# Three-Bean Artichoke Salad

**Prep time:** 7 min • **Yield:** 8 servings

| *Ingredients* | *Directions* |
|---|---|
| One 15-ounce can garbanzo beans, drained and rinsed | **1** In a large bowl, combine the beans, artichoke hearts, olive oil, and lemon juice. Sprinkle the mixture with salt and pepper to taste. Stir until well combined. |
| One 15-ounce can black beans, drained and rinsed | |
| 1 cup sliced fresh green beans | **2** Serve about ¾ cup of the bean mixture on a ½-cup bed of fresh arugula for each serving. |
| One 16-ounce can quartered artichoke hearts, drained | |
| 2 tablespoons olive oil | |
| 2 tablespoons lemon juice | |
| Salt and pepper to taste | |
| 4 cups fresh arugula | |

*Per serving:* Calories 110 (From Fat 37); Fat 4g (Saturated 1g); Cholesterol 0mg; Sodium 311mg; Carbohydrate 13g (Dietary Fiber 4g); Protein 5g; Iron 2mg; Calcium 42mg; Folate 58mcg.

*Note:* I'm not a fan of the typical vinegar-tasting dressings on bean salads, so I use a simple mix of olive oil and lemon in this recipe.

*Vary It!* If you like more veggies, add chopped red or green bell peppers and onions.

*Note:* Garbanzo beans also go by the name chickpeas.

# Chicken Hummus Pita

**Prep time:** 10 min • **Yield:** 1 serving

| *Ingredients* | *Directions* |
|---|---|
| **2 tablespoons prepared hummus (flavor of your choice)** | *1* Spread the hummus on the inside of the pita. |
| **½ whole-grain pocket pita** | *2* Fill the pita with the cold chicken breast, salad greens, tomato, cucumber, carrots, and black olives. |
| **2 ounces cold, cooked boneless chicken breast, sliced** | |
| **1 cup prewashed salad greens, rinsed** | |
| **½ small tomato, diced** | |
| **¼ cucumber, diced** | |
| **¼ cup shredded carrots** | |
| **2 tablespoons sliced black olives** | |

*Per serving:* Calories 286 (From Fat 73); Fat 8g (Saturated 2g); Cholesterol 48mg; Sodium 506mg; Carbohydrate 31g (Dietary Fiber 8g); Protein 25g; Iron 4mg; Calcium 87mg; Folate 121mcg.

*Tip:* Add a squeeze of fresh lemon before serving to bring the flavors together.

*Vary It!* Add your favorite sliced or shredded cheese for even more flavor.

*Tip:* If you want to save a little cash and not buy a package of presliced cooked chicken breast, just cut up some chicken breasts that are left over from a previous meal.

# Letting Flavor Stand Out in Quick Dishes

Just because you're using convenience foods and getting meals on the table in minutes doesn't mean you have to sacrifice taste. In fact, why not make flavor a star in your speedy recipes? Here's how:

- ✔ **Spice it up.** One of the best ways to add flavor in seconds is to explore your spice cabinet. For example, just a pinch of paprika or a dash of oregano can enhance the natural flavors of meats, vegetables, and grains. To see the magic of spice in action, try the Sautéed Summer Fruit over Ice Cream recipe in this section; the allspice in this dish really brings the flavor of the peaches to a new level.

    You can save a step by finding foods that are already flavored, like the dill-flavored Havarti cheese used in the Havarti Pear Grilled Cheese on Pumpernickel recipe.

- ✔ **Go fresh with herbs.** Fresh or pureed herbs can do wonders to enhance bland food. Case in point: Plain instant rice isn't so plain when you jazz it up with some chopped fresh parsley or cilantro. If you happen to have your own potted herb garden, you can pinch off those fresh herbs in a flash.

- ✔ **Extract it.** I'm addicted to almond extract. I put it in pancake mix (now my secret's out!), oatmeal, smoothies, coffee, and pretty much anything else I can add it to. If you're looking for a new twist on extract, try the Ricotta Parfait recipe in this section. The almond extract really brings out the flavor of the peaches. Instead of always using vanilla extract, play around with the many extract flavors available.

- ✔ **Embrace flavored vinegars and oils.** Flavored vinegars, such as balsamic, apple cider, and herb- or fruit-infused, are an excellent way to add flavor without calories or fat. Trust me, the first time you add a balsamic glaze to chicken or fish, you'll be hooked. Different oils provide different flavors, too. To see what I mean, try the Sesame Asparagus recipe, which uses sesame oil rather than olive oil. The sesame oil adds to the sesame seeds and soy sauce to give the veggies a real Asian flair.

I encourage you to branch out and try flavors other than your traditional standbys. You may be pleasantly surprised by the results. For example, the Grilled Bananas recipe in this section uses butterscotch chips rather than traditional chocolate chips for an enhanced flavor.

As you experiment more in the kitchen, you'll find your own tricks and secrets to enhancing flavor without adding calories or sacrificing nutrition.

# Havarti Pear Grilled Cheese on Pumpernickel

**Prep time:** 2 min • **Cook time:** 6 min • **Yield:** 1 serving

| Ingredients | Directions |
|---|---|
| 2 slices pumpernickel bread | *1* Heat a medium skillet over medium heat. Spread each slice of bread with 1 teaspoon of margarine. |
| 2 teaspoons trans-fat-free margarine spread | |
| 2 slices Havarti dill cheese | *2* Place one slice of prepared bread on the skillet (margarine side down) and top with one slice of cheese, the pear slices, and the second slice of cheese. Top the whole thing with the second slice of bread (margarine side up). |
| ¼ pear, sliced | |
| | *3* Cook the sandwich until it's crispy on one side, about 3 minutes. Carefully flip over the sandwich with a spatula and cook it until the other side is crispy, about 3 minutes. |

*Per serving:* Calories 373 (From Fat 191); Fat 21g (Saturated 11g); Cholesterol 46mg; Sodium 687mg; Carbohydrate 31g (Dietary Fiber 4g); Protein 15g; Iron 2mg; Calcium 344mg; Folate 45mcg.

*Tip:* Slice up the rest of the pear to have on the side or on a bed of greens for a quick salad.

*Vary It!* Use apple slices and cheddar or Swiss cheese on whole-wheat bread for a tasty variation of this sandwich.

*Tip:* You can use a panini maker (sandwich press) or indoor nonstick grill to make this sandwich in even less time because it allows you to heat both sides of the sandwich at once.

# Sesame Asparagus

**Prep time:** 2 min • **Cook time:** 8 min • **Yield:** 4 servings

| Ingredients | Directions |
|---|---|
| 1 pound asparagus spears, trimmed | **1** Preheat the oven to 450 degrees. |
| 1 tablespoon low-sodium soy sauce | **2** Place the asparagus on a baking sheet. Drizzle the asparagus with the soy sauce, sesame oil, and sesame seeds, and move the asparagus around on the baking sheet to cover it evenly. |
| 1 tablespoon sesame oil | |
| 1 tablespoon sesame seeds | |
| | **3** Bake the asparagus until it's tender, about 8 minutes. Halfway through cooking, gently stir the asparagus. |

*Per serving:* Calories 61 (From Fat 42); Fat 5g (Saturated 1g); Cholesterol 0mg; Sodium 157mg; Carbohydrate 3g (Dietary Fiber 1g); Protein 2g; Iron 4mg; Calcium 11mg; Folate 82mcg.

*Vary It!* If you don't want the Asian flair, just drizzle the asparagus with olive oil and sprinkle it with garlic salt and dried rosemary.

*Tip:* The asparagus cooks so fast because the oven is really hot. Make sure the oven is completely preheated when the asparagus goes in; otherwise, the cooking time will increase.

# Sautéed Summer Fruit over Ice Cream

**Prep time:** 7 min • **Cook time:** 3 min • **Yield:** 2 servings

| Ingredients | Directions |
|---|---|
| **1 tablespoon trans-fat-free margarine spread** | *1* Melt the margarine spread in a medium skillet over medium heat. |
| **1 large peach, peeled, pitted, and sliced** | *2* Add the peach slices to the skillet and sauté them for about 2 minutes, or until tender. Add the brown sugar, cinnamon, and allspice and cook for another minute. |
| **2 teaspoons brown sugar** | |
| **¼ teaspoon cinnamon** | |
| **¼ teaspoon allspice** | *3* In a small bowl, mix together the raspberries and sugar, coating the berries evenly. |
| **½ cup raspberries** | |
| **1 teaspoon sugar** | *4* Scoop ½ cup of ice cream into two separate dishes. Top each serving of ice cream with ½ of the peaches and raspberries. |
| **1 cup reduced-fat vanilla ice cream** | |

**Per serving:** *Calories 217 (From Fat 78); Fat 9g (Saturated 4g); Cholesterol 9mg; Sodium 118mg; Carbohydrate 34g (Dietary Fiber 4g); Protein 3g; Iron 1mg; Calcium 111mg; Folate 15mcg.*

***Vary It!*** Instead of peaches, use pineapple, apples, pears, bananas, or any fruit of your choice. Just cook it until it's tender.

***Tip:*** If you want to warm your raspberries, too, just add them to the peaches in the skillet with a minute left in cook time and delete the teaspoon of sugar.

***Note:*** If peaches aren't in season, you can use 8 slices of frozen peaches in place of the large fresh peach.

# Ricotta Parfait

**Prep time:** 5 min • **Yield:** 1 serving

| Ingredients | Directions |
|---|---|
| ½ **cup plain nonfat Greek yogurt** | *1* In a small bowl, stir together the yogurt, ricotta cheese, almond extract, and sugar. |
| ¼ **cup part-skim ricotta cheese** | |
| ½ **teaspoon almond extract** | *2* Pour half of the yogurt and ricotta mixture into the bottom of a parfait glass. Top with half of the cereal, berries, and almonds. Repeat these layers with the other half of the ingredients. |
| **1 teaspoon sugar** | |
| ½ **cup high-fiber bran cereal** | |
| ¼ **cup dried berry mix** | |
| ¼ **cup sliced, toasted almonds** | |

*Per serving:* Calories 438 (From Fat 156); Fat 17g (Saturated 4g); Cholesterol 25mg; Sodium 205mg; Carbohydrate 66g (Dietary Fiber 19g); Protein 23g; Iron 6mg; Calcium 333mg; Folate 107mcg.

*Tip:* Use a cereal like All Bran or Fiber One; they're super high in fiber! Fiber One stays crunchier, so use it if you like crunchy cereal.

*Vary It!* I like to use a dried berry mix with cranberries, blueberries, and cherries, but you can use dried pineapple, mango, coconut, figs, dates, or any fresh or canned fruit you have available.

*Note:* You find sliced almonds in bags in the baking aisle.

# Grilled Bananas

**Prep time:** 2 min • **Cook time:** 5–8 min • **Yield:** 2 servings

| Ingredients | Directions |
|---|---|
| 2 bananas (in peel) | **1** Preheat the grill to medium heat. |
| 2 tablespoons mini marshmallows | **2** With a knife, split through the banana peels lengthwise from top to bottom, cutting only halfway through the bananas so that you're creating a pocket in the fruit. |
| 2 tablespoons butterscotch chips | **3** Keeping the peels on, divide the marshmallows and butterscotch chips evenly between the two bananas and insert them into the split peels. |
| | **4** Wrap each banana loosely in aluminum foil and place the bananas split side up on the grill. Close the lid and cook them for 5 to 8 minutes. |
| | **5** Place the wrapped bananas on a plate and remove the foil. Open the peels a bit wider and serve with a spoon. |

*Per serving: Calories 176 (From Fat 34); Fat 4g (Saturated 3g); Cholesterol 0mg; Sodium 12mg; Carbohydrate 37g (Dietary Fiber 3g); Protein 2g; Iron 0mg; Calcium 11mg; Folate 23mcg.*

*Tip:* Stuff the marshmallows in before the butterscotch chips so they don't stick to the foil when you grill them. The banana peels will turn black. That's normal!

*Note:* This is a great dessert for any night you're grilling out. The grill's already hot, so you can just put the bananas on as soon as the meat comes off. Leave them on for longer than 8 minutes for them to caramelize even more. If you don't have a grill, you can bake the bananas in the oven at 350 degrees for 8 minutes.

*Vary It!* Use dark chocolate chips, white chocolate chips, peanut butter chips, coconut flakes, dried cranberries, or a spoonful of almond or peanut butter to mix up the taste of this dessert.

# Part IV

# What You May Not Be Thinking about but Should

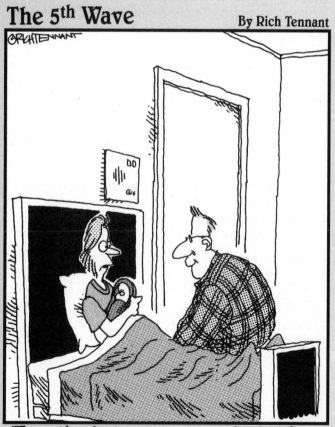

"Even the doctors were surprised at how involved you were in there. Especially right near the end when you turned on that CD of the 'William Tell Overture.'"

## In this part . . .

*B*ecause few pregnancies go according to any kind of textbook, this part has you covered if you end up with an unexpected medical issue that has nutritional implications, such as anemia or gestational diabetes. If you have food allergies, this part helps guide you in what to eat to make sure you're still getting the required nutrients you and your baby need.

Even though these nine months may feel long, the first few weeks and months after delivery fly by in the blink of an eye. To prepare you for your postpartum life, this part features a chapter devoted to feeding your baby and taking care of yourself after delivery, as well as a chapter that's all about helping you losing lingering pregnancy pounds when the time comes to get back into shape.

# Chapter 18

# Help Me, Doc! Situations That Require Medical Attention

. . . . . . . . . . . . . . . . . . . . . . . . . . . . . . . . . . . . . . . . . . . . . .

### In This Chapter

▶ Eating right and exercising to help control medical conditions you may face during pregnancy

▶ Surveying the nutrition concerns of mothers in special circumstances

. . . . . . . . . . . . . . . . . . . . . . . . . . . . . . . . . . . . . . . . . . . . . .

*A*lthough I hope that every pregnancy runs its course without a hitch, sometimes things get a tad complicated medically. Fortunately, good nutrition is one of the best ways to deal with these special situations. This chapter covers some of the common medical conditions women face during pregnancy, specifically those with nutritional implications, like gestational diabetes, high blood pressure, and anemia. It also addresses the specific nutritional concerns of teens, cancer survivors, and women carrying multiples.

# Using Diet and Exercise to Help Control Certain Medical Conditions

Good nutrition is vital during every woman's pregnancy, but certain health conditions require that you pay even closer attention to your diet to improve symptoms and reduce complications. In fact, the "prescription" for many pregnancy-related conditions (whether you develop them before or during pregnancy) is not medication, but rather lifestyle changes like eating right and exercising regularly.

If you have gestational diabetes, polycystic ovary syndrome, high blood pressure, preeclampsia, or anemia, you need to follow your doctor's advice on how to control your symptoms to reach the best possible outcome for you and your baby. But you may also want to seek out more specific, individualized advice from a registered dietitian (RD). An RD can sit down with you and map out the best nutrition plan possible to keep you and your baby healthy.

You can find an RD in your area by visiting www.eatright.org, clicking the Find a Registered Dietitian button, and typing in your zip code. (You can also search specifically for an RD who specializes in maternal nutrition.)

## Gestational diabetes

*Gestational diabetes,* a type of diabetes that can develop in the second half of pregnancy, affects how your body uses *glucose* (blood sugar). Scientists aren't entirely sure why some pregnant women develop gestational diabetes and others don't because pregnancy itself affects certain hormones that impact how insulin clears glucose out of the blood and gets it into cells. As your pregnancy progresses and your baby grows, the placenta produces hormones that block insulin, which may cause higher-than-normal glucose levels in the blood. Some women develop gestational diabetes in response to insulin's not working as efficiently during pregnancy.

Although anyone can develop gestational diabetes, you may be at a higher risk if you

- ✔ Have a family or personal history of diabetes or gestational diabetes (if you had gestational diabetes with a prior pregnancy, it's highly likely you'll have it again)
- ✔ Are overweight prior to pregnancy
- ✔ Are African American, Hispanic, Asian, or American Indian
- ✔ Are older than 25 years old

Most women with gestational diabetes don't experience the common symptoms of diabetes — unusual thirst, frequent infections (such as yeast and bladder), blurred vision, and weight loss. The only way to know for sure whether you have gestational diabetes is to undergo a glucose tolerance test, which your doctor will order when you're between 24 and 28 weeks.

During the one-hour glucose tolerance test, you have to drink a sugary solution and then wait an hour before having your blood tested. The doctor looks to see whether your body properly clears out the glucose or it leaves too much in your bloodstream. If your glucose level stays high, your doctor will likely recommend that you have a longer, three-hour glucose tolerance test to look in more detail at how your body is clearing glucose. If you fail that test, then you're among the estimated 4 percent of women who develop gestational diabetes.

If you're diagnosed with gestational diabetes, expect to make more frequent visits to your doctor. Also expect to have to monitor your own blood sugar levels at least once a day and very likely several times each day (first thing in the morning and after every meal) with a finger stick and a blood glucose meter.

# Myth buster: Sugar and diabetes

You've probably heard the myth that eating too much sugar causes you to get diabetes. Well, it's not true. Although reducing your intake of sugar helps control your glucose levels after you already have diabetes, no specific threshold of sugar actually causes you to have diabetes.

Now I'm not saying that you can eat all the gummy bears you want; you still need to watch your sugar intake while pregnant. After all, most high-sugar foods are low in nutrients and don't help nourish you or your baby.

If you're one of those women who gets to add "gestational diabetes" to her list of unpleasant pregnancy side effects, read on to find out about the complications that can arise from this condition and tips for how to manage it.

## Potential complications

With proper treatment, most women who have gestational diabetes go on to deliver healthy babies. They then return to a normal, nondiabetic state within six to eight weeks after delivering. If, however, you don't properly control your blood sugar through diet, exercise, and/or medications, the following complications can arise:

- ✔ **Risk of high blood pressure, preeclampsia, and eclampsia:** Mom is at higher risk of developing these conditions during pregnancy. (I give you the scoop on these conditions later in this chapter.)

- ✔ **High-birth-weight baby:** Because of Mom's high glucose levels, Baby makes extra insulin, causing her to grow bigger. In fact, women with gestational diabetes often deliver babies who weigh more than nine pounds.

- ✔ **Preterm labor:** A mother with gestational diabetes may naturally go into labor early, or her doctor may recommend early delivery because of the baby's large size.

- ✔ **Increased risk of cesarean delivery:** Because of the baby's large size, a cesarean delivery (also known as a *C-section*) is often necessary to deliver the baby.

- ✔ **Respiratory distress in Baby:** Many babies born to mothers with gestational diabetes have immature lungs and need help breathing until their lungs become stronger and more developed. These respiratory issues often happen in babies who are born preterm, but it can also occur in babies who aren't born early.

- ✔ **Jaundice in Baby:** Some babies born to diabetic mothers have immature livers that can't break down *bilirubin* (a yellow pigment that's created as a natural byproduct when the body breaks down red blood cells). Too much bilirubin leads to a yellowing of the skin and the whites of the eyes.

✔ **Low blood sugar in Baby after birth:** Some babies are at risk of having their blood sugar go too low because they produced more insulin during development in the womb. (Insulin naturally lowers blood glucose levels.) Low blood sugar can lead to shakiness, seizures, and trouble breathing for an infant.

✔ **Development of type 2 diabetes later in life:** Both Mom and Baby are at higher risk of developing diabetes later in life.

### Treating gestational diabetes with a carb-controlled diet and exercise

The universal treatment for gestational diabetes — whether you have a mild case or a severe one that requires daily insulin injections — is a diet that moderates your carbohydrate intake. As I explain in Chapter 3, carbohydrates are found mostly in grains, fruits, vegetables, and sweet foods. Although you shouldn't start following the Atkins diet (a diet that's very low in carbohydrates), you do need to use caution with portion sizes of carb-containing foods. Also try to avoid sugary foods, specifically liquid sources of sugar like regular soft drinks and even fruit juices, and limit portions of desserts, candy, and processed starches, like white bread, white rice, and many low-fiber cereals and crackers.

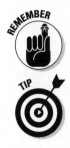

Fill up on foods that are high in fiber and protein to prevent spikes in your blood sugar.

If you're a carb lover, don't panic. Make an appointment with an RD who's also a Certified Diabetes Educator (CDE), and he or she can walk you through the best diet for you. Work with your RD to develop an individualized plan with the right amount of carbs, proteins, and fats that will nourish you and help you control your gestational diabetes at the same time.

Regular exercise is another part of the standard gestational diabetes treatment plan. Exercise can increase your body's sensitivity to insulin, meaning that your body doesn't need to produce as much of it to clear out the excess glucose. Check with your doctor for any limitations you may need to incorporate into your exercise routine.

## Polycystic ovary syndrome

*Polycystic ovary syndrome* (PCOS) is a common hormonal disorder that results in irregular menstruation, cysts on the ovaries, and overproduction of *androgens* (male hormones). PCOS is a leading cause of infertility, in part because many women with PCOS are overweight or obese. If you have PCOS and you're reading this, then congratulations on overcoming this pregnancy hurdle!

The exact cause of PCOS is unknown, but insulin levels that are too high (often due to the woman's being overweight or borderline diabetic) are thought to cause a spike in androgen production by the ovaries, leading to symptoms of PCOS. These symptoms include menstrual irregularities (prior to getting pregnant of course!), acne, or hair on your face or body. Testing includes blood tests for hormone or metabolic abnormalities in addition to a history and physical examination. (*Note:* Women don't usually get tested for PCOS while pregnant; they typically already know they have it.)

The big pregnancy complication for many women with PCOS is that PCOS can lead to insulin resistance, which results in high blood sugar and diabetes. If you have PCOS, alert your doctor as soon in your pregnancy as possible so that you can be screened earlier for gestational diabetes (see the preceding section for details). Follow your doctor's instructions on medications and life-style modifications, such as a carb-controlled diet and increased exercise, that are necessary to keep your blood sugar under control.

Depending on your pre-pregnancy weight, you may also be advised to adjust the desired amount of weight gain during your pregnancy (I share the average weight gain numbers in Chapter 5). I also recommend visiting an RD who specializes in pregnancy and PCOS to create an individualized nutrition plan for you.

## High blood pressure and preeclampsia

Even if you didn't have high blood pressure (also called *hypertension*) before you were pregnant, you may develop it while you're pregnant, particularly in the second or third trimester. This is especially true if you have a family history of high blood pressure or you're overweight prior to getting pregnant. Your doctor measures your blood pressure at every prenatal visit. Because you likely won't feel any symptoms if you have high blood pressure, it's extremely important that you attend all your prenatal appointments.

If high blood pressure goes undiagnosed, the risks for Baby and Mom are significant. High blood pressure can restrict the flow of blood to the placenta, potentially robbing your baby of the oxygen and nutrients carried in that blood and leading to *placental abruption* (when the placenta separates from the uterus), premature delivery, and/or a low-birth-weight baby. Risks to Mom include a higher risk of stroke or heart attack.

Sometimes high blood pressure leads to *preeclampsia,* a condition that's marked by a combination of high blood pressure, swelling, and excess protein in the urine (detected with a urine test your doctor may order). Preeclampsia can cause damage to the mother's liver, kidneys, and brain. It can also lead to fatal complications for the mother and baby. The only real cure for preeclampsia is delivery of the baby.

If you have high blood pressure, gestational diabetes, or a history of kidney or liver problems, you're at higher risk of developing preeclampsia. This condition occurs more often in women who are pregnant for the first time, especially those women who are over age 40. Multiple pregnancies (twins, triplets, or more) can also increase a woman's risk of developing this condition. Women typically develop preeclampsia in the second half of pregnancy.

Symptoms of preeclampsia include blurred vision, severe headaches that won't go away, fatigue, pain in the abdomen on the right side, shortness of breath, and infrequent urination. Gaining five or more pounds in a week can also be a sign of preeclampsia (from retaining fluid/swelling). Some swelling is normal in pregnancy, especially in the hands, feet, and face, but if you're concerned about your swelling or if you have any of the other symptoms (especially together), call your doctor.

Whether you have high blood pressure or preeclampsia, the primary nutrition recommendation is the same: Limit your intake of sodium to less than 2,300 mg per day. (Your doctor may want you to lower your intake to 1,500 mg if your case is more severe, so be sure to check with him or her to find out how much you need to modify your diet.) Chances are most of your daily sodium comes from processed and prepared foods, including soups, sauces (such as soy, BBQ, and tomato), condiments (think pickles and olives), cheese, processed meats (such as ham, pepperoni, and sausage), and restaurant food. Try to avoid these major sodium sources and read labels to see how much sodium is in the foods you're consuming.

Here are some additional diet-related ways to keep high blood pressure at bay:

- **Take in more potassium.** Potassium helps you maintain proper fluid balance in your body and has been shown to help with blood pressure control. Every fruit and vegetable has at least a little bit of potassium, but bananas, potatoes, and legumes (beans) have the most. Aim to consume at least five servings of fruits and vegetables every day to get your daily 4,700 mg.

- **Embrace dairy products.** Calcium has been shown to help keep blood pressure in check, so drink your milk and eat your yogurt (these foods are also good sources of potassium) or take a calcium supplement to get your 1,000 mg per day.

- **Avoid caffeine.** Caffeine can raise blood pressure, so avoid it if you have blood pressure issues.

- **Consider taking an omega-3 supplement.** Omega-3 fatty acids (DHA and EPA) have been found to help reduce blood pressure, so eat fatty fish such as salmon or take a fish-oil-based omega-3 supplement. Find out more about omega-3s in Chapter 3.

Along with adjusting your diet, you can make two other important lifestyle changes to help control your blood pressure: exercise and stress management. Check with your doctor to find out if you need to incorporate any limitations into your exercise routine and then head over to Chapter 5 for tips on adding exercise to your day. Controlling stress isn't easy, especially when you're preparing to bring a new life into the world, but getting plenty of rest and relaxation can help you keep it under control.

# Anemia

*Anemia,* or abnormally low levels of red blood cells, is fairly common in pregnancy because of the increased blood volume and the high demand for iron (the mineral that helps make red blood cells, which carry oxygen from the lungs to all parts of the body). To account for the increase in blood volume, pregnant women need to consume about 27 mg of iron per day.

You may be at risk of anemia if you entered pregnancy with low iron levels, or if you aren't getting enough iron in your diet now that you're pregnant. Your doctor will probably check your iron levels when you become pregnant and at least once more during your pregnancy. However, contact your doctor right away if you experience any of the following symptoms of anemia:

- ✔ Unusual weakness or fatigue
- ✔ Dizziness
- ✔ Numbness in the hands and feet
- ✔ Paleness of the skin
- ✔ Chest pain
- ✔ Irregular heartbeat

If you're anemic, you could have a low-birth-weight baby and/or preterm delivery. Low-birth-weight babies, especially those born preterm, can have learning disabilities, vision or hearing loss, respiratory problems, and heart defects. Studies on low-birth-weight babies have also shown a risk of chronic diseases such as high blood pressure, diabetes, and heart disease later on in life.

The best way to treat anemia is to consume more iron-containing foods; I introduce you to these foods in Chapter 3. Another way to get your daily dose of iron is to take a supplement. Your prenatal vitamin has some iron, but your doctor may recommend that you take even more iron in supplement form if your blood levels are too low. ***Note:*** Iron in supplements has been known to constipate some people, so eat high-fiber foods and drink plenty of water to prevent that unpleasant side effect.

# Nutrition Advice for Mothers with Special Considerations

As you probably already know, every pregnancy is different and every woman brings with her a unique set of genetics, habits, medical history, and circumstances. Parts I and II of this book present nutrition advice that applies to the average pregnant woman, but the following sections offer advice that's more specific to teenage mothers, mothers who've conquered cancer, and mothers carrying multiples.

## Nutritional concerns for teenage mothers

Pregnant teens bring a unique set of circumstances to pregnancy because they're often very busy with social events and school schedules and aren't always thinking about taking care of their bodies. Add to these issues erratic eating schedules with skipped meals and high-calorie, low-nutrient food choices and you have quite a challenge. To top it all off, a teenage body is still growing and needs nutrients to do so, and an unborn baby has to compete for those same nutrients. Teen pregnancies are considered high risk for all of these reasons, which is why it's important to go to all doctor's appointments throughout your pregnancy.

From a nutritional perspective, teenage mothers need four nutrients in higher amounts than adult mothers. Because teens are still in their bone-building years, they need 1,300 mg of calcium and 1,250 mg of phosphorus (a key component in bone and teeth). The other two nutrients teens need more of are magnesium (for bone health as well as enzyme production) at 400 mg a day and zinc (for tissue growth and immunity) at 12 mg a day.

If you're a pregnant teen, you absolutely must take a prenatal vitamin to ensure that you're getting many of your vitamins and minerals in supplement form. You may also need to take an extra calcium supplement that contains vitamin D and phosphorus to meet the increased demand for bone health, especially if you're not getting three to four servings of dairy foods (milk, yogurt, and cheese) every day. Talk to your doctor to find out how much and what kind of additional supplements you should take.

Pregnancy is not the time to restrict calories or worry about body image or weight gain; you need to eat plenty of nutritious foods to fuel your body and your baby. Generally speaking, pregnant teens under 18 years should gain 35 pounds during their pregnancy. If you're dealing with emotions that revolve around body image and not wanting to gain weight, talk with a therapist or your doctor about your feelings.

## *Nutritional concerns for mothers who are cancer survivors*

If you're a cancer survivor, you need to focus on fueling yourself with good food to help keep your body strong from the inside out. Your body has already gone through the trauma of cancer and treatment, which may have left you entering pregnancy with a less-than-ideal nutritional status. Aim to get 9 to 13 servings of fruits and vegetables every day (no, that's not a typo). Fruits and vegetables contain the most cancer-fighting nutrients and provide many of the nutrients you and your baby need.

Consult with an RD who can help you develop an eating plan that's right for you. Eat well-balanced meals that include whole grains, lean proteins, fruits, vegetables, and healthy fats so you can maintain or improve your nutritional status while pregnant. Always have healthy snacks handy so you can keep your body full of the energy you need. Talk to your doctor about your medical history to see whether she has any additional advice.

## *Nutritional concerns for mothers of multiples*

Carrying twins (or triplets or more!) is becoming more and more common. Women are having babies later in life, and one of the outcomes has been a higher rate of twins due to more than one egg being released in older women as a result of either hormonal changes or the use of fertility technologies. A multiple pregnancy is considered high risk, so expect that your doctor is going to want to see you more frequently to make sure you're not developing diabetes, high blood pressure, or preeclampsia or going into preterm labor.

If you started your pregnancy at a normal weight, you should shoot to gain 37 to 54 pounds if you're having twins. If you're having triplets, your doctor may recommend that you gain more weight. Basically, work with your doctor to come up with the right weight gain plan for you.

Gaining those extra pounds takes extra energy. Expect to eat a few hundred more calories for each child you're carrying. Try to get these extra calories through nutrient-rich foods. Chapter 11 provides you with some sample meal plans, but you may need to add a few snacks or increase portions of proteins to accommodate your increased needs. (Flip to Chapter 7 for some healthy snack ideas.) Your doctor may also tell you to take even more folic acid, calcium, or iron in addition to your prenatal vitamin.

When you're carrying multiples, your uterus is larger than that of a woman carrying a single child. Consequently, your stomach may feel less than inviting to more food. If you know exactly what I mean, spread your meals and snacks throughout the day so that you get consistent food in small-enough portions to prevent heartburn.

## Surviving bed rest without gaining too much weight

No woman goes into her pregnancy thinking she'll have to spend days on end in bed prior to delivery, but that's precisely what happens for some women. Doctors typically prescribe bed rest only when they're concerned about the placenta, premature dilation, preterm labor, or high blood pressure. The term *bed rest* can have varying meanings from complete rest in a hospital bed to modified bed rest on a couch or bed while at home. If your doctor recommends bed rest for you, ask for specific guidelines regarding things such as proper positions, bathroom breaks, baths, car rides (and driving), household chores, and sex.

Although right now you may welcome bed rest as a break from your crazy life, it gets old fast when you realize you can no longer go out to eat, go see a movie, or even go to the grocery store. When you're on bed rest, you're not only restricted from moving much (burning fewer calories) but you're also sitting around getting bored. Turning to food is one way to cut the monotony, but the result can be unwanted extra pounds of fat.

To keep yourself from gaining too much weight (and losing a lot of muscle tone) while on bed rest, try out these tips:

✔ Don't drown yourself in food because you're bored. Stay occupied with visiting with friends and family, watching movies, doing Sudoku and crossword puzzles, reading books and magazines, knitting, tweeting, blogging, scrapbooking . . . and anything else you can find to take your mind off the fact that you're confined to a bed.

✔ Ask your doctor if you can stretch or lift light weights (upper body only) to prevent blood clots and maintain strength. Just make sure you follow all your doctor's guidelines and limitations.

✔ Eat small, frequent meals and snacks to prevent heartburn.

✔ Eat less (fewer calories, smaller portions) than you would if you were active, but remember that you still need to take your prenatal vitamins and eat nutrient-rich foods.

✔ Ask your doctor about getting a prescription for physical therapy first while you're on bed rest to help prevent muscle loss and then after you deliver to help you regain your strength.

✔ Lay on your side but switch sides frequently to prevent skin sores and aches and to get some movement.

***Remember:*** Try not to dwell on the negatives of bed rest and remember that every day of bed rest keeps your baby in the womb where critical development is taking place.

# Chapter 19

# Mommy-and-Me Food Allergies

. . . . . . . . . . . . . . . . . . . . . . . . . . . . . . . . . . . . . . . . . . . . . . . . . . . . . .

### In This Chapter

▶ Discovering the most common food allergens

▶ Figuring out how to deal with a suspected allergy and prevent food allergies in your baby

. . . . . . . . . . . . . . . . . . . . . . . . . . . . . . . . . . . . . . . . . . . . . . . . . . . . . .

Food allergies are estimated to affect more than 12 million Americans, or 4 percent of the U.S. population. Children in particular have higher rates of food allergies during their first year or two of life due to their immature immune systems. After they reach age 5, many children outgrow food allergies, but some food allergies stay for a lifetime.

A food allergy occurs when your immune system mistakes the proteins in the food you eat for invaders and battles with them, causing a series of bodily reactions that may endanger your health. Currently, doctors don't have a cure for food allergies. Avoidance is the only strategy proven to prevent outbreaks.

In this chapter, I share substitutes for the eight most common food allergens so that if you have an allergy to one (or more) of these foods — or even if you merely suspect you may be allergic to one of them — you can be confident you're still ingesting the nutrients you and your baby need. I also let you know what to do if you think you may be allergic to a food, and I reveal some simple steps you can take to help reduce your child's risk of developing a food allergy.

## Identifying Common Food Allergens

Eight foods make up 90 percent of the food allergies people experience. If you're allergic (or suspect you're allergic) to one of the following foods, make sure you eat other foods that have similar nutrients so that you can avoid the food you're allergic to while still getting a balanced diet during your pregnancy. I offer suggestions for allergen substitutes in the following list:

## Symptoms of food allergies

Symptoms of food allergies can appear anywhere from minutes after consuming a food to about two hours afterward. Typical symptoms include the following:

- Tingling in the mouth or throat
- Swelling of the tongue and throat
- Rashes (eczema)
- Hives (swelling)
- Abdominal cramps, vomiting, and diarrhea
- Wheezing or difficulty breathing
- Loss of consciousness

- **Milk:** A key ingredient in cheese, yogurt, and ice cream, milk is rich in calcium and vitamin D, among other nutrients. Choose fortified soy-milk in place of regular milk, and look for dairy-free cheeses to get your calcium. If soymilk isn't your thing, take a calcium supplement (500 to 1,000 mg). Also take a vitamin D supplement because it's difficult to get through food.

- **Eggs:** Eggs are not only a breakfast staple but also an ingredient in a lot of other dishes, especially baked goods. Eggs are high in choline (I tell you all about this nutrient's importance in Chapter 3), so if you can't have eggs, incorporate beef, poultry, wheat germ, cauliflower, broccoli, and soy lecithin into your diet to make sure you're still getting enough choline. Read labels carefully and look for the words *egg, egg white,* and *albumin* in ingredient lists. Mayonnaise typically contains egg, as do flu and other vaccines.

- **Peanuts:** Peanuts are highly allergenic, so if you're allergic to them, don't touch them or let them touch your food. Read labels and avoid foods that say they're processed in a plant that also processes peanuts. Peanuts have monounsaturated fat, protein, fiber, folate, and other B vitamins. To get these same nutrients, you can eat tree nuts (if you're not allergic to them, that is), beans (garbanzo beans, navy beans, kidney beans, black beans, and so on), or lentils.

- **Tree nuts:** These nuts include walnuts, almonds, cashews, and pecans. They're full of protein, fiber, unsaturated fats, vitamin E, folate, and B vitamins. To get these nutrients if you're allergic to tree nuts, simply include some vegetable oils, avocados, and whole grains in your diet. Just as with peanuts, avoid touching tree nuts or eating foods processed in the same plant as tree nuts if you have an allergy.

- **Fish:** Fish, such as salmon, tuna, and cod, is an excellent source of protein and the best place to get the omega-3 fatty acids DHA and EPA.

If you're allergic to all fish, turn to other meats and meat alternatives for protein. To get your omega-3 fatty acids, your best bet is to take a fish-free DHA/EPA omega-3 supplement, like Ascenta NutraVege or Spectrum's Vegetarian DHA supplement.

✔ **Shellfish:** Shellfish, such as shrimp, lobster, and crab, is a lean protein that offers various vitamins and minerals, including selenium, vitamins D and B12, and zinc. You can get protein and many of these nutrients from other lean meats (lean beef, white-meat skinless poultry, or lean pork) or meat alternatives (soy foods and legumes), and you can take a vitamin D supplement and get selenium from chicken, eggs, nuts, and seeds. You can get your omega-3 fatty acids (DHA and EPA) from a shellfish-free supplement (check the label to make sure it's shellfish-free).

✔ **Soy:** Soy is the main ingredient in edamame (green soybeans), tofu, soy-milk, and many vegetarian meat and dairy alternatives. Manufacturers also add soy to many other foods, so read ingredient lists carefully and avoid foods with ingredients such as soy lecithin, soybean oil, miso, tamari, textured vegetable protein, and bean curd. Soy is a good source of protein and nutrients such as folate and other B vitamins, potassium, and iron. If you can't have soy, eat meat, eggs, or dairy to make sure you still get these nutrients.

✔ **Wheat:** You find wheat in a lot of grains, especially bread and bread products (bagels, English muffins, and so on), tortillas, cereals, and crackers. Wheat foods contain complex carbohydrates, folate, iron, B vitamins, and more. Look for wheat-free foods that provide similar nutrients, like rice, potatoes, and quinoa.

# What to Do If You Suspect a Food Allergy

If you suspect that you have a food allergy, keep a detailed food journal. Record not only the foods you eat but also the symptoms you experience and the timing of the symptoms as they appear. Keep in mind that some reactions can take several hours to appear. After you narrow down the food or foods that may be causing problems, avoid those foods for the duration of your pregnancy and talk to your doctor to find out how to deal with your allergies during pregnancy.

Read food labels carefully to look for any foods you may be allergic to. Become aware of all the different ways a particular food may be listed. For example, ingredient lists can list milk as yogurt, cheese, butter, cream, milk solids, whey, casein, lactose, and lactalbumin, just to name a few. Research each food you may be allergic to so you can avoid it at all costs.

## Distinguishing between food allergies and food intolerances

Food intolerances are different from allergies. Intolerances don't provoke an allergic reaction and aren't considered as dangerous. *Lactose intolerance* (the inability to digest *lactose,* or milk sugar) is the most common food intolerance. Some women find that they can't digest milk as easily when they're pregnant. If you're especially gassy or have loose stools after drinking milk or eating ice cream, don't be alarmed. Simply look for lactose-free milk (or use soymilk) and avoid cream-based foods. Hard cheeses, such as cheddar, mozzarella, and Swiss, are typically low in lactose and not as problematic.

Don't get tested for food allergies while pregnant. A positive reaction could result in less oxygen to you and your baby. Or you could go into *anaphylactic shock,* a severe allergic reaction that can come on quickly and cause death. The time to get tested for a food allergy is after your little one has safely entered the world.

# Preventing Food Allergies in Your Baby

About 3 million children in the United States have food allergies. Many children can outgrow food allergies, especially those from milk, soy, eggs, and wheat. However, allergies to peanuts, tree nuts, fish, and shellfish often last a lifetime. The following sections offer guidance on the steps you can take to prevent your child from developing a food allergy, starting before he's born and continuing throughout his first year.

Smoking has been linked to an increased risk of food allergies, so make sure you avoid smoking when pregnant and stay away from anyone who's smoking around you to decrease your exposure to second-hand smoke.

## Deciding whether you need to avoid certain foods while pregnant

The science around preventing food allergies is still fairly controversial and inconclusive. Years ago, the general consensus was that all pregnant women should completely avoid potentially allergenic foods to help reduce allergies in their kids. However, more recent evidence shows that complete avoidance isn't necessary. In fact, eating potentially allergenic foods may be beneficial because doing so exposes the baby to those foods early on.

If you, your partner, or one of your older children has a food allergy, your baby has a higher risk of developing a food allergy. Obviously, if you're allergic to a particular food, you need to avoid it during your pregnancy. But if your partner or an older child is allergic to a certain food, you may also want to avoid that allergen, especially during the third trimester.

Then again, because the science is still evolving and no one's really sure whether complete avoidance is necessary for high-risk mothers, you can opt to reduce your intake (instead of completely eliminating the food from your diet). For example, if your toddler is allergic to peanuts, you may decide to eat peanuts during this pregnancy but reduce your daily PBJ to once a week or twice a month.

Antioxidant vitamins C, E, and beta carotene, as well as vitamin D, have been shown to help with allergy prevention. Omega-3 fatty acids are also good for allergy prevention because they assist in reducing inflammation and promote development of a healthy nervous system (find out more about omega-3 fatty acids in Chapter 3). Probiotics encourage good bacteria in the digestive tract, and some studies have found that taking them while pregnant may help with mild reduction of allergies in babies. You find probiotics in supplement form or in foods like yogurt and kefir.

## Recognizing the role breast-feeding plays in allergy prevention

After your baby arrives, you can take a major step toward reducing his risk of developing food allergies by breast-feeding him exclusively for the first four to six months of his life. Breast milk contains your natural antibodies to strengthen your baby's immune system, helping him fight off allergies and sickness those first few months of life when his immune system is weaker. In addition to getting important immune-building factors from your milk, your baby also avoids the common allergens found in cow's milk and soy-based formulas.

Avoiding potential food allergens while breast-feeding is more necessary if you have a baby who's at high risk of developing allergies. If you, your partner, or an older child has an allergy to a specific food, simply avoid that food while breast-feeding. But don't feel like you have to avoid all eight of the most common food allergens (I list these earlier in the chapter).

If you don't have allergies in your family, you can eat moderate amounts of all potentially allergenic foods while breast-feeding. Just be aware that your baby may have a reaction to one (or more) of those foods. Watch for signs that your baby isn't tolerating your milk. These signs include extraordinary fussiness, unusual stools, bloody diarrhea, hives, eczema, or trouble breathing. Seek medical help from your baby's pediatrician and consult with a registered dietitian who specializes in pediatric allergies.

## Creating taste preferences in your baby

Have you ever wondered why some babies accept their broccoli and green beans with no complaint while others spit them out, shuddering up and down?

Along with your baby's heart and lungs, the areas of her brain that are associated with taste and smell are also developing while she's in the womb. Your amniotic fluid, which your baby inhales and swallows, has different flavors and smells, depending on what you eat. So what you eat can literally shape your baby's palate.

You have five taste senses: sweet, sour, salty, bitter, and umami (savory). Your body's natural instinct is to reject bitter and sour and to accept sweet, umami, and salty tastes. Most vegetables contain natural bitter-tasting compounds, so if you want your baby to accept her veggies, you have to introduce her to those flavors very early on in life. Role modeling healthy eating behaviors literally starts while your baby is in the womb.

If you can't breast-feed or are simply uninterested in breast-feeding and food allergies tend to run in the family, use a hypoallergenic formula.

# Introducing food allergens to your child

The best way to reduce allergic reactions in any child is to delay introducing solid foods until she's 4 to 6 months old. Scientists used to think that delaying solid foods for longer than six months was beneficial in allergy prevention, but more recent recommendations from the American Academy of Pediatrics (AAP) show that 4 to 6 months old is a good time to begin introducing babies to solid foods. For the best results, start with low-allergy foods, such as rice cereal and bland fruit and vegetable purees (green beans, squash, and applesauce, for example). The AAP has also found no current convincing evidence to delay the introduction of foods that are considered to be highly allergenic, such as fish, eggs, and peanuts.

Allergic responses typically don't occur after just one exposure to food. Offer only one new food every few days so that you can determine which food caused the reaction if your baby has one. After your baby has a nice repertoire of foods, vary the routine to provide different foods that provide a variety of flavors (and nutrients) on a regular basis.

Excessive exposure to foods can cause allergic reactions. For instance, common allergens in other countries vary from those in the United States because their staple foods are different. Rice is a common allergen in Japan, whereas chickpeas are a common allergen in India. To avoid overexposure to the common allergens in your culture, offer a variety of foods to your infant.

# Chapter 20

# After the Arrival: Caring for You and Your Baby

*In This Chapter*

▶ Eating right after delivery to help speed up your recovery

▶ Considering the benefits of nursing

▶ Knowing what to eat while you nurse

▶ Feeding your baby (with breast milk or formula) to ensure proper growth

Congratulations on your new arrival! You've been carrying your gorgeous new bundle for the past 40 weeks or so, and now you're able to enjoy the fruits of your labor (literally!). Whether you had a 30-hour labor or a planned C-section delivery, childbirth takes a lot out of you, but good nutrition can help restore your body to what it once was. This chapter tells you all about the nutrients you need as you recover from childbirth. And because choosing to breast-feed comes with its own set of nutrition rules, this chapter also helps you make the decision about nursing and introduces you to the basics of nursing nutrition. Last but not least, it gives you a quick crash course in feeding your little one, whether you opt for breast milk or formula.

## Getting the Nutrients You Need to Fuel Your Recovery

Good nutrition is important all throughout your life, but it's critical when you're recovering from childbirth — the first two to four weeks (or so) after vaginal delivery and eight to ten weeks (or so) after C-section delivery. The nutrients provided in healthy foods aid your body in repairing and rebuilding after pregnancy and delivery. In fact, your recovery time could be longer if your body doesn't get the proper nourishment. So make sure you nourish your body with lean proteins, whole grains, fruits, vegetables, and dairy.

Certain nutrients are especially important during the recovery period. Make sure you get plenty of the following in your post-delivery diet:

- **Iron:** Due to the blood loss during delivery (you lose some blood with both vaginal and C-section deliveries), make sure you're still getting plenty of iron — 27 grams (g) — during the recovery period after giving birth. After your recovery period, you can drop down to the pre-pregnancy iron intake level of 18 g per day as long as your doctor hasn't determined that you're anemic or recommended a higher level. Find out how to add more iron to your diet in Chapter 3.

- **Protein:** Protein has the amino acids your body needs to help it build and repair cells and muscles that were damaged during childbirth, especially if you had a C-section. Try to get the 71 g per day (the same you needed during pregnancy) throughout the recovery period following delivery. No need to go out of your way to eat large steaks; just focus on getting protein from meats, seafood, dairy, eggs, beans, soy, or nuts at every meal. See Chapter 3 for more on adding protein to your diet.

- **Vitamin C:** Vitamin C is good for wound healing whether you delivered vaginally or via C-section. Aim to get 85 milligrams (mg) during the recovery period by drinking your 100 percent fruit juice, eating some strawberries or kiwi, and eating plenty of other fruits and vegetables.

- **Fiber:** Many women complain of constipation in the weeks following delivery. To avoid becoming one of them, drink lots of fluid and eat 28 g of fiber per day during the recovery period. (Refer to Chapter 3 for ideas on adding more fiber to your diet.)

You may also find that taking a probiotic supplement on a regular basis helps relieve constipation. If you get really constipated and don't have a bowel movement for several days, use a natural laxative or stool softener every few days until you become regular again. Moving your body with some daily physical activity can also help keep your bowels moving.

Keep taking a multivitamin after you deliver to help fill in any nutrient gaps in your diet. If you're nursing, continue taking your prenatal vitamins until you stop nursing. If you're going the formula route and still have some prenatal vitamins left, finish them off and then switch over to a general women's multivitamin.

Don't be afraid to ask friends and family to help you in your recovery by preparing nutritious meals. If you're cooking for yourself, cook more than you need and freeze the extra to use on a difficult day when you don't have the time or energy to cook.

## Adding caffeine and alcohol back into your diet

Did you pack Champagne or wine in your hospital bag? Tempted to order a double espresso in the recovery room?

You've been so good during your pregnancy, and now you want to celebrate with some caffeine and alcohol, right? Enjoying a drink of either is okay, but be careful about how much you drink if you're nursing (they both pass into breast milk). Keep in mind that you may get jittery or not sleep well if you drink too much caffeine

at once, so ease back into your caffeine routine with half regular/half decaf coffee. As for alcohol, limit yourself to half of an alcoholic drink while you build up your tolerance again, and, of course, don't drink heavily when you're caring for your child. (Moderate drinking guidelines suggest women stick to no more than one drink per day all the time, not just after pregnancy.) See the section "Being smart about alcohol and caffeine" for details about consuming these substances when nursing.

# To Nurse, or Not to Nurse?

Deciding to breast-feed instead of feeding your baby formula has implications for both parties starting soon after your little one makes her debut, so you need to make your choice before giving birth. The following sections provide you with some points of consideration to aid you in the decision-making process.

The choice not to breast-feed has already been made for some women. If you have an infection like tuberculosis or human immunodeficiency virus (HIV), are on certain medications or treatment for cancer (like those for chemotherapy or radiation), or are drinking heavily or using drugs, do not breast-feed. If you've had breast implants, you should be able to breast-feed, but you may not produce quite as much milk and may need to supplement with formula to make sure your baby gets enough to eat.

## Benefits of nursing for Mom

You may be surprised to find out that your baby isn't the only one who benefits from nursing. You get quite a few benefits, too:

✔ **Breast milk is the most nutritious food you can give your child.** A healthy baby is a happy baby, and a happy baby makes for a happy mom! (I review all the benefits of breast milk for your baby in the next section.)

✔ **Producing milk requires a lot of calories, and many of those calories come from your body as it breaks down its fat stores.** Translation: Good-bye lingering pregnancy pounds — provided you don't exceed your calorie needs. (In other words, you can't overeat and expect to lose weight.)

✔ **Nursing gives you a chance to develop a special bond with your child.** Your baby is physically depending on you for nourishment, and the time you spend together on the recliner or couch feeding is special time.

✔ **Nursing can help improve your mood.** Most women experience some mood swings after giving birth; hormones, a brand new lifestyle, and a lack of sleep all contribute. Studies have shown that women who breast-feed have lower incidence of postpartum depression, mainly because of the hormone oxytocin, which signals milk production in the body. Oxytocin has also been linked to reduced levels of anxiety, leaving you more relaxed and able to bond with your baby.

✔ **Nursing may protect your health in the future.** Some studies show a lower incidence of ovarian and breast cancer in women who breast-fed their infants.

✔ **Nursing is free (or at least a lot cheaper than expensive formula).** Breast pumps, if you need them, aren't cheap, but compared to the cost of formula, they're a small investment to make.

✔ **Nursing requires that you sit down numerous times every day to relax.** It's a great time to read, meditate, or get caught up on your favorite TV shows with your feet up. I read more books while I was nursing than I had in the previous three years!

## How long should I nurse?

Breast milk can provide all the nutrition your baby needs for the first six months of life. At four to six months, you can start introducing solid foods, but keep in mind that breast milk or formula will continue to be your baby's primary nutrition until about a year when he starts eating a larger portion of solids.

So exactly how long should you plan to breast-feed? The American Academy of Pediatrics recommends breast-feeding for one year. The World Health Organization recommends doing so for two years. How long you go is up to you and your baby. I nursed for one year with each of my boys. Right when we got to the end of that year, I could tell they were ready to move onto solids and bottles, and I was very happy that I had met my goal of lasting the full year.

If the thought of nursing for a year or more is scary, just remember that any amount of time you nurse is better than no time at all. Whether you nurse for one week, three months, six months, or two years, your baby is still getting all the benefits from your breast milk that I describe in this chapter.

## Can I nurse if I had multiples?

Nursing multiples is definitely a possibility. Even if you can't provide all of their nutrition after birth, partial nursing for each baby still offers benefits. Some women are able to exclusively breast-feed multiples successfully for a short period of time; others have to rely on supplementation with formula. Just keep in mind that you need more fluid and nutrition if you're producing more milk (see the "Practicing Good Nutrition When You're Nursing" section for guidelines on a nursing mom's nutrient needs).

# *Benefits of breast milk for Baby*

Breast-feeding is as good for your baby as it is for you; it offers the following benefits:

- ✔ Breast milk contains just the right proportion of carbohydrates, proteins, fats, vitamins, and minerals that your baby needs for healthy growth (as long as you continue to eat right while nursing).

- ✔ Breast milk is full of antibodies and immune properties that help protect your baby against infections and illnesses and that are impossible to mimic in formula. More immune properties translate to fewer doctor visits and sick days and reduced risk of allergies.

- ✔ Breast milk is easy to digest, clean, and safe. After all, you don't have to worry about whether you cleaned your bottles all the way or whether the water you're using with the formula is safe and free of bacteria. Plus, the breast milk is fresh out of the breast, whereas formula may sit out for a while before your baby drinks it.

- ✔ Breast milk reduces your baby's chances of developing many chronic diseases later in life: obesity, diabetes, heart disease, asthma, certain cancers, and intestinal diseases. Researchers think that what babies are fed early in life has a specific *metabolic programming effect,* meaning that the nutrition early in life programs a person's metabolism and health for the future.

- ✔ Some studies suggest that breast-fed babies have higher IQ test scores later in life due to the unique fatty acids found in breast milk as well as the emotional bonding that may contribute to brain health.

# *Overcoming obstacles of breast-feeding*

Even though I firmly believe nursing is the best thing for you and your baby, before you make your decision, you need to realize that breast-feeding does have its difficulties:

✔ **Nursing requires a certain level of commitment.** Whether you're in the middle of making or eating dinner, enjoying time with friends, or getting precious sleep, if your baby's hungry, you have to stop what you're doing to feed her.

Many times as my husband watched me lugging my pump everywhere or missing out on social events because I was in the back room nursing, he would say, "I'll make sure those boys know the commitment you made to nurse them."

✔ **Nursing in public can be awkward.** Depending on your comfort level of nursing in public, you may find yourself sitting in the car or bathroom a lot more often. If you do nurse in public, bring along a drape or big blanket to be as discreet as possible.

✔ **Nursing requires that you continue to pay close attention to what you eat and drink.** The nutritional do's and don'ts for nursing (outlined in the next section) are somewhat of a continuation of those for pregnancy. Seeking out nutritious foods to build the nutrient content of your milk and avoiding those foods and drinks that can be harmful in your milk are still on the top of the priority list.

✔ **You have to plan when and where to pump.** If you're a working mom and are still nursing when you go back to work, a breast pump is a necessity. I highly recommend a hands-free pumping bra (to be used only when you're pumping) so you can be free to flip through a magazine or work on the computer while you're pumping. Create a checklist so that you don't forget to pack any of the pump parts each day. Clean your pump between pumping sessions and keep the milk cold in the refrigerator or in a cooler with ice packs to keep it safe.

# Practicing Good Nutrition When You're Nursing

Rule number one of nursing nutrition: You have to eat some additional calories per day to help your body produce milk. In fact, nursing women need to consume about 330 to 400 more calories than they did before pregnancy. The more active you are and the more milk you produce, the more calories you need.

If you're trying to lose weight and nurse at the same time, don't consume fewer than 1,800 calories a day. If you do, your milk production may suffer. Later in this chapter, you find some sample meal plans that are based on getting 2,200 calories per day, an amount that supports milk production but can also promote a small amount of weight loss (depending on your caloric needs).

As for what you should eat to get the calories your body needs, treat your *lactation,* or nursing, diet pretty much the same as your pregnancy diet. Continue to fill your plate with nutritious foods and limit your intake of those foods that provide little nutritional value and a lot of excess calories. The next sections break down the specific nutrients you need to pay attention to when you're nursing, provide some sample menus so you can see how to incorporate them into your diet, and offer some advice for consuming caffeine and alcohol.

## Focusing on carbohydrates, proteins, and fats

Carbohydrates are your body's source of energy, and when you're nursing, you need about 300 g of carbs per day to support milk production. Your body also needs 29 g of fiber, the part of complex carbohydrates that doesn't get digested, per day, so load up on those whole grains, beans, fruits, and vegetables. As for protein, aim to get the same amount per day as you did when you were pregnant: about 20 percent of your calories. For example, if you're eating 2,200 calories per day, aim to get 110 g per day.

Fat is necessary in everyone's diet. Focus on the healthier monounsaturated and polyunsaturated fats found in nuts, seeds, olive or canola oil, and avocados. Limit your intake of the artery-clogging saturated and trans fats. Aim to get about 73 g of fat (that's 30 percent of your daily calories for a 2,200-calorie nursing diet). Fats in your diet help you absorb certain nutrients (including vitamins A, D, E, and K, as well as some phytonutrients) that are important for you and your baby.

You can read more about where to get carbohydrates, fiber, protein, and fats in Chapter 3.

## Highlighting other important nutrients

Most of the nutrients you need to pay special attention to when you're nursing are the same ones you focused on during pregnancy, but the amounts you take in may actually be greater than they were when you were pregnant. Believe it or not, creating milk requires more energy and nutrients than growing a baby!

Following are some of the nutrients you need to focus on if you're a nursing mom, arranged in order of importance:

✔ **DHA and EPA:** These omega-3 fatty acids help with heart health, and DHA, in particular, helps your baby's brain development and vision. Aim to get at least 300 mg of DHA and 220 mg of EPA per day from fish or supplemental fish oil.

✔ **Vitamin D:** Vitamin D is necessary for bone health and overall disease prevention for your baby. Some studies suggest that lactating women take 1,000 to 6,000 international units (IU) of supplemental vitamin D to sustain an adequate amount of vitamin D in their breast milk. Because most women don't have adequate vitamin D levels in their breast milk, the American Academy of Pediatrics recommends giving at least 400 IU of supplemental vitamin D drops per day to all breast-fed infants up to the age of 1 year. (Note that infant formula provides adequate vitamin D, so drops aren't necessary for formula-fed babies.)

✔ **Vitamin A:** Vitamin A promotes healthy vision, immunity, and cell and tissue growth in your baby's body. Your vitamin A needs almost double compared to pre-pregnancy. Aim to get 4,333 IU (1,300 micrograms, or mcg) each day by eating fruits and vegetables that are dark orange or green (like sweet potatoes, carrots, cantaloupe, papaya, and spinach) or liver.

✔ **Choline:** Choline assists with development of the hippocampus, the memory center of the brain. Aim to get 550 mg each day from egg yolks, fish, beef, poultry, pork, or wheat germ.

✔ **Vitamin C:** Vitamin C helps build connective tissue, heals wounds, and boosts immunity in your baby. Aim to get 120 mg of vitamin C, which is found in fruits and vegetables and is especially high in citrus fruits, strawberries, kiwi, bell peppers, and potatoes.

✔ **Potassium:** Potassium helps maintain the right fluid balance and blood pressure in your baby. You need 5,100 mg daily, and you find it in bananas, beans, fish, potatoes, tomatoes, almonds, and more.

✔ **Chromium:** Chromium helps to keep blood sugar in proper range by working in insulin. The amount of chromium you need while breast-feeding (45 mcg) is almost double what you needed pre-pregnancy. You find chromium in beef, poultry, pork, whole grains, and cheese.

Continue taking your prenatal vitamin as long as you nurse. The prenatal vitamin helps you meet the increased nutrient needs of nursing even on days when your diet isn't quite perfect.

## Staying hydrated

To create a liquid in your body, you need to add extra liquid to your diet — 128 ounces (or 3.8 liters or 16 cups) of liquid per day to be exact. Not all of that liquid has to be water (other fluids can hydrate, too), but do try to get at last half of your total 128 ounces from water. See Chapter 3 for some helpful hydration tips.

To help you get all the fluid you need in a 24-hour period, keep a bottle of water near where you nurse and drink up while your baby drinks from you. When I was nursing, I always put an insulated mug of ice water on the table next to the recliner I sat in while nursing before I went to bed at night. That way, I could hydrate while nursing even in the middle of the night!

## Sampling some meal plans for nursing moms

I created the following sample meal plans so you can see how to put this chapter's nursing nutrition recommendations into action. Both plans provide you with 2,200 calories. Not only does this amount of calories give you the extra calories you need for nursing, but it also promotes gradual weight loss. (For more information on losing excess pregnancy pounds the healthy way, see Chapter 21.)

### Day 1

*Breakfast*

⅔ cup of Homemade Maple Berry Crunch Granola (Chapter 12)

6 ounces of lowfat or nonfat Greek yogurt

*Snack 1*

1 orange

*Lunch*

Spinach, Date, and Blue Cheese Chicken Panini (Chapter 14)

10 baby carrots with 2 tablespoons of light ranch dressing

*Snack 2*

½ cup of lowfat cottage cheese with ½ cup of canned pineapple (canned in juice)

*Snack 3*

100-calorie, high-fiber muffin top, like VitaTop (or other fiber-rich nutrition bar)

*Dinner*

4 ounces of skinless turkey breast cutlet cooked in 1 tablespoon of olive oil

½ cup of cooked quinoa

1 cup of cooked broccoli

*Snack 4*

8 ounces of lowfat chocolate milk

Enjoy your chocolate milk cold or heat it up to make it hot chocolate! Oh, in case you were wondering, chocolate milk does contain a very small amount of caffeine, but it's not enough to keep you awake or to pass into your breast milk.

### Day 2

#### Breakfast

2 frozen whole-grain waffles

1 tablespoon of peanut butter

½ of a banana

1 tablespoon of maple syrup

#### Snack 1

1 cup of frosted shredded wheat cereal (dry or with ½ cup of lowfat milk)

#### Lunch

White Bean and Portobello Salad (Chapter 13)

#### Snack 2

1 cup of frozen or canned low-sodium vegetable soup

#### Snack 3

2 fresh Medjool dates

#### Dinner

1 Italian Stuffed Steak Roll (Chapter 14)

1 cup of cooked, quartered roasted potatoes

1 cup of cooked sugar snap peas

#### Snack 4

1 cup of light or lowfat ice cream

## Being smart about alcohol and caffeine

Alcohol and caffeine pass into breast milk, which means that if you're taking in these substances, your baby is, too. Alcohol can interrupt a baby's sleep, and large amounts passed to a newborn on a regular basis can cause problems with brain development. Alcohol may also affect your ability to produce milk because it suppresses oxytocin, the hormone that signals milk production in your body.

## What's your flavor?

You may have heard people say that you shouldn't eat garlic, onions, beans, or spicy foods while nursing because they may upset the baby. Well, every baby is different, but some do get fussy or particularly gassy when they get certain foods through your milk. For example, my son spit up more than usual after I ate artichokes, so I cut them out of my diet for the rest of the time I nursed him. If you suspect that certain foods are causing problems for your baby, keep a diary of the foods you're eating and the symptoms your baby is having and see if you can find a connection.

Your baby experiences different flavors based on the foods you eat. So if you want a child who's more likely to eat fruits and vegetables, start introducing him to these flavors early on through your breast milk. (No guarantees it'll work, though!)

Ideally, you'll continue to avoid alcohol throughout the entire time you're nursing, but if you feel the need to have an occasional (once or twice a week or less) alcoholic drink, try to have it right after a feeding. Alcohol isn't stored in your milk, so as long as you wait two to three hours after you have one drink to feed your baby, the amount of alcohol that passes to your baby will be very small. You can also pump and discard (pump and dump) your milk to avoid passing alcohol to your baby. Keep in mind, though, that if you don't have pumped milk from a previous session stored, you may need to feed your baby formula to make up for the dumped milk.

As for caffeine, even small amounts of this stimulant can leave a baby jittery and irritable, cause interrupted sleep, increase her heart rate, and affect her breathing.

In general, limit yourself to no more than 200 to 300 mg of caffeine per day. (To see the typical amounts of caffeine in foods and beverages, see Chapter 2.) If you notice that your baby seems to be feeling the effects of the caffeine you're taking in, cut out caffeine from your diet. Your baby will be most sensitive for the first six months, but it's best to limit caffeine the whole time you're nursing.

# Feeding Baby

Your baby's stomach is only the size of a thimble when he's born. With such a tiny stomach, he needs to eat frequently to get all the nutrition he needs in a day. You have two options for feeding your newborn: breast milk or formula. I cover breast milk earlier in this chapter. *Formula* is food that's specially designed to simulate and be a proper substitute for breast milk. The sections that follow cover the basics of feeding your baby with either option.

Regardless of what you choose to feed your baby, be sure to take him in for his regularly scheduled checkups so that your pediatrician can monitor his growth. The best way to find out if your baby is getting enough nutrition is to see whether he's growing at the proper pace with his length, weight, and head circumference. By the time he's a few days old, he should have six or more wet diapers and one or more dirty diapers each day, and you should be feeding him about 8 to 12 times per day.

## With breast milk

The first milk your baby receives from you is called *colostrum*. It's typically yellow in color and is chock-full of antibodies that help build your baby's immune system. (Colostrum is almost like your baby's first immunization — only a lot less painful!) Colostrum lasts for two to four days after delivery.

After colostrum is gone, your milk comes through in two stages. First, you have the transitional milk, which comes in between two and five days and lasts until about 14 days after birth. Transitional milk is creamy and provides the fat your baby needs during these first few weeks. After transitional milk, you have mature milk, which is thinner and more watery. You'll produce this type of milk until you stop nursing; it provides the sole source of nutrition for your baby for the first four to six months of life.

The sooner you start breast-feeding and the more often you offer the nipple, the more likely your baby is to latch on. Your nipples will be sore for a week or two, but the soreness will pass quickly and the benefits far outweigh a few weeks of pain. (See the earlier section "Benefits of breast milk for Baby" for details.)

While nursing, you can hold your baby in three main positions: the traditional cradle position, the lying down position, or the football hold. Figure 20-1 shows an example of each position. Choose the position that works for you and allows your baby to breathe. Always make sure his nose isn't pressed against your skin to the point where he can't breathe.

If you ever feel significant pain in one of your breasts, feel around for a lump. You probably have a clogged duct. Apply warm compresses and gently massage it while your baby is nursing to try to unplug it. Call your doctor if the pain progresses and you feel achy, feverish, and have reddened areas on your breast. You probably have mastitis and will need an antibiotic to relieve the infection. The good news is that you can keep nursing because the infection won't pass to your baby.

Allow your baby to tell you when he's done eating. Initially, you may be nursing for 10 to 15 minutes on each side, poking him awake as he falls asleep on the breast. After a while, though, he'll become a pro and will suck you dry in a few minutes so he can get back to the important task of playing.

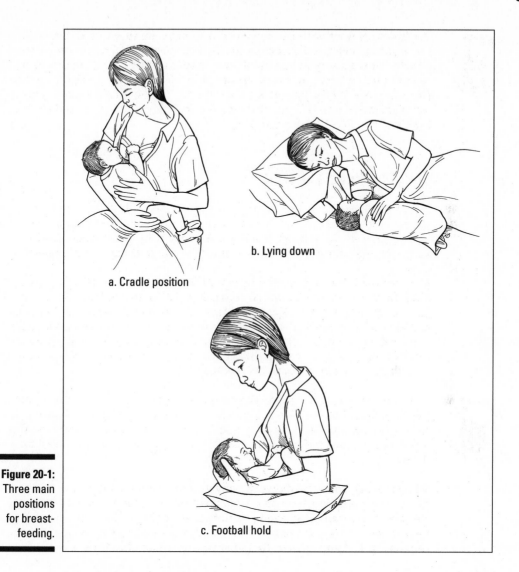

a. Cradle position

b. Lying down

c. Football hold

**Figure 20-1:** Three main positions for breast-feeding.

# With formula

Millions of research dollars have gone into making formulas with just the right mix of vitamins, minerals, carbohydrates, proteins, fats, and calories for infants. Most infant formula also has omega-3 fatty acids added, and some have *probiotics* (healthy bacteria to boost immune and digestive health). Formula comes in a few different varieties:

✔ **Ready-to-use liquid:** This is the most convenient type of formula because it doesn't require any mixing or measuring. You just open it up and serve. It's typically also the most expensive.

✔ **Concentrated liquid:** This type of formula requires you to mix it with water to bring it to the right concentration for your infant. The good news is that it mixes easily since it's already in liquid form.

✔ **Powdered formula:** This formula type requires you to mix it with water. It's the most economical choice of formula type and also takes up the least amount of storage space in your pantry. If you go this route, just make sure you mix it well to prevent lumps.

If your baby can't handle these regular formulas, you can also find cow's milk–based, soy-based, lactose-free, and hydrolyzed varieties. In addition, you can find special formulas for premature babies and a hypoallergenic variety for those at risk of allergies. Ask your pediatrician if you're not sure which kind of formula is right for your baby.

Don't try to make your own formula or use regular soy or cow's milk as formula. Your baby has very specific needs in the first year of life, and formulas have been designed to meet those nutritional needs. Also, make sure you mix and use your formula according to the package directions. Don't add olive oil, baby cereal, or anything extra to formula. If you add other foods, your baby will fill up on those foods and potentially miss out on the essential nutrients in the formula.

Substituting generic formula for its more expensive name-brand counterpart is perfectly fine as long as you trust the generic brand to have the same nutritional quality as the name brand.

To prepare a bottle of formula, make sure everything — from the surfaces you use to prepare the bottle to your hands and the bottle itself — is clean. If you have to add water to the formula, use boiled, cooled water to make sure it's bacteria-free. Test the temperature of the bottle by dripping one droplet of milk on the inside of your wrist. If it's too warm, let the bottle cool in cold water for a few minutes. Throw away the unused contents of a prepared bottle if your baby doesn't finish the bottle within two hours. You may be tempted to put it back in the refrigerator for later, but the safest thing to do is to throw it out and prepare a new bottle for the next feeding.

When feeding your baby with a bottle, cradle his head, keeping him in a semi-upright position (laying him flat may cause ear infections). Tilt the bottle so that the entire nipple area of the bottle is filled with milk to keep him from swallowing air. Allow your baby to drink as much as he wants, not forcing him to finish the whole bottle. If he finishes it and wants more, make another fresh bottle and offer him more. Finally, burp him by gently patting his back while he's over your shoulder or on your lap.

# Chapter 21

# Losing Those Lingering Pounds

. . . . . . . . . . . . . . . . . . . . . . . . . . . . . . . . . . . . . . . . . . . . . . . . . . . .

## In This Chapter

▶ Creating realistic goals for weight loss after pregnancy

▶ Figuring out how many calories you need and what you should eat to get them

▶ Fitting exercise into your new routine

▶ Getting your body ready for another pregnancy

. . . . . . . . . . . . . . . . . . . . . . . . . . . . . . . . . . . . . . . . . . . . . . . . . . . .

*L*osing all your pregnancy weight can easily take nine months to a year. If you gained a lot of weight, shedding those excess pounds can take even longer. So don't aspire to be like your favorite celebrities who bounce right back into shape after having a baby. If you do, you'll be setting yourself up for certain failure. Why? Because returning to your pre-pregnancy weight in just a few weeks isn't realistic — unless of course you have a trainer, chef, nanny, and housekeeper, and your full-time job is having an ideal image. Also, many celebrities take the weight off quickly by losing it the wrong way, and you don't want to do that either.

This chapter focuses on helping you get your pre-pregnancy body back the healthy way — by eating good-for-you foods, watching portion sizes, and exercising, not getting sucked into some fad diet. I share diet and exercise advice aimed at getting you slimmed down and full of good energy to spend with your new family. I also present tips for getting your body ready to start trying for another child when the time is right.

If you're reading this chapter while you're still pregnant and find yourself dreaming about getting your body back, remember that the best way to lose the pregnancy pounds is to avoid gaining an excessive amount of weight while you're pregnant. Turn to Chapter 5 to find the recommended weight gain based on your pre-pregnancy weight.

# Setting Yourself Up for Success with Realistic Expectations

The first step to successfully losing weight after your babe is born is to have realistic expectations based on the amount of weight you gained throughout the past 40 or so weeks. During the average pregnancy, the momma-to-be gains anywhere from 25 to 35 pounds. Approximately 10 of these pounds come off right after you deliver your baby and the placenta. Within one to two weeks after delivery, you'll likely lose another 5 (or more) pounds as the fluid balance in your body starts to return to normal.

Before you start worrying about losing the rest of your pregnancy pounds, remember that your body just went through a lot carrying your baby and delivering him safely into the world. Give yourself a few weeks of rest and recovery and enjoy this time with your new baby before you start restricting calories and working out. After all, you can't care for your baby if you don't care for yourself, and doing too much too soon is a surefire way to add unnecessary physical and emotional stress.

The following sections give you an idea of how long your belly will continue to look pregnant and how quickly you should strive to lose the extra weight.

## Knowing how long your belly will stay

The stories of women who walk out of the hospital in their pre-pregnancy-sized jeans are exaggerated. The reality is that your pregnancy belly sticks around for a while (for example, I left the hospital after delivery looking like I was still about five months pregnant). It's not fat that's overstaying its welcome; it's your uterus or, more accurately, the size of your uterus.

Your uterus takes about four weeks to contract back down to its normal size. Every day of those four weeks, your uterus shrinks just a little bit more. Need proof? Check your panties. Bleeding is a sign that your uterus is indeed shrinking, and you can expect to bleed for about ten days after delivery. *Warning:* If you're concerned that your bleeding may be abnormal, call your doctor right away.

You can help speed up your uterus's shrinking act by breast-feeding. Nursing your baby releases hormones that help shrink the uterus.

If you're like me and can't stand the thought of wearing your maternity clothes any longer but can't yet fit into your pre-pregnancy clothes, consider buying a few inexpensive pairs of pants that are a size or two larger than your normal size. These transitional pieces can get you through until your pre-pregnancy clothes fit again.

After your uterus shrinks back to its normal size, you'll notice that you still have some skin and fat remaining. The skin should shrink back on its own, but it'll take time to adjust to your body's new shape. The excess fat, on the other hand, won't go away by itself. But don't worry; by following the nutrition and exercise strategies I outline later in this chapter, you can shrink the excess fat back to its pre-pregnancy level.

## Understanding proper rates of weight loss

If you gained the recommended 25 to 35 pounds during your pregnancy, aim to lose about 1 pound per week beginning about one month after delivery. Bear in mind that the more weight you gained during your pregnancy, the faster it may come off. So if you happened to gain 50 or 70 pounds during your pregnancy, healthy weight loss could be more like 2 pounds per week. Say you have an extra 12 to 20 pounds still hanging on a month or so after delivery. Losing that weight at a rate of 1 pound per week will take about three to five months. Note that if you're nursing, you will probably still weigh a few more pounds than pre-pregnancy due to the weight of the milk and storage of calories required to produce milk (in the form of body fat).

Although you want to lose your excess pregnancy weight at a reasonable rate, try your best to get down to your pre-pregnancy size by your baby's first birthday. Many women who don't get the weight off within the first year after childbirth struggle to get it off for the rest of their lives, which can lead to health risks associated with being overweight, such as type 2 diabetes, hypertension, heart disease, and joint problems.

# Fueling Your Body the Right Way

I've seen many people exercise themselves into the ground and not lose weight because they've ignored their diet. What, when, and how you eat can easily determine how much weight you lose post-pregnancy. After all, half of the weight-loss equation has to do with the calories you consume in the food you eat. If you don't pay attention to your diet, you can exercise a ton and still not experience any weight loss.

If you treated pregnancy as a time to clean up your diet and fill your plate with nutritious foods, stay on that path after you deliver to lose excess weight and increase your energy level. If, while pregnant, you chose to "treat" yourself to an assortment of high-calorie foods in large quantities, now's the time to clean up your food choices and focus on getting yourself healthier. After all, you're not just doing this for yourself; you have your baby to think about now!

If you were taught to clean your plate from a young age, you've likely continued to do so as an adult out of habit. Well, you need to break this habit if you want to have an easier time losing your pregnancy weight. Instead of worrying about cleaning your plate, pay attention to your body's hunger cues so that you can recognize the difference between feeling satisfied and feeling stuffed. In doing so, you can determine when to push the plate away and when to keep eating. (I help you discover how to read your body's hunger signals in Chapter 7.)

Another part of the weight-loss equation is not allowing yourself to become ravenously hungry. If you do, you'll be much more likely to succumb to temptation and eat too much too quickly; not to mention you'll probably eat food that's not the healthiest for you. So to keep your hunger at bay, eat small snacks throughout the day that are high in either fiber or protein. For a list of satisfying snack ideas, see Chapter 7.

## *Focusing on nutrient-dense foods*

Nutrient-dense foods provide your body with the nutrients it needs to function; as a bonus, they're often low in calories, too. Beginning right after delivery, start focusing on foods that contain the following filling components (see Chapter 3 for more details on each one):

- ✔ **Fiber:** Fiber is literally indigestible plant matter. Your body tries to digest it but can't, so it keeps you feeling full longer (and also helps keep you regular). Eat a minimum of 25 grams of fiber per day.

- ✔ **Protein:** Protein also takes longer to digest, keeping you feeling satisfied for a longer period of time. Aim to get 75 grams of protein per day (that's 20 percent of your calories, based on a 1,500-calorie weight-loss diet; see the next section for details on how many calories you should be getting).

- ✔ **Fat:** Focus on eating healthy fats, like those found in fish, olive oil, nuts, seeds, and avocados. Eat about 50 grams of fat per day (that's 30 percent of your calories, based on a 1,500-calorie weight-loss diet; skip to the next section for more on how many calories you need).

- ✔ **Water:** Drinking water before and during meals aids in digestion and helps fill you up a bit, even if only temporarily. Drink 91 ounces of total fluid (a little more than eleven 8-ounce cups, or 2.7 liters) per day, with the majority of that coming from water.

Aim to reduce or eliminate your intake of foods that don't fill you up and that don't give you any nutritional value, especially while you're trying to lose those lingering pregnancy pounds. Consume items like alcohol, sweets and desserts, fried foods, and regular soft drinks occasionally (as in, not frequently) and in small, reasonable quantities.

# Creating a calorie deficit

To lose weight, you need to consume fewer calories than you burn. Sounds easy enough, right? The problem is that you don't have a gas gauge that tells you exactly how much fuel you're burning at different times throughout the day. So instead of knowing exactly how many calories you need to consume each day, you have to guesstimate.

 If you're nursing, I recommend that you consume between 1,800 and 2,200 calories per day. If you go much lower, you may compromise your body's milk production. If you're not nursing, I recommend that you consume between 1,500 and 1,800 calories per day, depending on your metabolism. If you go lower than that, you'll have a hard time getting all the nutrients you need in a day.

 To help you determine just how many calories you need to support weight loss, keep track of what you eat and drink for a week. You can do so by logging into one of the many calorie-tracking websites (like www.fitday.com) or smartphone applications (like Lose It!) or by using a food journal such as *Calorie Counter Journal For Dummies* (written by Rosanne Rust and Meri Raffetto and published by John Wiley & Sons, Inc.). Tracking what you eat and drink is extremely eye-opening. In fact, studies have proven that people who keep track of what they eat lose twice as much weight as those who don't pay any attention.

As you track what you eat, focus on where your calories come from. Be aware that you can end up with 500 or more extra calories at a meal just by having bread and butter or olive oil and an alcoholic or sugary drink. Add an extra appetizer or dessert — or both — and you can easily pile on an extra 1,000 calories!

After you track your food and drink for a week, you'll have a rough idea of how many calories you consume per day. Say that number is 2,600 calories on average. For most women, that's too many and is probably leading to weight gain. For the next week, focus on eating 300 to 400 fewer calories than what you're currently eating and try to burn an extra 100 to 200 calories in exercise (see the later section "Incorporating Exercise into Your Post-Delivery Routine" for details). Doing so gives you a sum deficit of about 500 calories per day, which should help you lose about a pound per week. (It takes about 3,500 calories to lose 1 pound of fat. If you divide 3,500 calories by 7 days a week, you get 500, which is the calorie deficit per day you need to lose 1 pound per week.)

 Don't drop your calorie intake down to 1,500 calories (or 1,800 calories, if you're nursing) until about a month after delivery so that you can recover from childbirth before you start restricting your intake. Right after delivery, focus on eating nutrient-dense foods, not reducing calories (see the preceding section and Chapter 20 for more on what to eat during the recovery period). Your body needs good nutrition to recover, and if you just reduce your calorie intake (and don't focus on what you eat), you risk getting sick or injured from too much restriction too soon.

Anytime you restrict calories, you should also take a multivitamin supplement. You can continue taking your prenatal vitamin until it runs out and then switch to a regular women's multivitamin (unless you're nursing, in which case you should stick with the prenatal until you stop nursing). However, don't rely solely on that supplement to give you everything you need! Fill your plate with nutrient-rich foods that will provide your body with the things it needs to function at its best.

## Sampling some meal plans to help you lose weight

The following sample meal plans provide you with 1,500 calories per day. (Note that if you're nursing, you need to take in at least 1,800 calories per day; turn to Chapter 20 for sample meal plans just for nursing moms.) By following the examples set in these plans, you can get the nutrients you need to keep your strength up while also losing weight.

### Day 1

**Breakfast**

Ricotta Parfait (Chapter 17)

**Snack 1**

12-ounce decaf skim latte

**Lunch**

Frozen meal with fewer than 300 calories (such as Healthy Choice, Kashi, Amy's, Meals to Live, Lean Cuisine, or Smart Ones)

**Snack 2**

6 ounces of lowfat or nonfat Greek yogurt

**Snack 3**

1 whole red pepper or other raw vegetable(s), cut into slices

**Dinner**

3 ounces of lean steak (like sirloin or round steak)

½ cup of mashed potatoes (made with skim milk and just a little bit of added fat)

1 cup of cooked green beans

**Snack 4**

¾ cup of frozen grapes

# Myth buster: Foods that burn calories

You've probably heard people say that celery, grapefruit, cucumbers, lettuce — the list goes on and on — all burn more calories than they contain. Unfortunately, this myth isn't true. Yes, part of your metabolism (the number of calories you burn in a day) is attributed to the *thermic effect of food,* or in layman's terms, the calories needed to digest your food. However, the number of calories that you burn while chewing and that your intestines burn while digesting is actually very small. If you enjoy eating very low-calorie foods, keep them in your diet, but if you dip that celery into ranch dressing, all bets are off!

Frozen grapes are an excellent low-calorie treat to eat in place of ice cream at night! Plus, they take longer to eat because you can savor them one at a time.

## Day 2

### Breakfast

6 ounces of low-sodium tomato juice

2 egg whites plus 1 whole egg

1 light whole-grain English muffin

### Snack 1

1 SOYJOY nutrition bar (or other nutrition bar that has about 130 to 150 calories)

### Lunch

1½ cups of Black Bean Chili (Chapter 15)

1½ cups of a mixed greens salad with 2 tablespoons of light salad dressing

### Snack 2

2 pieces of Laughing Cow light cheese (or any lowfat, pasteurized cheese that has about 70 calories total) with 1 ounce of whole-grain crackers

### Snack 3

1 peach

### Dinner

3 ounces of skinless chicken breast

½ cup of whole-wheat spaghetti

½ cup of meatless marinara sauce

½ cup of cooked spinach

### Snack 4

Mixed Berry Frozen Yogurt (Chapter 16)

# Incorporating Exercise into Your Post-Delivery Routine

After giving birth, many women think they have a free pass that says they either shouldn't or don't have to exercise. Not true! Sure, you need a few weeks or months (depending on your individual circumstances) to recover from childbirth, but don't let too much time pass before you reap the benefits of getting active and staying fit. If you do, you'll miss out on these great benefits of post-pregnancy exercise:

- ✔ A reduced risk of postpartum depression or lessened symptoms
- ✔ Stress relief
- ✔ Improved concentration
- ✔ The loss of pregnancy fat stores
- ✔ The ability to be a good example of being active to your child(ren)

One of the best gifts you can give your children is the gift of good health, both for them and you. If you're not healthy, you're at risk of chronic conditions and premature death, and you may not have the good energy required to properly care for your children. If losing the pregnancy pounds isn't a big enough motivator to get you moving, think about the boundless love you have for your new baby and stay fit for her.

The next sections offer advice for beginning your post-delivery exercise routine and suggestions for the types of exercise you should focus on.

Check with your doctor before starting any post-delivery exercise, especially if you had a complicated pregnancy or delivery. So if you want to start exercising before your postpartum follow-up appointment (usually six weeks after delivery), be sure to call your doctor first.

## Getting started

As soon as you have the green light from your doctor, slowly start incorporating exercise back into your routine. Aim for three 30-minute sessions each week and build from there. If you're short on time, remember that even brief bouts of exercise can be beneficial. Do five or ten minutes of exercise several times throughout the day when your baby is sleeping to squeeze some fitness into your day.

As you begin to exercise post-pregnancy, keep in mind the following serious considerations:

✔ **Don't push yourself too hard, even if you were in good shape before and during your pregnancy.** If you do, you may wind up with a serious injury because your joints are more elastic for several months following delivery. (This increased elasticity is due to a hormone called *relaxin* that's released during pregnancy.) Case in point: I was active during both of my pregnancies, running or doing the elliptical machine and lifting light weights until the day I delivered. I got back on the treadmill two weeks after having my first child. I started with walking but soon brought it up to running within a few days. Unfortunately, I ended up injuring my hip because I did too much too soon. Within a month after giving birth, I started running at levels I was doing pre-pregnancy, not realizing that my bone structure, especially the alignment of my hips, had changed. I urge you to learn from my mistake; don't do too much too soon!

✔ **If you had a C-section, make sure you wait the required eight weeks before you climb any stairs or do any heavy lifting (anything heavier than your baby), running, or other form of exercise.** If you don't let your body recover fully from major abdominal surgery (a process that takes at least eight weeks) before you start exercising again, you risk causing permanent damage to your body.

✔ **Wait about four to eight weeks after giving birth to start doing heavy abdominal exercises (like abdominal crunches), especially if you've noticed a gap in your abdominal muscles.** Start slowly when you do add abdominal exercises into your routine. Stop exercising and see a doctor if you notice excessive bleeding, have pain, are unusually exhausted or short of breath, or have soreness in your muscles that doesn't go away after a few days.

Consider starting out with simple walking. Meet other new moms for stroller walks, walk on a treadmill, or go out by yourself for some alone time to de-stress. Even if you're not a jogger, you may want to invest in a jogging stroller, which has bigger wheels and is ideal for long exercise walks. If you want to exercise with other moms and your stroller, search for a Stroller Strides class in your area at www.strollerstrides.com.

Other good activities to start with include using elliptical trainers, cycling, swimming, and participating in low-impact aerobics, Pilates, and yoga classes. Look for a postnatal exercise class where newborns are welcome either to sleep in the car seat while you work out or to be part of the exercise.

If you're nursing, feed your baby (or pump) before you exercise because your milk may have a sour taste to your baby for a period of time after you've finished intense exercise due to a high lactic acid content. Also be sure to drink plenty of water before, during, and after exercise to keep yourself well hydrated, and don't forget to buy a supportive exercise bra in your new nursing size. (For pointers on proper nutrition while nursing, see Chapter 20.)

# Fitting in all three types of exercise

Exercise comes in three types: aerobic (cardiovascular), strength training (weight lifting), and stretching (flexibility). Try to incorporate all three in your post-pregnancy workout so that you have a well-rounded routine that strengthens your muscles, heart, and lungs while preventing injuries.

- ✔ **Aerobic exercise:** Anything that requires you to move major muscle groups and causes your heart to pump at a higher rate for a sustained length of time. Aerobic exercise burns the most calories quickly; after all, you can burn 300 or more calories in one 30-minute aerobic session, depending on the intensity of exercise. Examples of aerobic exercise include walking, running, hiking, cycling, swimming, stair stepping, cross-country skiing, and participating in aerobic classes. When you first start out, aim to get at least 30 minutes of aerobic exercise three times per week; then work up to doing some aerobic exercise most days of the week. Extend your exercise time as you get more fit.

- ✔ **Strength training:** Anything that requires challenging your muscles to grow. You can do strength training with weight machines, dumbbells, resistance bands, and even your own body weight. The advantage of strength training is that it helps build strong bones and muscles. The more muscle you have, the more calories you burn all the time, whether you're exercising, sleeping, or rocking your baby. Strength training also helps stabilize your core muscles, reducing your risk of injury. Aim to spend two 20- to 30-minute sessions doing strength training each week and do your best to work all your major muscle groups. Find a challenging weight that you can lift for 8 to 12 repetitions before you tire and try to do two sets of each exercise.

One of my favorite strength-training workouts doesn't use a single piece of equipment — except for my own body! I use a set of workout cards called Powerhouse Hit The Deck. I pick a workout card and do that exercise for 30 seconds and then pick another card for my next exercise. I love this workout because you can do it anywhere and you can choose as many cards (exercises) as you have time for. (Check out www.power houseperformancecoaching.com/hit-the-deck for more details on this particular workout.)

- ✔ **Stretching:** Anything that elongates the muscle to improve its elasticity and flexibility. Stretching is best to do after you've exercised when your muscles are still warm; it's a great way to prevent injuries. As part of your stretching routine, start by stretching all your major muscle groups, including your quadriceps, hamstrings, chest, and back, and then move on to your smaller muscles, including your biceps, triceps, and calves. Hold each stretch for at least 15 to 30 seconds and do each stretch twice for maximum benefit. Don't bounce around while you stretch, but rather hold the pose steady while you feel mild discomfort.

In addition to aerobic exercises, strength training, and stretching, make sure you find time to do your Kegel exercises to strengthen your pelvic floor muscles. You can do these exercises by squeezing the muscles inside your vagina that stop the flow of urine. Aim to do three sets of ten exercises, squeezing for ten seconds and relaxing for ten seconds for each one, daily.

# Preparing for the Next Baby Bump

Some women are so overwhelmed with their new baby that they can't even think about having another one; others fall so deeply in love that they start planning the next one right away. If you're ready to bring another little one into this world, make sure you properly prepare your body before becoming pregnant again. The next sections tell you how to do so.

If you were carrying excess pounds before or gained too much during your first pregnancy, take some time to lose weight before trying to get pregnant again. Losing excess weight before you get pregnant decreases your chances of developing gestational diabetes, high blood pressure, and preeclampsia, as well as reduces the odds that you'll need a C-section. (Find out more about the risks of carrying excess weight in Chapter 5.)

## Deciding how soon to start trying again

To give your next baby the best chance at good health, try to wait a minimum of 11 to 18 months before getting pregnant again. The ideal time to wait (according to research on optimal pregnancy outcomes) is between 18 months and 2 years. Note that this range is the time span from delivery of the first baby to pregnancy with the next one, not delivery of the next baby.

Why wait? Here are just a few good reasons:

- Your hormones (specifically, those that affect ovulation) are still stabilizing for the months (up to a year) after you've had a baby. Because getting pregnant is highly dependent on hormonal reactions, your chances of getting pregnant will be higher after you reach proper hormone levels.

- Pregnancy definitely takes a lot out of you physically, emotionally, and nutritionally.

- You need some time to adjust to having a new baby in the house; in other words, you need to adjust to not getting proper sleep and rest.

- If you've been nursing, producing milk can deplete your body's nutritional stores, especially if you're not eating a balanced, healthy diet. (By the way, it's a myth that you can't get pregnant while nursing. Pregnancy is less likely but still possible. Consider using some form of birth control to prevent an earlier-than-desired pregnancy. Your doctor can recommend birth control methods that are safe while nursing.)

Studies have found that a short gap (especially less than six months) between pregnancies has been associated with preterm delivery, low weight for gestational age, early infant death, birth defects, and even maternal death. On the other hand, waiting longer than five years between pregnancies has also been associated with premature delivery.

## Restoring your nutritional status

In order to best restore your nutritional status — in other words, in order to fill up your vitamin, mineral, and protein stores — keep eating as you were during pregnancy, minus the extra calories. Minimize your intake of empty-calorie foods and fill your plate with fruits, vegetables, lean proteins, lowfat dairy, beans, nuts and seeds, and whole grains.

During pregnancy, your body can become depleted in many nutrients, particularly the following ones:

- ✔ **Iron:** You need more iron during pregnancy due to increased blood volume. Your doctor can check your iron levels with a simple blood test and give you recommendations as to whether you need to supplement or not. You can help keep your iron levels high by continuing on a prenatal vitamin between pregnancies.

- ✔ **Folate:** This nutrient is necessary in those preconception months because the moment you become pregnant it's used to help form critical parts of your baby, like the neural tube, which is part of the brain stem and spinal cord. Make sure you eat foods that are high in folate (see Chapter 3) and take your prenatal vitamin.

- ✔ **Protein:** Protein helps your body build and repair muscles and tissue. It also keeps you feeling fuller longer, so it may help you shed some of those extra pregnancy pounds between babies. Aim for eating some form of protein (think meats, seafood, dairy, soy, beans, and nuts) at each meal and incorporate it into snacks.

Taking supplements between babies is a good idea. So continue taking your prenatal vitamin, extra vitamin D, and an omega-3 supplement that contains DHA and EPA fatty acids. Limit alcohol and caffeine so you don't have to cut it out/reduce it after you find out you're pregnant again.

# Part V
# The Part of Tens

The 5th Wave                                    By Rich Tennant

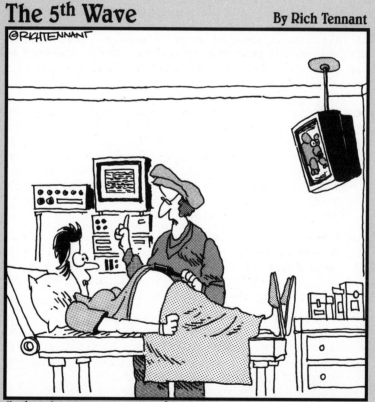

"That's a telecast of parade balloons used in the Macy's Thanksgiving Day Parade. Your ultrasound images are over here."

# In this part . . .

Who doesn't love a top ten list? This part gives you two of 'em. First, I give you a concise list of foods that I've identified to be ultra healthful and packed with pregnancy-critical nutrients. Next up is a list of ten key strategies to help you lose the pregnancy pounds when you're ready to get back to your pre-pregnancy weight.

# Chapter 22

# More Than Ten Nourishing Foods for Your Whole Pregnancy

*In This Chapter*

▶ Discovering foods that provide essential nutrients for you and your baby

▶ Branching out to try some potentially new-to-you nutritious foods

The best way to meet the extra nutrient demands of you and your baby is to incorporate nutrient-dense foods into your daily meal plan (which includes both meals and snacks). In this chapter, I list eleven such nutrient-dense pregnancy superfoods that are not only nutritious but also delicious. (What can I say? I couldn't resist throwing a bonus food into the mix.)

## Asparagus

Asparagus is the leading vegetable source of folate. It's also high in several other B vitamins, iron, vitamin K, vitamin A, and fiber. Coming in at about 40 calories per cup cooked, asparagus is one of the best nutritional bargains a pregnant woman can get. I personally love sautéing asparagus in a dash of olive oil with some fresh garlic — yum! You may also like the Sesame Asparagus recipe in Chapter 17.

Asparagus contains a sulfur compound called *methyl mercaptan* that makes some people's urine smell funny as soon as 15 minutes after they eat asparagus. Have you ever noticed this? Some of you are nodding yes while the rest of you are thinking, "She's gone off the deep end, talking about smelly urine!" But I assure you, this compound is real! Not everyone has the gene to break it down, so only some people have smelly urine. So if you try asparagus for the first time during your pregnancy, don't panic if your urine smells funny afterward!

# Avocado

Avocados often get a bad rap for being high in fat, but the fat they contain is actually the heart-healthy monounsaturated kind that your body needs a bit of during pregnancy. These fruits also boast 20 essential vitamins and minerals, including pregnancy-necessary folate, potassium, vitamin C, vitamin K, and a bit of choline, iron, and zinc. As a nutritious bonus, a whole avocado also contains 13 grams of fiber. How can that creamy and delicious fruit pack in all those nutrients? Only nature knows.

One ounce (or three slices) of avocado is just 45 calories, so you can enjoy this pregnancy superfood without having to worry about going overboard on your calorie intake. The next time you entertain, try the Avocado Shrimp Martinis in Chapter 13 for something a little different.

# Beef

Most people think of beef as a protein source, and although it certainly is one, beef is also a nutritional powerhouse of iron, zinc, vitamins B6 and B12, niacin, selenium, and choline — all in high doses. Before you start worrying about beef being too fattening to eat during pregnancy, realize that the government has labeled 29 different cuts of beef as *lean*. All 29 lean cuts are actually lower in fat than skinless chicken thighs.

Turn to Chapter 14 for some excellent beef recipes, like the tasty Cocoa-Rubbed Grilled Steaks — how can you not love chocolate and beef together? If you're not a steak lover, try using ground beef in tacos, spaghetti with meat sauce, or Nana's Moussaka (a unique recipe with eggplant that I include in Chapter 14).

# Berries

Berries are generally high in antioxidants and vitamin C, and they offer some potassium, manganese, and fiber. However, each kind of berry has at least one nutritional standout:

- ✔ Strawberries have 98 milligrams of vitamin C and 40 micrograms of folate.
- ✔ Raspberries and blackberries each have 8 grams of fiber per cup.
- ✔ Blueberries are highest in antioxidants and have 29 micrograms of vitamin K.

A 1-cup serving of berries costs you only 50 to 84 calories, depending on which berry you choose. Try them out in the berry good Berries and Cream French Toast in Chapter 12 for breakfast, the Fruity Poppy Seed Salad in Chapter 13 for lunch, or the Mixed Berry Frozen Yogurt in Chapter 16 for dessert.

# Edamame

If you're looking for a nutritional powerhouse, look no further than the green soybean called *edamame*. Every 1-cup serving of edamame contains 17 grams of protein plus 8 grams of fiber and loads of folate, iron, vitamin K, choline, potassium, and zinc. If you haven't tried it, now is the perfect time to branch out.

You often find edamame as an appetizer at Japanese restaurants, but you can also get it in the produce or frozen section of all major grocery stores and natural health food stores. Edamame looks like sugar snap peas, but unlike pea pods, edamame pods aren't edible. So when you eat edamame, pop the beans into your mouth and discard the shell. Some stores carry already-shelled edamame that's ready to eat out of the package or add to your favorite dish. I share several fun edamame recipes in Chapters 13 and 15.

Along with edamame, other soy foods like tofu, tempeh, soymilk, and soy nuts are good ways to get plant-based protein throughout your pregnancy. Soy is a complete protein, which means it contains all the essential amino acids (the building blocks of protein) that you and your baby need.

# Eggs

I've included eggs in this superfood list not only because they're a good source of high-quality protein but also because they're one of the best food sources of choline. Choline isn't the easiest thing to get in your diet, but it's vital for brain development. Eggs also provide selenium, riboflavin, and vitamin B12, a bit of iron and zinc, and a good deal of lutein and zeaxanthin, which help with vision. Look for the DHA-enriched eggs to get an extra dose of *docosahexaenoic acid* (DHA), the omega-3 fatty acid that's vital for brain health.

The important thing about eggs is that most of these nutrients are found in the yolk. Years ago people were dumping the yolks due to cholesterol concerns, but now researchers know that an egg every day doesn't raise cholesterol levels when it's part of an overall lowfat diet. So don't dump the yolk or order egg white omelets while you're pregnant because you'll be missing out on a lot of the beneficial nutrients eggs have to offer.

Need another reason to love eggs? They're inexpensive and versatile. Of course, they work great in breakfast; turn to Chapter 12 for some great recipes. But you can also eat hard-boiled eggs as snacks or in salads and use eggs to whip up yummy desserts.

For safety reasons, always cook your eggs until they're firm — no runny yolks!

# Greek Yogurt

Most yogurt contains "good" live-culture bacteria that help with digestion and boost the immune system. All yogurt varieties can be beneficial during pregnancy because of their calcium, vitamin B12, riboflavin, potassium, and phosphorus, but I especially like Greek yogurt because it generally has twice as much protein as regular yogurt. I also find that most Greek varieties have less sugar. Greek yogurt is strained differently than American-style yogurt, providing a rich, creamy, thick texture and a tangy taste, so don't be alarmed when you try it for the first time.

Traditional Greek yogurt is extremely high in fat, specifically artery-clogging saturated fat. Read yogurt labels carefully and look for the numerous 0% or 2% fat varieties of Greek yogurt available on the market.

I typically have one serving of lowfat or nonfat Greek yogurt every day for my midmorning snack. You find three very different (but yummy!) ways to use Greek yogurt in Chapter 17: Dill and Chive Veggie Dip, Decaf Mocha Smoothie, and Ricotta Parfait.

# Legumes

One of my former coworkers used to call me the "Bean Queen" because I told all my clients to eat more beans (also known as *legumes*)! The legumes food category includes lentils, black-eyed peas, split peas, as well as black, red, kidney, pinto, soy, garbanzo, and cannellini beans. Legumes, in general, are one of the most nutritious foods because they provide carbohydrates, fiber, and plant-based protein. But they also have folate, potassium, iron, calcium, and zinc.

If you want the numerous health benefits of beans without all the legwork, think canned. Instead of soaking them overnight (like you have to do with dried beans), all you have to do with canned beans is pop open a can of 'em, drain 'em, and rinse 'em in a colander (to get one-third of the sodium off and potentially reduce the gassy feelings you have after eating them). Then they're ready to go in any recipe. I'm such a bean fan that I sometimes eat garbanzo beans (also called *chickpeas*) right out of the can!

Throughout Part III, you find soup, salad, pasta, sandwich, and even dessert recipes that all contain beans. See whether you can find the dessert recipe in Chapter 16 that calls for beans and give it a try!

# Milk

Drinking milk is one easy way to get your recommended three servings of dairy a day. Every 8-ounce glass of milk supplies 30 percent of your daily calcium and 8 grams of protein, as well as riboflavin, vitamin B12, and vitamin D. (In fact, milk is one of the only food sources of vitamin D, and it's not even in milk naturally. It's fortified into it.) Milk comes in several varieties. I recommend sticking with lowfat (1%) or fat-free (skim) to avoid the artery-clogging saturated fat found in 2% and whole milk.

You can enjoy milk simply by drinking a glass of it with a meal or snack, but you can also use it in smoothies, on cereal, in oatmeal, or in treats like hot chocolate or pudding. In addition to drinking it plain, you may find that you enjoy chocolate milk; after all, it's a sweet and nutritious treat!

Milk contains a natural sugar called *lactose*. If you're *lactose intolerant* (in other words, if you get gassy or experience diarrhea after drinking milk), look for *lactose-free* on the labels of the milk you buy. You get the same benefits without the lactose and the unpleasant side effects.

# Quinoa

Quinoa (pronounced *keen*-oh-wa) has been around for thousands of years; in fact, the Incas considered it to be the "mother of all grains." What is it? Quinoa is a gluten-free whole grain that comes in red and white varieties. Vegetarians love it because it's high in protein and contains all the essential amino acids that are typically found in animal proteins. Quinoa is also loaded in nutrients, especially those essential pregnancy nutrients, like fiber, folate, iron, potassium, and a nice array of B vitamins.

Before you cook quinoa, be sure to rinse the seeds thoroughly to remove bitter compounds. Then you can cook it in about 15 minutes on the stovetop. Once prepared, it has a light and fluffy texture and a mild and almost nutty flavor, which makes it a great addition to both savory and sweet dishes.

The crunchy texture promotes its use in cold salads or as a nice alternative to rice in side or main dishes. You can also make quinoa as a hot cereal, just like cream of wheat. Check out the Quinoa Nut Mix in Chapter 13 for a great quinoa snack.

# Salmon

Salmon is one of the best available food sources of DHA omega-3 fatty acids. During pregnancy and early childhood, DHA is critical for brain and nervous system development, so if you want your child to be smart, get plenty of DHA when you're pregnant. Along with DHA, salmon also contains protein, vitamins B6 and B12, niacin, and phosphorus.

If you're worried about getting too much mercury from fish, salmon is a great option for you because it's considered to be a low-mercury fish. Plus, it's easy to find in restaurants and grocery stores everywhere. Watch out for smoked salmon, though, because it can harbor dangerous bacteria. (For more information on foods to steer clear of throughout your pregnancy, see Chapter 4.)

Skip on over to Chapter 14 for a delicious salmon recipe with a nice mango and avocado salsa. Or try poached salmon served cold on top of a green salad. If you make a lot of quick meals, consider making canned salmon a staple in your pantry.

# Chapter 23

# Ten Tricks for Getting Back to Your Pre-Pregnancy Weight

## In This Chapter

▶ Eating smaller portions and paying attention to what (and how much) you're eating

▶ Exercising to burn calories and build muscle mass

▶ Getting the sleep you need and taking time for yourself

Admittedly, losing weight is never easy, especially when you're still physically recovering from childbirth and mentally and emotionally adjusting to life with a new baby. But you don't have to be one of those women who never loses her lingering pregnancy pounds.

This chapter arms you with ten tricks for getting rid of the extra pregnancy weight. If you implement these tricks, you can return to your pre-pregnancy weight and have the energy you need to care for your new bundle of joy.

Don't expect the weight to come off overnight or even in a few weeks. Some people say it takes nine months to grow a baby and nine months to get your body back after pregnancy. Although it may seem like forever now, nine months isn't a bad goal to shoot for. After all, the slower the weight comes off, the more likely it is to stay off because you're not following fads or gimmicks or starving yourself and putting yourself at risk of malnutrition. Have patience with yourself and be persistent in your efforts to lose that excess pregnancy weight.

## Listen When Your Belly Says It's Full

Your belly always tells you when it's had enough. So instead of cleaning your plate every time you sit down to a meal, listen to what your belly is saying. I assure you there's a distinct difference between feeling satisfied and feeling stuffed. When you push the plate away at satisfied, you leave room for your body to use stored fat as energy so you can get the weight loss you desire. (For help becoming more in tune with your body's hunger and fullness signals, flip to Chapter 7.)

If you do clean your plate, wait at least 15 to 20 minutes before going back for seconds. Why? Because it takes about that long for your stomach's fullness signal to reach your brain. If you wait, you may find that you're not hungry for seconds after all. Eating your meals slowly also helps with this delay so you can stop before you overeat, only to feel stuffed 15 minutes later when your brain catches up to your stomach.

## Don't Starve Yourself

Starving yourself is *not* the way to get your pre-pregnancy body back. Skipping meals only leads to deprivation and an invitation to binge when your willpower finally caves in. If you starve yourself, you risk ending up with a pan of brownies or bag of chips calling your name.

If you're formula-feeding, don't eat less than 1,500 calories a day while you're recovering from childbirth; if you're nursing, don't eat less than 1,800 calories. If you eat too few calories, your body senses that it's starving and goes into crisis mode, lowering your metabolism to conserve its fat stores. The other major disadvantage to eating too few calories is that you could become malnourished. Getting the carbohydrates, proteins, essential fats, vitamins, and minerals you need is hard to do when you're eating so few calories.

## Eat Small Portions and Eat Frequently

One easy way to control your calorie intake is to control your portion sizes. Chapter 8 offers some tips for managing portion size when dining out, but you also need to pay attention to portion size at home. Consider eating from smaller plates until you have a better idea of the appropriate single-serve portion sizes of different foods. Drinking a glass of water before and with your meals can also help you eat less.

Eating smaller portions goes hand in hand with eating frequently. The snacks you eat in between meals help curb your appetite so you don't become ravenously hungry and eat everything in sight. They also give you something to look forward to in between meals so that you can more easily push the meal plate away. After all, not stuffing yourself during mealtime is easier to do when you know you have a snack waiting for you later.

Choose snacks with fiber and protein to help keep you feeling full longer. Flip to Chapter 7 for some healthy and satisfying snack suggestions and Chapter 13 for a few tasty snack recipes. Just make sure you measure out snacks like nuts, crackers, and ice cream so you don't end up eating the entire container!

# Be Mindful of What You're Eating

Being mindful of what you're eating means avoiding distractions, slowing down, and being aware of exactly what you're eating and how much you truly need. This level of awareness can help you feel fully satisfied with smaller amounts of food, which often leads to weight loss. Food is one of the many pleasures in life, and you should enjoy it to its fullest capacity. So try to appreciate every calorie you eat.

Instead of eating while standing at the kitchen counter or sitting in front of the TV, use the Plate-Chair-Table rule. Put your food on a plate (doing so helps ensure that you eat a reasonable portion) and always sit down in a chair at a table so that you can fully appreciate your food.

Are you a nighttime snacker? For many people, the most dangerous time of day for mindless eating is after dinner. Having a snack in the evening can actually be a good idea, but keep the snack at about 150 calories and account for your nighttime snack calories in your daily calorie budget. If you find yourself munching mindlessly or going from one food to the next in the evenings, brush your teeth! If you're anything like me, you'll stop eating just so you don't have to brush your teeth a second time in one night. Plus, most foods don't taste as good when your mouth is full of mint!

# Get Moving

You've heard it before: To lose weight, the number of calories going into your body must be less than the number of calories going out. Obviously, cutting back on what you eat can help reduce the calories you take in, but being more active can help you expend more calories.

Being active doesn't have to mean "exercising," especially during the first few weeks after you give birth. You can be more active simply by parking farther away from the store, taking the stairs rather than the elevator, or walking your baby around the room rather than sitting in the rocking chair.

Talk to your doctor about when it's safe for you to start adding exercise (beyond a little extra movement in your daily activities) back into your routine. Find tips for how to start exercising again in Chapter 21.

After your doctor clears you to exercise again postpartum, you can start working more traditional exercise — like walking, running, and cycling — back into your daily routine. Any amount of exercise is better than none, so start out by getting 10 minutes of exercise each day and work up to 30 minutes most days of the week. No matter what you do for exercise, it's a great way to relieve stress, give you a break away from your baby, and, of course, burn calories.

A good time to exercise is while your baby is sleeping, but you can also have someone else watch the little guy while you take a quick exercise break. If you go this route, try to exercise outside or away from home so that you're not tempted to give up midway through your workout if your baby starts fussing.

# Increase Your Muscle Mass

The more muscle you have in your body, the more calories you burn when you're doing any activity, whether it's exercising or sleeping. Muscle is constantly active, burning a few calories even at rest.

You build muscle by engaging in strength training (weight lifting). This type of exercise not only burns calories while you're doing it but also continues burning them for a period of time afterward. Your body has to build and repair the muscles you just used, and that process requires that you burn more calories.

While you were pregnant, you probably gained a little bit of muscle. After all, the more weight you have on your body, the more muscle you need to carry it. So if you gained 30 pounds during your pregnancy, your legs had to carry those extra 30 pounds everywhere — when you climbed the stairs, when you got up from sitting, when you walked down the block . . . you get the idea. Now that you weigh less, you need to do resistance exercise if you want to keep that extra muscle.

You can do strength training with weight machines, dumbbells, resistance bands, or even your own body weight. Anything that challenges your muscles helps strengthen them and ultimately leads to burning more calories.

# Breast-feed to Burn More Calories

Depending on how much milk you produce, you can actually burn more calories while breast-feeding than you did while growing your baby in your womb. Breast-feeding (or nursing) is really the best-kept secret for losing weight postpartum. Of course, because you still need to balance the calories you're eating with the calories you're burning, I can't guarantee you'll lose weight simply by nursing. However, even without all the benefits breast milk offers your baby (many of which I outline in Chapter 20), nursing is worth the hard work simply to mobilize some of the extra fat your body stored during pregnancy.

Breast milk is naturally high in fat because your baby needs those essential fats during her first few years of life, especially for brain development. How does your milk get so high in fat? You guessed it — by breaking down excess fat from your body! Pregnancy hormones signal your body to store fat while pregnant, but your body gladly mobilizes that fat into breast milk after you deliver. Isn't nature wonderful?

# Get Enough Sleep

A good seven or eight hours of sleep can do wonders for your body weight. Don't buy it? Studies of sleep-deprived individuals have shown that these people are heavier than those who get the recommended seven or eight hours of sleep a night.

Two specific hormones are to blame for the excess weight in sleep-deprived folks: leptin and ghrelin. *Leptin* is produced in your fat cells, and it's responsible for telling your brain when you're full when eating a meal. *Ghrelin* is produced in your gastrointestinal tract, and its job is to tell your brain when you're hungry. When you're sleep deprived, your body decreases production of leptin and increases production of ghrelin. The result is one tired mommy who's hungry and can't get satisfied and keeps on eating — not exactly the best scenario for weight loss.

Perhaps you're laughing at the mere thought of getting a decent night's sleep considering such a thing is quite difficult to achieve when you have a new baby, especially if you're nursing. If you have trouble getting enough sleep, create rituals at bedtime (like taking a relaxing bath, meditating, or reading quietly) so that you fall asleep easily when you do go to bed. Talk to your partner about your need for sleep, and ask him or her to help you discipline yourself to get to bed at a decent hour in the evening. (***Note:*** If you're a napper, steal a refreshing 20-minute nap each day, but don't nap any longer than that or else you risk disrupting your nighttime sleep, which is more important.)

# Make Time for Yourself

Taking time for yourself can help lead to weight loss for two key reasons:

- ✔ The time you take for yourself can relieve stress, which can help cut back on emotional eating by decreasing the release of stress hormones that promote overeating.
- ✔ You can use the time you carve out for yourself to get uninterrupted exercise time by going to the gym or taking a nice long walk.

Focusing on yourself may be difficult when you have a new little bundle of love to focus all your attention on. However, you can't be the best mom you can be if you don't take care of yourself. Even carving out 15 minutes (or more) of uninterrupted time each day to soak in the tub, read a magazine, surf the Internet, or go for a walk can refresh you and renew your energy.

# Remember Why You're Trying to Lose Weight — For Baby

Now that you have a beautiful child to love, keeping yourself at a healthy weight is even more important than it was before if you want to be around for all the significant and special times that lie ahead in your child's life.

If you ate healthier while you were pregnant because you wanted to fuel your baby with the right nutrients to grow and develop in your womb, then guess what? Those same healthy foods that were good for your baby are just what you need to stay energized and healthy. Keep eating all those fruits, vegetables, whole grains, lean proteins, lowfat dairy products, and healthy fats that became your staples during pregnancy. (I tell you all about these delicious but nutritious foods in Chapter 3.)

When you don't feel like taking the stairs or popping in that workout DVD, think of your sweet babe's face and all the moments you have to look forward to together. That's some serious motivation to get moving!

# Appendix

# Metric Conversion Guide

- - - - - - - - - - - - - - - - - - - - - - - - - - - - - - - - - - - - - - - - - - - - - -

*N**ote:* The recipes in this book weren't developed or tested using metric measurements. There may be some variation in quality when converting to metric units.

| Common Abbreviations | |
|---|---|
| *Abbreviation(s)* | *What It Stands For* |
| cm | Centimeter |
| C., c. | Cup |
| G, g | Gram |
| kg | Kilogram |
| L, l | Liter |
| lb. | Pound |
| mL, ml | Milliliter |
| oz. | Ounce |
| pt. | Pint |
| t., tsp. | Teaspoon |
| T., Tb., Tbsp. | Tablespoon |

## Volume

| U.S. Units | Canadian Metric | Australian Metric |
|---|---|---|
| ¼ teaspoon | 1 milliliter | 1 milliliter |
| ½ teaspoon | 2 milliliters | 2 milliliters |
| 1 teaspoon | 5 milliliters | 5 milliliters |
| 1 tablespoon | 15 milliliters | 20 milliliters |
| ¼ cup | 50 milliliters | 60 milliliters |
| ⅓ cup | 75 milliliters | 80 milliliters |
| ½ cup | 125 milliliters | 125 milliliters |
| ⅔ cup | 150 milliliters | 170 milliliters |
| ¾ cup | 175 milliliters | 190 milliliters |
| 1 cup | 250 milliliters | 250 milliliters |
| 1 quart | 1 liter | 1 liter |
| 1½ quarts | 1.5 liters | 1.5 liters |
| 2 quarts | 2 liters | 2 liters |
| 2½ quarts | 2.5 liters | 2.5 liters |
| 3 quarts | 3 liters | 3 liters |
| 4 quarts (1 gallon) | 4 liters | 4 liters |

## Weight

| U.S. Units | Canadian Metric | Australian Metric |
|---|---|---|
| 1 ounce | 30 grams | 30 grams |
| 2 ounces | 55 grams | 60 grams |
| 3 ounces | 85 grams | 90 grams |
| 4 ounces (¼ pound) | 115 grams | 125 grams |
| 8 ounces (½ pound) | 225 grams | 225 grams |
| 16 ounces (1 pound) | 455 grams | 500 grams (½ kilogram) |

## Length

| Inches | Centimeters |
|--------|-------------|
| 0.5 | 1.5 |
| 1 | 2.5 |
| 2 | 5.0 |
| 3 | 7.5 |
| 4 | 10.0 |
| 5 | 12.5 |
| 6 | 15.0 |
| 7 | 17.5 |
| 8 | 20.5 |
| 9 | 23.0 |
| 10 | 25.5 |
| 11 | 28.0 |
| 12 | 30.5 |

## Temperature (Degrees)

| Fahrenheit | Celsius |
|------------|---------|
| 32 | 0 |
| 212 | 100 |
| 250 | 120 |
| 275 | 140 |
| 300 | 150 |
| 325 | 160 |
| 350 | 180 |
| 375 | 190 |
| 400 | 200 |
| 425 | 220 |
| 450 | 230 |
| 475 | 240 |
| 500 | 260 |

# Index

## • Numerics •

7-Up, caffeine in, 25
10-minute cooking. *See* quick recipes
2,000-calorie meal plan, 151–153
2,300-calorie meal plan, 153–154
2,450-calorie meal plan, 155–156

## • A •

Ace-k (acesulfame K) sweetener, 122
acupressure, treating nausea with, 77
ADI (acceptable daily intake), 122–125
aerobic exercise, 70–71, 326
agave nectar, avoiding, 50, 123
alcohol
  adding after delivery, 305
  avoiding, 20, 50, 60–61
  controversy, 24
  coping strategies, 61–62
  impact on fertility, 24
allergies. *See* food allergies
almonds, protein in, 36
anaphylactic shock, 300
anemia, 15, 293
animal protein, impact on ovulation, 23
anthocyanins, 265
antioxidants
  in eggs, 166
  in fruits, 265
  in grains, 160
  in red beans, 233
  sources of, 176, 254
appetizer recipes. *See also* snack recipes
  Asian-Style Chicken Wings, 187
  Avocado Shrimp Martinis, 183
  Chicken Lettuce Wraps, 189
  Dill and Chive Veggie Dip, 274
  Fig and Olive Bruschetta, 184
  Minty Watermelon Salsa, 181
  Sausage-Stuffed Baked Potato Skins, 188
  Steamed Artichoke with Garlic-Herb Dipping Sauce, 185
  Sun-Dried Tomato and Ricotta Stuffed Mushrooms, 186
  White Chicken and Pineapple Flatbread, 190

appetizers, dealing with, 108–109
Apple Cinnamon Crêpes, 269
Apple Cinnamon Trail Mix, 177
apples
  fiber in, 45
  pesticide residue, 120
Apricot Oatmeal Bake, 163
Artichoke Salad, Three-Bean, 277
Artichoke with Garlic-Herb Dipping Sauce, 185
Asian Chicken Spinach salad, 198
Asian-Style Chicken Wings, 187
asparagus
  benefits, 331
  pesticide residue, 120
  sesame, 281
aspartame, 123
avocado
  benefits, 332
  pesticide residue, 120
Avocado Shrimp Martinis, 183

## • B •

B vitamins, folic acid, 18
babies
  breast-feeding, 314–315
  creating taste preferences in, 302
  evaluating amount of nutrition in breast milk versus formula, 314–316
  introducing flavors to, 313
  preventing food allergies in, 300–302
baby weight, gaining, 11. *See also* losing pregnancy weight; weight
baby's growth (illustration), 32
back tension, relieving, 73
bacon, substitution for, 144
bacteria
  *Campylobacter*, 54
  *Clostridium botulinum*, 125
  *E. coli*, 50, 54
  foods with, 50–52
  growth of, 142
  *Listeria*, 50–52, 55
  *Salmonella*, 50, 52, 55–56
Baked Ziti with Tofu, 240

baking foods, 146
Banana Chocolate Chip Muffins, 161
Banana Mini Trifle, 257
bananas
 fiber in, 45
 grilled, 284
bean dishes
 Beef and Bean Quesadillas, 205
 Black Bean Chili, 232
 Broccoli, Beans, and Feta Pasta, 250
 Giant Beans with Spinach and Feta, 237
 Quinoa Tabbouleh with Garbanzo
  Beans, 235
 Ratatouille with Cannellini Beans, 234
beans. *See also specific recipes*
 benefits of, 233
 fiber in, 45
 snacking on, 99
bed rest, controlling weight gain, 296
beef. *See also specific recipes*
 avoiding undercooked, 10, 50
 benefits, 202, 332
 cooking temperature, 141
 safety guidelines, 202
 storing, 136–137
beef recipes
 Beef and Bean Quesadillas, 205
 Beef Empanadas, 204
 Cocoa-Rubbed Grilled Steaks, 209
 Good to the Last Lick Casserole, 203
 Indian Lentil Slow Cooker Beef Stew, 207
 Italian Stuffed Steak Rolls, 208
 Nana's Moussaka, 206
Beet and Pistachio Salad, 196
bell peppers, pesticide residue, 120
berries, benefits, 332–333
Berries and Cream French Toast, 164
Berry Frozen Yogurt, 255
Bikram yoga, avoiding, 72
Black Bean Chili, 228, 232
black beans, protein in, 36
blackberries
 benefits of, 332
 fiber in, 45
blood, water content in, 46
blood pressure, controlling with calcium, 40.
  *See also* high blood pressure
blood sugar, 19. *See also* diabetes;
  gestational diabetes

blueberries
 benefits, 332
 pesticide residue, 120
BMI (body mass index), 26–27
bologna, being cautious of, 51
bones, protecting, 42
bottles, feeding babies with, 316
botulism (illness), 50
BPA (biphenol A), 58
brain development
 choline and, 40
 fat and, 37
 iodine and, 43
braising foods, 146
bread
 fiber in, 45
 storing in freezer, 137
 substitution for, 145
breadcrumbs, substitution for, 144
breakfast
 grains, 160
 importance of, 159
 preparing in 5 minutes or less, 174
breakfast recipes
 Apricot Oatmeal Bake, 163
 Banana Chocolate Chip Muffins, 161
 Berries and Cream French Toast, 164
 Broccoli Hash-Brown Quiche, 171
 Cottage Cheese Pancakes, 165
 Greek Omelet, 170
 Maple Berry Crunch Granola, 162
 Sausage Asparagus Frittata, 169
 smoothies, 171–174
 Southwest Avocado Breakfast Burrito, 167
 Spinach, Egg, and Cheese Sandwich, 168
breast-feeding. *See* nursing
breasts, feeling pain in, 314
Broccoli, Beans, and Feta Pasta, 250
broccoli, fiber in, 45
Broccoli Cheese Soup, 230
Broccoli Hash-Brown Quiche, 171
Broccoli with Mustard Sauce and
  Cashews, 243
broiling foods, 146
brownies, Fudgy Peppermint Black Bean, 260
buffets, dealing with, 109
burping, reducing, 82–83
burrito recipe for breakfast, 167

butter
  storing in refrigerator, 136
  substitution for, 144
  use in recipes, 2

• *C* •

cabbage, pesticide residue, 120
caffeine
  adding after delivery, 305
  being cautious of, 51
  in chocolate, 25
  in coffee, 25, 112
  controversy with, 24
  coping strategies, 61–62
  effects of, 61
  in energy drinks, 25
  impact on fertility, 24
  limiting intake of, 20, 61
  in soda, 25
  in tea, 25
cake recipes, Chocolate Butterscotch Chip
    Bundt Cake, 264
calcium
  blood pressure control, 40
  in eggs, 166
  in grains, 160
  in prenatal vitamins, 40
  sources of, 40, 176, 254
  in vegetarian lifestyle, 48
caloric intake
  daily, 35, 37
  first trimester, 30
  for 40 weeks of pregnancy, 33
  second trimester, 31–32
  third trimester, 33–34
calorie deficit, creating after delivery,
    321–322
calories. *See also* meal plans
  balancing, 10
  carbohydrates, 35–36
  consuming, 13
  fat, 37
  protein, 36–37
  sources of, 34–37
calorie-tracking websites, 321
*Campylobacter* bacteria, 54
cancer survivors, nutritional concerns, 295

cantaloupe, pesticide residue, 120
carbohydrates
  impact on ovulation, 23
  simple versus complex, 36
  as source of energy, 35–36
  sources of, 36
casseroles, cooking temperature for, 141
celery, pesticide residue, 120
cell building and repair
  antioxidants, 265
  fatty acids, 41
  protein, 36–37
  vitamin A, 43
  zinc, 43
Celsius, Fahrenheit equivalent, 345
centimeters, equivalent in inches, 345
cereal
  fiber in, 45
  snacking on, 99–100
cesarean (C-section) delivery
  exercising after, 16
  increased risk of, 21, 42
  recovery period, 325
Champagne mocktail, 182
cheese, 2
  avoiding soft, 51
  reducing amounts of, 145
  snacking on, 99
  storing, 136–137
  unpasteurized, 11
chemicals, limiting exposure to, 59
cherries, pesticide residue, 120
chicken
  avoiding in salads, 50
  avoiding undercooked, 10
  cooking, 141, 216
  storing in refrigerator, 137
chicken recipes
  Asian Chicken Spinach Salad, 198
  Asian-Style Chicken Wings, 187
  Chicken Hummus Pita, 278
  Chicken Kabobs, 224
  Chicken Lettuce Wraps, 189
  Crispy Lime Chicken Tenders, 223
  Curry Chicken Salad, 222
  Mixed Greens with Chicken, Cantaloupe,
    & Red Grapes Salad, 192
  Peachy Chicken Barley Pilaf, 225

chicken recipes *(continued)*
  Rosemary Chicken on Asparagus
    Risotto, 221
  Spinach, Date, and Blue Cheese Chicken
    Panini, 226
  White Chicken and Pineapple Flatbread, 190
Chili, Black Bean, 228
chips (whole grain), snacking on, 101
chocolate
  caffeine in, 25
  dark, 259
  nutrients in, 259
  snacking on, 99
chocolate recipes. *See also* White Chocolate
    Berry Oatmeal Cookies
  Chocolate Banana Blast Smoothie, 173
  Chocolate Butterscotch Chip Bundt Cake, 264
  Chocolate Lover's Sippable Sundae, 262
  Dark Chocolate Cherry Pistachio Bark, 261
  Fudgy Peppermint Black Bean
    Brownies, 260
  Peanut Butter Chocolate Chip Pie, 263
cholesterol
  good versus bad, 37
  managing, 22
choline, sources of, 40
cider, avoiding unpasteurized, 51
clams, avoiding raw, 50
"Clean 15" foods, 119–120
cleaning supplies, choosing, 59
*Clostridium botulinum* bacteria, 125
Cocoa-Rubbed Grilled Steaks, 209
coffee. *See* caffeine
Coke, caffeine in, 25
cold cuts, being cautious of, 51
collard greens, pesticide residue, 120
colostrum, defined, 314
conception troubles. *See* fertility
constipation, overcoming, 11–12
convenience foods, 272–273
cookies, White Chocolate Berry Oatmeal, 270
cooking
  healthy methods, 143–147
  process, increasing comfort of, 147–148
  techniques, 145–147
  temperatures, 140–142
corn, sweet, 120
cottage cheese, snacking on, 99
Cottage Cheese Pancakes, 165
countertops, keeping clean, 139

crackers, snacking on, 101
Cranberry Gelatin Salad, 200
Cranberry Twist mocktail, 182
cravings
  controlling, 13
  managing, 103–104
  *pica* condition, 103
  reasons, 102
cream, substitution for, 144
cream cheese, storing in refrigerator, 136
cream soups, substitution for, 144
Creamy Grape Salad, 199
Crispy Lime Chicken Tenders, 223
crêpes, Apple Cinnamon, 269
Crunchy Garbanzo Beans, 179
C-section delivery (cesarean)
  exercising after, 16, 21
  increased risk of, 42
  recovery period, 325
cupcakes, Lemon Raspberry, 268
Curry Chicken Salad, 222
cutting board, keeping clean, 139

• *D* •

dairy products
  impact on ovulation, 23–24
  shopping for, 133
  substitution for, 144
Dark Chocolate Cherry Pistachio Bark, 261
Decaf Mocha Smoothie, 274
Deconstructed Greek Salad, 197
defrosting food, 142
dehydration from vomiting, 78–79
deli meats
  being cautious of, 51, 129
  storing in refrigerator, 136
dentist, prenatal visit to, 19
dessert recipes. *See also* chocolate recipes
  Apple Cinnamon Crêpes, 269
  Banana Mini Trifle, 257
  Fruit Cookie Pizza, 266
  Grilled Bananas, 284
  Kiwi Custard Pie, 256
  Lemon Raspberry Cupcakes, 268
  Mango Coconut Rice Pudding, 258
  Mixed Berry Frozen Yogurt, 255
  Pineapple Spice Loaf with Cream Cheese
    Frosting, 267

Ricotta Parfait, 283
Sautéed Summer Fruit over Ice Cream, 282
White Chocolate Berry Oatmeal
    Cookies, 270
desserts, eating out, 113–114
DHA (docosahexaenoic acid), 41–42, 125
    source of, 336
    in vegetarian lifestyle, 48
diabetes. *See also;* gestational diabetes
    blood sugar, 19
    managing, 21
    predisposition to, 43
diet, impact on fertility, 22–25
diet and exercise. *See also* exercise
    anemia, 293
    gestational diabetes, 288–290
    high blood pressure, 291–293
    PCOS (polycystic ovary syndrome), 290–291
    preeclampsia, 291–293
dietician, visiting, 22
digestive tract, 80–85
Dill and Chive Veggie Dip, 275
dining out
    appetizers, 108–109
    beverages, 112–113
    buffets, 109
    desserts, 113–114
    food safety, 114–116
    healthy choices, 107
    high-fat foods, 106–107
    high-sodium foods, 106
    oversized portions, 109–111
    placing orders, 107–108
    reading menus, 105–106
    travel tips, 111
"Dirty Dozen" foods, 119–120

● **E** ●

*E. coli* bacteria, 50–51, 53
eating
    amounts of food, 12
    feeling full, 96
    for energy, 87–88
    hunger cues, 31, 33
    knowing when to stop, 97
    small amounts, 93
eating for two, concept of, 29–30
eating out. *See* dining out

eating plan, pursuing, 22
edamame, 233, 241, 333
Eggplant, Olive, and Goat Cheese Pizza, 251
eggplant, pesticide residue, 120
eggs, 2
    allergic reaction to, 298
    avoiding raw, 11, 50
    avoiding runny, 11
    being cautious of, 52
    benefits, 166, 333–334
    choline in, 40
    cooking, 142
    protein in, 36
    storing in refrigerator, 136
empanadas, beef, 204
energy, getting from carbohydrates, 35–36
energy drinks, caffeine in, 25
EPA (eicosapentaenoic acid), 41–42, 125
Equal sweetener, 123
espresso, caffeine in, 25
estrogen, impact on digestive tract, 80
EWG (Environmental Working Group),
    57, 119–120
exercise. *See also* diet and exercise
    aerobic, 70–71
    avoiding, 74
    benefits, 68
    core temperature, 70
    doing daily, 27
    heart rate, 69
    Kegel, 327
    lifting light weights, 71–72
    monitoring intensity, 69
    Physical Activity Guidelines for Americans, 68
    post-pregnancy, 324–327
    prenatal, 18–19
    safety guidelines, 68–69
    strength training, 71–72
    "talk test," 69
    weekly amount, 68
    yoga, 72–73

● **F** ●

Fahrenheit, Celsius equivalent, 345
farting, reducing, 82–83
FAS (fetal alcohol syndrome), 60
Fat Cal per serving, 37
fathers, fertility nutrition for, 28

fatigue
  eating for energy, 87–88
  overcoming, 11–12, 86–87
fats, 36–37. *See also* high-fat foods
  daily consumption, 37
  impact on ovulation, 23
  monounsaturated, 37
  nervous system development, 37
  polyunsaturated, 37
  saturated, 37
  tracking grams of, 37
  trans, 37
  types of, 37
FDA (Food and Drug Administration), 122
fertility. *See also* ovulation
  impact of diet on, 22–25
  maintaining BMI for, 26
  nutrition for fathers, 28
fiber
  adding to daily diet, 45–46
  benefit of, 44
  daily requirement, 44
  in eggs, 166
  on food labels, 45
  in fruit, 254
  getting after delivery, 304
  in grains, 160
  sources of, 44–45, 176
Fig and Olive Bruschetta, 184
first trimester (weeks 1-13)
  caloric intake, 30
  meal plans for, 151–153
fish. *See also* seafood dishes
  allergic reaction to, 298–299
  avoiding mercury in, 18
  avoiding undercooked, 10
  being cautious of, 125–126
  benefit of, 125
  cooking, 141–142
  food safety, 210
  high-mercury, 50
  recommendations, 126–127
  smoked, being cautious of, 52
  sources of omega-3s, 41
  storing in freezer, 137
flatulence, reducing, 82–83
flavors, introducing babies to, 313
flaxseed, fiber in, 45
flour, 2, 145

fluids. *See also* hydration; water
  daily requirement, 46
  sources of, 46–47
folate, 39
  depletion of, 328
  in eggs, 166
  in fruit, 254
  in grains, 160
  impact on ovulation, 24
  source of, 176, 331
folic acid, 10, 18. *See also* folate
  impact on ovulation, 24
  prenatal amounts of, 20
  sources of, 39
food
  defrosting, 142
  measuring, 343–345
  refrigerating, 143
food allergens, introducing children to, 302
  eggs, 298
  fish, 298–299
  milk, 298
  peanuts, 298
  shellfish, 299
  soy, 299
  tree nuts, 298
  wheat, 299
food allergies, 15
  getting tested for, 300
  versus intolerances, 300
  preventing in babies, 300–302
  risk factors, 300
  role of breast-feeding in, 301–302
  supplements for, 301
  suspecting, 299
  symptoms, 298
Food and Drug Administration (FDA), 122
food labels, reading, 37, 45, 130–132
food safety, 14, 51–52, 130
foodborne illnesses, 53–56
foods
  to avoid, 10–11, 50–51
  to be cautious of, 51–52
  grab-and-go, 128–129
formula, feeding babies with, 313–316
freezer, storing food in, 137, 142
French toast recipe for breakfast, 164
Fresh Mozzarella, Tomato, and Pepper
    Salad, 195

frittata recipe for breakfast, 169
frozen meals, choosing, 127–128
Frozen Strawberry Lemonade mocktail, 182
Frozen Yogurt, Berry, 255
fruit, snacking on, 99
Fruit Cookie Pizza, 266
fruit desserts. *See* dessert recipes
fruits
  benefits, 254
  blue and purple, 265
  freezing and canning, 242
  green, 265
  orange and yellow, 265
  precut, 272
  red, 265
  rinsing, 140
  shopping for, 133
  storing in freezer, 137
Fruity Poppy Seed Salad, 193
Fudgy Peppermint Black Bean Brownies, 260

## • *G* •

garbanzo bean recipes, 179, 235
Garden Fresh Paella, 215
gas, reducing, 11–12, 82–83
GERD (gastroesophageal reflux disease), 80
germs, guarding against, 140
gestational diabetes. *See also* diabetes
  blood sugar, 19
  complications, 289–290
  diagnosis, 15, 288
  explained, 21, 288
  glucose tolerance test, 288
  risks of, 42, 288
  treating, 290
Giant Beans with Spinach and Feta, 237
ginger, treating nausea with, 77
glucose
  processing, 19
  tolerance test, 288
Good to the Last Lick Casserole, 203
go-to pregnancy snack list, 99–101
Gnocchi with Pesto, 249
grains
  benefits of, 160, 176
  protein in, 36
  shopping for, 133

granola recipe for breakfast, 162
Grape Fizz mocktail, 182
Grape Salad, Creamy, 199
grapefruit, pesticide residue, 120
Grapefruit Salad, Honey Orange, 276
grapes
  eating frozen, 323
  pesticide residue, 120
Greek Omelet, 170
Greek salad, 197
Greek Spinach Pie (Spanakopita ), 245
Greek yogurt, 36, 100, 334
greens, kale and collard, 120
Grilled Bananas, 284
grilling foods, 146
grocery lists, using, 133–134
grocery shopping, 13–14
  cutting costs, 129
  following meal plans, 130
  reading food labels, 130
  using lists, 130
ground beef
  cooking temperature, 141
  storing, 136–137
  substitution for, 144
gums, bleeding, 19

## • *H* •

ham
  avoiding in salads, 50
  being cautious of, 51
  cooking temperature, 141
  storing in freezer, 137
hands, washing, 140
Havarti Pear Grilled Cheese on
    Pumpernickel, 280
HDL cholesterol, 37
health conditions
  diabetes, 21
  high blood pressure, 21
  high cholesterol, 22
  hypertension, 21
  PCOS (polycystic ovary syndrome), 21
healthy choices, making, 13–14, 107
healthy cooking, 143–147
heart disease, predisposition to, 43

heartburn
  avoiding, 80–82
  causes of, 80
  overcoming, 11–12
heart-healthy compounds, source of, 265
hemorrhoids, dealing with, 11–12, 84–85
herbal products, being cautious of, 52
herbs, 2, 279
HFCS (high-fructose corn syrup), 123
high blood pressure
  controlling 21, 40, 292–293
  diet adjustments for, 15, 292–293
  risks of, 291
high-fat foods, spotting on menus, 106–107.
    *See also* fats
high-sodium foods, spotting on menus, 106.
    *See also* salt
honey, 2, 50, 124
Honey Orange Grapefruit Salad, 276
honeydew melon, pesticide residue, 120
hormone production, 43
hormones
  ghrelin, 341
  impact on digestive tract, 80
  leptin, 341
hot dogs, being cautious of, 51
hummus
  Chicken Hummus Pita, 278
  fiber in, 45
  prepared, 273
hunger, physical versus psychological, 103
hunger cues, 31, 33. *See also* eating
hunger gauge, using, 94–96
hydration. *See also* fluids; water
  importance of, 46–47
  while nursing, 310–311
hyperemesis gravidarum, 78–79
hypertension, managing. *See* high blood
    pressure

• *I* •

ice cream
  avoiding homemade, 52
  choosing, 254
  Sautéed Summer Fruit recipe, 282
immune system, protecting, 42–43, 265
inches, equivalent in centimeters, 345
Indian Lentil Slow Cooker Beef Stew, 207

ingredients, substituting, 144–145
insulin, using, 19
iodine, 43
iron
  absorption, 39
  deficiency, 39–40
  depletion of, 328
  in eggs, 166
  getting after delivery, 304
  in grains, 160
  impact on ovulation, 24
  increased need for, 39–40
  nausea caused by, 38
  sources of, 39, 176
  in vegetarian lifestyle, 48
Italian Stuffed Steak Rolls, 208

• *J* •

juice
  avoiding unpasteurized, 51
  use in recipes, 2

• *K* •

kale, pesticide residue, 120
Kegel exercises, doing, 327
ketchup
  storing in refrigerator, 136
  using, 247
kitchen, keeping clean, 139–140
kiwi, pesticide residue, 120
Kiwi Custard Pie, 256

• *L* •

labor, inducing, 148
lacto-ovo vegetarian, 48
Lasagna, Vegetable, 250
laxatives, avoiding, 84
LDL cholesterol, 37
leftovers
  convenience of, 150
  cooking temperature, 141
  keeping safe, 115–116
  reheating, 142
legumes, benefits, 23, 233, 334–335
lemon juice, use in recipes, 2

Lemon Raspberry Cupcakes, 268
lemon scents, treating nausea with, 77
lemon water, 112
lentils
    fiber in, 45
    Indian Lentil Slow Cooker Beef Stew, 207
    Sloppy Lentil Joes, 236
lime juice, use in recipes, 2
*Listeria* bacteria, 50–51, 55
liver, being cautious of, 52
losing pregnancy weight. *See also* weight
    avoiding starvation, 338
    for babies, 342
    being active, 339–340
    belly, 318
    breast-feeding, 341
    calorie deficit, 321–322
    diet and exercise, 319–320
    drinking water to aid digestion, 320
    fat, 320
    fiber, 320
    frequency of eating, 338
    getting full, 337–338
    getting sleep, 341–342
    increasing muscle mass, 340
    meal plans for, 322–323
    mindfulness of eating, 339
    nutrient-dense foods, 320
    portion sizes, 338
    process of, 317
    protein, 320
    rate of, 319
    setting expectations, 318
    snacking, 339
    strength training, 340
    taking time for self, 342
    uterus shrinking, 318
lycopene, 247

## • M •

Mango Avocado Salmon, 212
Mango Coconut Rice Pudding, 258
mangos, pesticide residue, 120
Maple Berry Crunch Granola, 162
margarine
    storing in refrigerator, 136
    substitution for, 2, 144
mayonnaise, storing in refrigerator, 136

meal plans. *See also* calories
    2,000 calories, 151–153
    2,300 calories, 153–154
    2,450 calories, 155–156
meals
    planning, 150–151
    size of, 12
measurements, metric, 343–345
meat spreads, being cautious of, 52
meat temperatures, 141
meat thermometer, using, 10, 141–142
meatless dishes. *See* vegetarian lifestyle;
        *specific recipes*
meats
    avoiding in salads, 50
    avoiding undercooked, 50
    being cautious of, 51
    precooked, 273
    preportioned, 273
    presliced, 273
    white, 216
medications, reviewing, 21
melon, honeydew, 120
memory, improving, 265
menus, reading, 105–106
mercury, avoiding in fish, 18, 50, 57–58,
        125–126
metabolism, defined, 323
metric conversion table, 343–345
microwave, using, 273
milk
    allergic reaction to, 15, 298
    avoiding unpasteurized, 51
    benefits of, 335
    protein in, 36
    storing in refrigerator, 137
    unpasteurized, 11
    use in recipes, 2
milkshakes, 113
Minty Watermelon Salsa, 181
miscarriage, myth busters, 57
Mixed Berry Frozen Yogurt, 255
Mixed Greens with Chicken, Cantaloupe &
        Red Grapes salad, 192
mocktails
    Champagne, 182
    Cranberry Twist, 182
    Frozen Strawberry Lemonade, 182
    Grape Fizz, 182

mocktails *(continued)*
  Orange Pineapple Slush, 182
  Shirley Temple, 182
  Virgin Daiquiri, 182
monounsaturated fats, 37
morning sickness. *See* nausea
moussaka (recipe), 206
Mozzarella, Tomato, and Pepper Salad, 195
muffin recipe for breakfast, 161
multiples
  carrying, 295–296
  nursing, 307
multivitamins. *See also specific vitamins*
  prenatal, 10
  taking before and during pregnancy, 10, 38
  taking after delivery, 304
mushroom recipe, 186
MyPlate guidelines, 34–35, 150

### • N •

Nana's Moussake, 206
nausea
  causes of, 75–76, 78
  dealing with, 76–78
  iron as cause of, 38
  medical intervention, 78–79
  overcoming, 11–12
  severe, 78–79
nectarines, pesticide residue, 120
nervous system, 37
neural tube, formation of, 18, 40
nursing
  alcohol, 312–313
  benefits for babies, 307
  benefits for Mom, 305–306
  caffeine, 312–313
  caloric intake, 321
  committment, 308
  duration of, 306
  exercising, 325
  hydration, 310–311
  losing weight while, 16, 308
  meal plans, 311–312
  multiples, 307
  nutritional concerns, 16, 308–309
  overcoming obstacles, 307–308
  positions, 314–315
  in public, 308
  pumping, 308

role in allergy prevention, 301–302
  spicy foods, 313
  time per feeding, 314
nursing nutrients
  carbohydrates, 309
  choline, 310
  chromium, 310
  DHA and EPA, 310
  fats, 309
  potassium, 310
  proteins, 309
  vitamin A, 310
  vitamin C, 310
  vitamin D, 310
nut butters, snacking on, 100
nut mixes, snacking on, 100, 178
Nutrasweet, 123
nutrients
  calcium, 40
  carbohydrates, 35–36
  choline, 40
  fats, 37
  folate, 39
  folic acid, 39
  getting enough, 38
  impact on fertility, 22–24
  iodine, 43
  iron, 39–40
  omega-3 fatty acids, 41–42
  protein, 36–37
  vitamin A, 43
  vitamin D, 42–43
  zinc, 43
nutrition
  for dad-to-be, 28
  link between mother and child, 43
  prior to pregnancy, 10
nutrition bars, snacking on, 100
Nutrition Facts panel, reading, 131–132
nutrition shakes, snacking on, 100
nutritious options, picking, 13–14
nuts, 23
  prechopped, 272
  snacking on, 100

### • O •

oatmeal
  fiber in, 45
  snacking on, 100

Oatmeal Cookies, White Chocolate Berry, 270
oatmeal recipe for breakfast, 163
obesity, predisposition to, 43
OB/GYN (obstetrician/gynecologist), 19
oils
  flavored, 279
  substitution for, 144
olive oil, use in recipes, 2, 299
omega-3 fatty acids, 125
  DHA (docosahexaenoic acid), 41–42
  fish-free supplements, EPA
    (eicosapentaenoic acid), 41–42
  restoring post-pregnancy nutrition
    status, 328
  source of, 336
omelet recipe for breakfast, 170
onions, 2, 120
Orange Pineapple Slush mocktail, 182
organic foods
  animal foods, 118
  considering, 119–121
  Dirty Dozen, 119
  labels, 118–119
  pesticide residue, 120
  produce, 118
  pros and cons, 121
osteoporosis, reducing risk of, 40
ovulation. *See also* fertility
  impact of diet on, 23–24
  improving by losing weight, 26
oysters, avoiding raw, 50

● *p* ●

paella recipe, 215
pancake recipe for breakfast, 165
pantry, storing foods in, 137–138
Parmesan-Herb-Crusted Pork Chops, 218
pasta, substitution for, 145
pasta recipes
  Broccoli, Beans, and Feta, 250
  Gnocchi with Pesto, 249
  Vegetable Lasagna, 248
PCOS (polycystic ovary syndrome),
    21, 290–291
peaches, pesticide residue, 120
Peachy Chicken Barley Pilaf, 225
Peanut Butter Chocolate Chip Pie, 263
peanut butter, protein in, 36
peanuts, allergic reaction to, 298

pears, fiber in, 45
Pecan-Crusted Tilapia with Pear and Fig
    Chutney, 213
pepper (black), use in recipes, 2
peppers, coring and seeding, 172
Pepsi, caffeine in, 25
perishable foods, storing, 143
pesticide residue, 58, 119–120
phthalates, 58–59
Physical Activity Guidelines for
    Americans, 68
phytonutrients, source of, 265
*pica* condition, 103
pies
  Kiwi Custard, 256
  Peanut Butter Chocolate Chip, 263
pineapple, pesticide residue, 120
Pineapple Spice Loaf with Cream Cheese
    Frosting, 267
pizza
  Fruit Cookie Pizza, 266
  making healthier, 247
  Roasted Eggplant, Olive, and Goat
    Cheese Pizza, 251
PKU (phenylketonuria), 123
plant proteins, 23. *See also* protein foods
plastics, 58–59
poaching foods, 146
polyunsaturated fats, 37
Pomegranate Power Smoothie, 174
popcorn
  fiber in, 45
  recipe, 180
  snacking on, 100
pork
  avoiding undercooked, 10, 50
  cooking, 141, 216
  storing, 136–137
pork recipes
  Parmesan-Herb-Crusted Pork Chops, 218
  Super Easy Pulled Pork, 217
portion sizes, 110–111
post-pregnancy, 15–16
  adding alcohol, 305
  adding caffeine, 305
  exercise, 324–327
  nutrients, 304
  strength training, 326
  stretching, 326
  walking, 325

potassium
  in eggs, 166
  in fruit, 254
  in grains, 160
  sources of, 176
potatoes
  fiber in, 45
  pesticide residue, 120
  sweet, 120
poultry
  avoiding undercooked, 50
  cooking temperature, 141
  storing, 137
pounds. *See* weight
powdered sugar, use in recipes, 2
Powerhouse Hit The Deck workout cards, 326
preeclampsia, 15
  explained, 291
  increased risk of, 42
  nutrition recommendation, 292
  risk factors, 292
  symptoms, 292
pregnancies, intervals between, 327–328
pregnancy
  first trimester, 30
  restoring nutritional status after, 328
  second trimester, 31–32
  third trimester, 33–34
"pregnancy 50," avoiding, 66–67
prenatal care
  avoiding alcohol, 20
  dentist, 19
  family doctor, 19
  folic acid, 20
  limiting caffeine, 20
  OB/GYN (obstetrician/gynecologist), 19
  prescriptions, 21
  quitting smoking, 20
  weight management, 20
prenatal vitamins, calcium in, 40
prepared foods, being cautious of, 129
prescriptions, reviewing, 21
probiotics
  benefits of, 84
  in formula, 315
produce, fresh, 242

progesterone, impact on digestive tract, 80
protein
  complete, 233
  depletion of, 328
  digesting, 37
  in eggs, 166
  getting enough after delivery, 304
  in grains, 160
  sources of, 176, 254
  in vegetarian lifestyle, 48
protein foods
  almonds, 36
  black beans, 36
  eating post-pregnancy, 15
  eggs, 36
  grains, 36
  impact on ovulation, 23
  meat, 36
  milk, 36
  peanut butter, 36
  shopping for, 134
  tofu, 36
  yogurt, 36
Pulled Pork, Super Easy, 217

• *Q* •

Quesadillas, Beef and Bean, 205
quiche recipe for breakfast, 171
quick recipes, 272–273
  Chicken Hummus Pita, 278
  Decaf Mocha Smoothie, 274
  Dill and Chive Veggie Dip, 275
  enhancing flavor in, 279
  Grilled Bananas, 284
  Havarti Pear Grilled Cheese on
    Pumpernickel, 280
  Honey Orange Grapefruit Salad, 276
  Ricotta Parfait, 283
  Sautéed Summer Fruit over Ice Cream, 282
  Sesame Asparagus, 281
  Three-Bean Artichoke Salad, 277
quinoa, benefits of, 335–336
Quinoa Nut Mix, 178
Quinoa Tabbouleh with Garbanzo Beans, 235

## • R •

raspberries, benefits of, 332
Ratatouille with Cannellini Beans, 234
RD (registered dietitian), visiting, 22
recipes. *See also specific recipes*
  guidelines for, 2
  making healthier, 144–145
recovery. *See* post-pregnancy
red beans, benefits of, 233
refrigerator
  keeping clean, 140
  storing food in, 136–137
resistance training, 71–72
rice (white), substitution for, 145
Rice Pudding, Mango Coconut, 258
Ricotta Parfait, 283
RLS (restless leg syndrome), 88
RMR (resting metabolic rate), increase in, 33
Roasted Beet and Pistachio Salad, 196
Roasted Eggplant, Olive, and Goat Cheese
  Pizza, 251
roasting foods, 146
Rosemary Chicken on Asparagus Risotto, 221

## • S •

saccharin, 52, 124
salads
  snacking on, 100
  pairing with meals, 191
salad dressing
  storing in refrigerator, 137
  substitution for, 144
salad recipes
  Asian Chicken Spinach, 198
  Cranberry Gelatin, 200
  Creamy Grape, 199
  Deconstructed Greek, 197
  Fresh Mozzarella, Tomato, and Pepper, 195
  Fruity Poppy Seed, 193
  Honey Orange Grapefruit, 276
  Mixed Greens with Chicken, Cantaloupe &
    Red Grapes, 192
  Roasted Beet and Pistachio, 196

  Three-Bean Artichoke, 277
  White Bean and Portobello, 194
salmon, benefits of, 336
Salmon, Mango Avocado, 212
*Salmonella* bacteria, 50, 55–56
salsa, storing in refrigerator, 137
salt. *See also* high-sodium foods
  reducing amounts of, 145
  table, 2
sandwiches, snacking on, 100
saturated fats, 37
Sauerkraut and Turkey Sausage Pasta
    Bake, 220
Sausage Asparagus Frittata, 169
Sausage-Stuffed Baked Potato Skins, 188
Sautéed Summer Fruit over Ice Cream, 282
sautéing foods, 146
Scallops with Noodles, Thai, 214
seafood. *See* fish
seafood dishes
  Garden Fresh Paella, 215
  Mango Avocado Salmon, 212
  Pecan-Crusted Tilapia with Pear and Fig
    Chutney, 213
  Spaghetti with Clam Sauce, 211
  Thai Scallops with Noodles, 214
seasoned salt, substitution for, 145
second trimester (weeks 14-27)
  caloric intake, 31–32
  meal plans, 153–154
Sesame Asparagus, 281
Sesame Noodle Salad, 239
shellfish
  allergic reaction to, 299
  avoiding raw, 50
Shirley Temple mocktail, 182
shortening, substitution for, 144
side effects, avoiding, 11–12
Sierra Mist, caffeine in, 25
sleep, getting enough of, 88–89, 341
Sloppy Lentil Joes, 236
smoked seafood, being cautious of, 52
smoking, quitting, 20
smoothies
  boosting nutritional value, 172
  Chocolate Banana Blast, 173

smoothies *(continued)*
  Decaf Mocha, 274
  Pomegranate Power, 174
  snacking on, 100, 113
snack recipes. *See also* appetizer recipes
  Apple Cinnamon Trail Mix, 177
  Crunchy Garbanzo Beans, 179
  Quinoa Nut Mix, 178
  Truffle-Flavored Popcorn, 180
snacks
  beans, 99
  cereal, 99–100
  cheese, 99
  chips (whole grain), 101
  chocolate, 99
  cottage cheese, 99
  crackers, 101
  determining number of, 101
  eating, 27
  fruit, 99
  guidelines for smart snacking, 98
  nut butters, 100
  nut mixes, 100
  nutrition bars and shakes, 100
  nuts, 100
  oatmeal, 100
  planning, 150
  popcorn, 100
  salads, 100
  sandwich (half), 100
  scheduling, 101
  smoothies, 100
  veggies and hummus, 100
  yogurt (Greek), 100
soda, caffeine in, 25
sodium. *See* high-sodium foods; salt
soft drinks, 112
soups
  Black Bean Chili, 228
  Broccoli Cheese, 228, 230
  Souped-Up Split Pea, 228
  Tomato Bulgur, 228–229
Southwest Avocado Breakfast Burrito, 167
soy, allergic reaction to, 299
soy-based foods, 23

soybeans, benefits of, 233
Spaghetti with Clam Sauce, 211
Spanakopita (Greek Spinach Pie), 245
spinach
  fiber in, 45
  pesticide residue, 120
Spinach, Date, and Blue Cheese Chicken
    Panini, 226
Spinach, Egg, and Cheese Sandwich, 168
spinal cord, formation of, 18
Splenda, 125
Split Pea Soup, Souped-Up, 231
Sprite, caffeine in, 25
sprouts, avoiding raw, 50
starches, 36
Steak Rolls, Italian-Stuffed, 208
Steamed Artichoke with Garlic-Herb Dipping
    Sauce, 185
Steamed Broccoli with Mustard Sauce and
    Cashews, 243
steaming foods, 147
stevia, 125
strawberries
  benefits of, 332
  fiber in, 45
  pesticide residue, 120
strength training, 71–72, 326
stretching, post-pregnancy, 326
Stroller Strides class, 325
stuffing and gravy, being cautious of, 52
sucralose, 124
sugar, 2, 145
Sun-Dried Tomato and Ricotta Stuffed
    Mushrooms, 186
Sunett sweetener, 122
Super Easy Pulled Pork, 217
supplements, taking, 38
sushi, eating, 10
Sweet 'N Low, 124
sweet peas, pesticide residue, 120
Sweet Potato Hash, 246
sweet potatoes, pesticide residue, 120
sweeteners, 122–125
swelling, dealing with, 89
swimming, 70

## • T •

takeout food, reheating, 115
tapas-style meals
  Artichoke with Garlic-Herb Dipping Sauce, 185
  Asian-Style Chicken Wings, 187
  Avocado Shrimp Martinis, 183
  Chicken Lettuce Wraps, 189
  Fig and Olive Bruschetta, 184
  Sausage-Stuffed Baked Potato Skins, 188
  Sun-Dried Tomato and Ricotta Stuffed Mushrooms, 186
  White Chicken and Pineapple Flatbread, 190
tea
  caffeine in, 25
  unsweetened, 112
teenage mothers, nutritional concerns, 294
teeth, taking care of, 19
temperatures, 2
  for cooking meat, 141
  danger zone, 143
  degrees, 345
  safety of, 10
Thai Scallops with Noodles, 214
third trimester (weeks 28-40)
  caloric intake, 33–34
  meal plans, 155–156
Three-Bean Artichoke Salad, 277
Tilapia, Pecan-Crusted with Pear and Fig Chutney, 213
tofu, 233
  Baked Ziti with Tofu, 240
  protein in, 36
Tofu Vegetable Stir-Fry, 238
Tomato Bulgur Soup, 228–229
tomatoes, lycopene in, 247
Total Fat listing, 37
toxins
  mercury, 57–58
  pesticides, 58
  plastics, 58–59
*Toxoplasma* parasite, 56
trail mix recipe, 177
trans fats, 37
tree nuts, allergic reaction to, 298

trimesters
  first (weeks 1-13), 30, 151–153
  second (weeks 14-27), 31–32, 153–154
  third (weeks 28-40), 33–34, 155–156
triplets, carrying, 295–296
Truffle-Flavored Popcorn, 180
Truvia sweetener, 125
tuna
  avoiding in salads, 50
  being cautious of, 51
turkey
  being cautious of, 51
  cooking, 216
turkey recipes
  Sauerkraut and Turkey Sausage Pasta Bake, 220
  Turkey Cheeseburger Chowder, 219
twins, carrying, 295–296

## • U •

USDA (United States Department of Agriculture), 118–119
utensils, keeping clean, 139
uterus, shrinking, 16, 318
UTIs (urinary tract infections), avoiding, 85–86

## • V •

Vegetable Lasagna, 248
vegetable recipes. *See specific recipes*
vegetables
  benefits, 242
  canned, 272
  freezing and canning, 242
  frozen, 272
  precut, 272
  preparing safely, 14
  rinsing, 140
  shopping for, 133
  storing in freezer, 137
vegetarian lifestyle
  calcium, 48
  continuing, 18, 47–48
  DHA (docosahexaenoic acid), 48

vegetarian lifestyle *(continued)*
  iron, 48
  lacto-ovo, 48
  protein, 48
  vegan, 48
  vitamin B12, 48
  vitamin D, 48
  zinc, 48
Veggie Dip, Dill and Chive, 275
veggies and hummus, snacking on, 100
*Vibrio* bacteria, 50
vinegars, flavored, 279
Virgin Daiquiri mocktail, 182
vision
  developing in babies, 43
  improving, 265
vitamin A, 43, 52
vitamin B12, 48
vitamin C, 304
vitamin D, 42–43, 48
vitamins, prenatal, 38. *See also* multivitamins
vomiting, risk of, 78–79

## • *W* •

water. *See also* fluids; hydration
  percentage in blood, 46
  as source of hydration, 46–47
watermelon, pesticide residue, 120
watermelon salsa recipe, 181
websites
  American Dietetic Association, 22
  food safety, 51–52
  MyPlate guideline, 35, 150
  nutrient data for snacks, 98
  portion sizes, 110
  Powerhouse Hit The Deck workout cards,
    326
  Stroller Strides class, 325
weeks 1-13 (first trimester)
  caloric intake, 30
  meal plan, 151–153
weeks 14-27 (second trimester)
  caloric intake, 31–32
  meal plans, 153–154

weeks 28-40 (third trimester)
  caloric intake, 33–34
  meal plans, 155–156
weight. *See also* losing pregnancy weight
  avoiding "pregnancy 50," 66–67
  calorie tracking, 321
  complications from excess, 66
  gaining gradually, 11, 63–65
  impact on fertility, 26
  importance of, 26–27
  losing, 26–27, 65
  losing post-pregnancy, 16
  losing to improve ovulation, 26
  normal, 64
  obese, 64
  overweight, 64
  prenatal management, 20
  pre-pregnancy, 30, 64
  preventing excess gain, 11, 65–67
  range, 64, 319
  underweight, 64
weights, lifting, 71–72
wheat, allergic reaction to, 15, 299
Wheat Berry Edamame with Dried Fruit, 241
wheat germ, fiber in, 45
White Bean and Portobello salad, 194
White Chicken and Pineapple Flatbread, 190
White Chocolate Berry Oatmeal Cookies, 270.
    *See also* chocolate recipes

## • *y* •

yoga, 72–73
yogurt (Greek), 36, 100, 334

## • *Z* •

zinc, 43, 48
Ziti with Tofu, Baked, 240
Zucchini Patties, 244

## Apple & Macs

iPad For Dummies
978-0-470-58027-1

iPhone For Dummies,
4th Edition
978-0-470-87870-5

MacBook For Dummies, 3rd
Edition
978-0-470-76918-8

Mac OS X Snow Leopard For
Dummies
978-0-470-43543-4

## Business

Bookkeeping For Dummies
978-0-7645-9848-7

Job Interviews
For Dummies,
3rd Edition
978-0-470-17748-8

Resumes For Dummies,
5th Edition
978-0-470-08037-5

Starting an
Online Business
For Dummies,
6th Edition
978-0-470-60210-2

Stock Investing
For Dummies,
3rd Edition
978-0-470-40114-9

Successful
Time Management
For Dummies
978-0-470-29034-7

## Computer Hardware

BlackBerry
For Dummies,
4th Edition
978-0-470-60700-8

Computers For Seniors
For Dummies,
2nd Edition
978-0-470-53483-0

PCs For Dummies,
Windows
7 Edition
978-0-470-46542-4

Laptops For Dummies,
4th Edition
978-0-470-57829-2

## Cooking & Entertaining

Cooking Basics
For Dummies,
3rd Edition
978-0-7645-7206-7

Wine For Dummies,
4th Edition
978-0-470-04579-4

## Diet & Nutrition

Dieting For Dummies,
2nd Edition
978-0-7645-4149-0

Nutrition For Dummies,
4th Edition
978-0-471-79868-2

Weight Training
For Dummies,
3rd Edition
978-0-471-76845-6

## Digital Photography

Digital SLR Cameras &
Photography For Dummies,
3rd Edition
978-0-470-46606-3

Photoshop Elements 8
For Dummies
978-0-470-52967-6

## Gardening

Gardening Basics
For Dummies
978-0-470-03749-2

Organic Gardening
For Dummies,
2nd Edition
978-0-470-43067-5

## Green/Sustainable

Raising Chickens
For Dummies
978-0-470-46544-8

Green Cleaning
For Dummies
978-0-470-39106-8

## Health

Diabetes For Dummies,
3rd Edition
978-0-470-27086-8

Food Allergies
For Dummies
978-0-470-09584-3

Living Gluten-Free
For Dummies,
2nd Edition
978-0-470-58589-4

## Hobbies/General

Chess For Dummies,
2nd Edition
978-0-7645-8404-6

Drawing
Cartoons & Comics
For Dummies
978-0-470-42683-8

Knitting For Dummies,
2nd Edition
978-0-470-28747-7

Organizing
For Dummies
978-0-7645-5300-4

Su Doku For Dummies
978-0-470-01892-7

## Home Improvement

Home Maintenance
For Dummies,
2nd Edition
978-0-470-43063-7

Home Theater
For Dummies,
3rd Edition
978-0-470-41189-6

Living the
Country Lifestyle
All-in-One
For Dummies
978-0-470-43061-3

Solar Power Your Home
For Dummies,
2nd Edition
978-0-470-59678-4

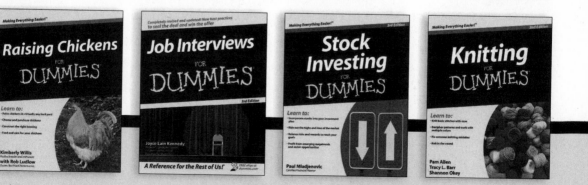

...ng For Dummies,
...Edition
8-0-470-61996-4

eBay For Dummies,
6th Edition
978-0-470-49741-8

Facebook For Dummies,
3rd Edition
978-0-470-87804-0

Web Marketing
For Dummies,
2nd Edition
978-0-470-37181-7

WordPress
For Dummies,
3rd Edition
978-0-470-59274-8

## Language & Foreign Language

French For Dummies
978-0-7645-5193-2

Italian Phrases
For Dummies
978-0-7645-7203-6

Spanish For Dummies,
2nd Edition
978-0-470-87855-2

Spanish
For Dummies,
Audio Set
978-0-470-09585-0

## Math & Science

Algebra I
For Dummies,
2nd Edition
978-0-470-55964-2

Biology For Dummies,
2nd Edition
978-0-470-59875-7

Calculus For Dummies
978-0-7645-2498-1

Chemistry For Dummies
978-0-7645-5430-8

## Microsoft Office

Excel 2010 For Dummies
978-0-470-48953-6

Office 2010 All-in-One
For Dummies
978-0-470-49748-7

Office 2010 For Dummies,
Book + DVD Bundle
978-0-470-62698-6

Word 2010 For Dummies
978-0-470-48772-3

## Music

Guitar For Dummies,
2nd Edition
978-0-7645-9904-0

iPod & iTunes For
Dummies, 8th Edition
978-0-470-87871-2

Piano Exercises
For Dummies
978-0-470-38765-8

## Parenting & Education

Parenting For Dummies,
2nd Edition
978-0-7645-5418-6

Type 1 Diabetes
For Dummies
978-0-470-17811-9

## Pets

Cats For Dummies,
2nd Edition
978-0-7645-5275-5

Dog Training For Dummies,
3rd Edition
978-0-470-60029-0

Puppies For Dummies,
2nd Edition
978-0-470-03717-1

## Religion & Inspiration

The Bible For Dummies
978-0-7645-5296-0

Catholicism For Dummies
978-0-7645-5391-2

Women in the Bible
For Dummies
978-0-7645-8475-6

## Self-Help & Relationship

Anger Management
For Dummies
978-0-470-03715-7

Overcoming Anxiety
For Dummies,
2nd Edition
978-0-470-57441-6

## Sports

Baseball
For Dummies,
3rd Edition
978-0-7645-7537-2

Basketball
For Dummies,
2nd Edition
978-0-7645-5248-9

Golf For Dummies,
3rd Edition
978-0-471-76871-5

## Web Development

Web Design
All-in-One
For Dummies
978-0-470-41796-6

Web Sites
Do-It-Yourself
For Dummies,
2nd Edition
978-0-470-56520-9

## Windows 7

Windows 7
For Dummies
978-0-470-49743-2

Windows 7
For Dummies,
Book + DVD Bundle
978-0-470-52398-8

Windows 7 All-in-One
For Dummies
978-0-470-48763-1

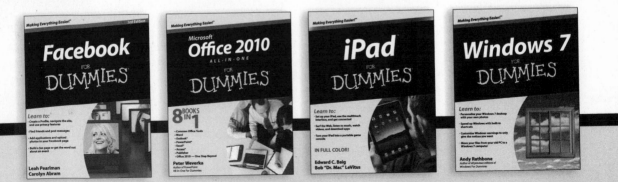